Implementing the Grand Challenge of Reducing and Preventing Alcohol Misuse and its Consequences

'Reducing and Preventing Alcohol Misuse and Its Consequences' is one of the American Academy of Social Work and Social Welfare's Grand Challenges for Social Work, a program launched in 2012. This book reports on the work of many social work and allied professions scholars, describing current strategies for achieving the ambitious goals identified in this Grand Challenge.

The chapters in this book fall into two broad categories: 'general' pieces, and those which address specific workforce development issues for meeting the Grand Challenge. The contributors cover the problem of alcohol misuse from a number of perspectives, including racial/ethnic disparities in alcohol treatment services; adolescents and emerging adults; and trauma/PTSD. The book also explores both technology-based interventions for reducing alcohol misuse and its consequences, and various models for preparing the workforce by effectively engaging in screening, brief intervention, and referral to treatment (SBIRT), for those experiencing alcohol-related problems complicated by other social and behavioral health problems. The book concludes with two interviews, focused global initiatives, and fetal alcohol spectrum disorders.

This book was originally published as a special issue of the *Journal of Social Work Practice in the Addictions*.

Audrey L. Begun is Professor of Social Work at Ohio State University, USA.

Diana M. DiNitto is Professor of Social Work at the University of Texas-Austin, USA.

S. Lala Straussner is Professor of Social Work at New York University, USA.

Implementing the Grand Challenge of Reducing and Preventing Alcohol Misuse and its Consequences

Edited by
Audrey L. Begun, Diana M. DiNitto and S. Lala Straussner

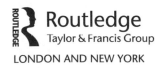

Routledge
Taylor & Francis Group

LONDON AND NEW YORK

First published 2018 by Routledge

2 Park Square, Milton Park, Abingdon, Oxon OX14 4RN
605 Third Avenue, New York, NY 10017

Routledge is an imprint of the Taylor & Francis Group, an informa business

First issued in paperback 2021

Publisher's Note

The publisher has gone to great lengths to ensure the Quality of this reprint but points out that some imperfections in the original copies may be apparent.

British Library Cataloguing in Publication Data
A catalogue record for this book is available from the British Library

ISBN 13: 978-1-138-57288-1 (hbk)
ISBN 13: 978-0-367-52995-6 (pbk)

Typeset in ITC Garamond Std
by RefineCatch Limited, Bungay, Suffolk

Publisher's Note
The publisher accepts responsibility for any inconsistencies that may have arisen during the conversion of this book from journal articles to book chapters, namely the possible inclusion of journal terminology.

Disclaimer
Every effort has been made to contact copyright holders for their permission to reprint material in this book. The publishers would be grateful to hear from any copyright holder who is not here acknowledged and will undertake to rectify any errors or omissions in future editions of this book.

Contents

Citation Information

The chapters in this book were originally published in the *Journal of Social Work Practice in the Addictions*, volume 17, issue 1–2 (January–June 2017). When citing this material, please use the original page numbering for each article, as follows:

Introduction to the Special Issue:
Implementing the Grand Challenge of Reducing and Preventing Alcohol Misuse and Its Consequences
Audrey L. Begun and Diana M. DiNitto
Journal of Social Work Practice in the Addictions, volume 17, issue 1–2
(January–June 2017), pp. 1–9

Chapter 1
The Grand Challenge of Reducing Gender and Racial/Ethnic Disparities in Service Access and Needs Among Adults with Alcohol Misuse
Jennifer I. Manuel
Journal of Social Work Practice in the Addictions, volume 17, issue 1–2
(January–June 2017), pp. 10–35

Chapter 2
Impact of Race on the Implementation of Empirically Supported Treatments in Substance Abuse Treatment
Carissa van den Berk-Clark, David A. Patterson Silver Wolf (Adelv Unegv Waya), and Sha-Lai Williams
Journal of Social Work Practice in the Addictions, volume 17, issue 1–2
(January–June 2017), pp. 36–56

Chapter 3
Recovery Schools Rise to the Challenge: Shifting Alcohol Norms and Behaviors in Youth and Emerging Adults
Lori Holleran Steiker and Julie McElrath
Journal of Social Work Practice in the Addictions, volume 17, issue 1–2
(January–June 2017), pp. 57–74

Chapter 10

Complementing SBIRT for Alcohol Misuse with SBIRT for Trauma: A Feasibility Study
James Topitzes, Lisa Berger, Laura Otto-Salaj, Joshua P. Mersky, Fiona Weeks, and Julian D. Ford
Journal of Social Work Practice in the Addictions, volume 17, issue 1–2 (January–June 2017), pp. 188–215

Chapter 11

NIAAA and the Global Challenge: An Interview with Dr. Margaret (Peggy) Murray, Director, Global Alcohol Research Program, National Institutes of Health, National Institute of Alcohol Abuse and Alcoholism
Audrey L. Begun
Journal of Social Work Practice in the Addictions, volume 17, issue 1–2 (January–June 2017), pp. 216–223

Chapter 12

Fetal Alcohol Spectrum Disorders: An Interview with Dr. Shauna Acquavita, Assistant Professor, University of Cincinnati
Diana M. DiNitto
Journal of Social Work Practice in the Addictions, volume 17, issue 1–2 (January–June 2017), pp. 224–235

For any permission-related enquiries please visit:
http://www.tandfonline.com/page/help/permissions

Notes on Contributors

Jon Agley is Assistant Research Scientist at the Department of Applied Health Science, Indiana University, USA. He is also an Evaluation Specialist at the Indiana Prevention Resource Center at the same institution.

Melanie Barker is the Executive/Clinical Director of the SDSU Center for Alcohol & Drug Studies & Services', USA, Driving Under the Influence (DUI) Program.

Audrey L. Begun is Professor of Social Work at the College of Social Work, Ohio State University, USA. Her research interests include addiction science, incarcerated women, and sibling relationships.

Suzanne Brown is Assistant Professor at the School of Social Work, Wayne State University, USA.

Taylor Berens Crouch is a Postdoctoral Fellow of Behavioral Medicine at the Medical University of South Carolina, USA.

Lisa Berger is Professor of Social Work at the School of Social Welfare at the University of Wisconsin-Milwaukee, USA. Her research interests include alcohol assessment and alcohol intervention in medical and workplace settings.

Suzanne Borys is Assistant Division Director of Research, Evaluation and Prevention at the New Jersey Division of Mental Health and Addiction Services, USA.

Charlotte Bright is Associate Professor at the School of Social Work, University of Maryland, USA.

Joan M. Carlson is Assistant Professor at the School of Social Work, Indiana University, USA.

Cali-Ryan Collin is Director of Clinical Training at the School of Social Work, Simmons College, USA.

David Crabb is Professor of Medicine at Indiana University School of Medicine, USA. He has been involved in alcoholism and liver research since the early 1980's.

Rebecca M. Cunningham is Professor of Emergency Medicine and Associate Chair in the Department of Emergency Medicine, University of Michigan Medical School, USA.

Carlo DiClemente is Professor at the Department of Psychology, University of Maryland-Baltimore County, USA.

Diana M. DiNitto is Professor of Social Work at the School of Social Work, the University of Texas-Austin, USA. Her research and teaching interests are in social welfare policy, alcohol and drug problems, and violence against women.

Lindsay Emery is a Graduate Fellow at the Department of Psychology, University of Maryland-Baltimore County, USA.

Julian D. Ford is Professor at the Department of Psychiatry, University of Connecticut, USA.

Jodi Frey is Associate Professor at the University of Maryland, School of Social Work, USA.

Ruth A. Gassman is Associate Research Scientist at the Department of Applied Health Science, Indiana University, USA. She is also Executive Director of the Indiana Prevention Resource Center at the same institution.

Kristen Gilmore Powell is Assistant Research Professor at the School of Social Work, Rutgers University, USA. She is also Associate Director of the Center for Prevention Science.

Sarah L. Gold is a doctoral candidate at the School of Social Work, Rutgers University, USA. Her research interests include: housing assistance, social policy, poverty, inequality, children, and families.

Donald Hallcom is Director of Prevention and Early Intervention at the New Jersey Division of Mental Health and Addiction Services, USA.

Melinda Hohman is Director and Professor at the School of Social Work, San Diego State University, USA.

Lori Holleran Steiker is Distinguished Professor at the University of Texas-Austin, USA. Her research interests include substance abuse prevention, culturally grounded social work practice, adult and adolescent substance abuse and recovery, and social work with groups.

Khadija Khaja is Associate Professor at the School of Social Work, Indiana University, USA. Her interests include international social work practice and curriculum development, ethnographic qualitative research, cultural competency, child welfare, women's health, online student centered teaching, and multicultural teaching pedagogy.

Adele Levine is Senior Project Manager at Brigham and Women's Hospital, Boston, USA.

James J. Lister is Assistant Professor at the School of Social Work, Wayne State University, USA.

Jennifer I. Manuel is Assistant Professor at the Silver School of Social Work, New York University, USA.

Julie McElrath is the Executive Director of University High School, USA. She has facilitated Dialectical Behavior Therapy (DBT) groups for adults and adolescents, and provided individual therapy at a drug and alcohol residential treatment facility.

Angela M. McNelis is Professor and Associate Dean for Scholarship, Innovation and Clinical Science at the George Washington University School of Nursing, USA.

Joshua P. Mersky is Associate Professor of Social Work at the School of Social Welfare, University of Wisconsin-Milwaukee, USA.

Melissa Moreland is a Research Assistant at the University of Maryland School of Social Work, USA.

Kimberly H. M. O'Brien is an Instructor in Psychiatry at Harvard Medical School, USA. She is also a Research Scientist at the Education Development Center and at Boston Children's Hospital.

Steven J. Ondersma is Associate Professor at the Merrill Palmer Skillman Institute for Child and Family Development, Wayne State University, USA.

Laura Otto-Salaj is Associate Professor of Social Work at the School of Social Welfare, University of Wisconsin-Milwaukee, USA.

David A. Patterson, Silver Wolf (Adelv Unegv Waya), is Associate Professor at the Brown School of Social Work, Washington University in St Louis, USA. He investigates best practice implementation in human services organizations, specifically investigating worker and organizational characteristics and their roles in implementing and disseminating empirically-supported treatments.

N. Andrew Peterson is Professor with the School of Social Work at Rutgers University, USA. His research examines the mechanisms through which community organizations promote empowerment and community change. His work also focuses on preventing community-level problems that contribute to social and health disparities.

Jennifer M. Putney is Assistant Professor at the School of Social Work, Simmons College, USA.

Stella M. Resko is Associate Professor in the School of Social Work, Wayne State University, USA.

Paul Sacco is Associate Dean for Research and Associate Professor at the School of Social Work, University of Maryland, USA. His research focuses primarily on behavioral health and addictions with an emphasis on life course development.

Rhonda Schwindt is Assistant Professor at the George Washington University School of Nursing, USA. Her research is focused on reducing the disproportionate impact of tobacco use among high risk populations.

S. Lala Straussner is Professor of Social Work at New York University, USA. Her current research focuses on "wounded healers" or wellness issues of social workers.

Laura Ting is Associate Professor at the School of Social Work, University of Maryland, USA. Her research interests include domestic violence, victims and abuse treatment, and motivational interviewing techniques.

James Topitzes is Associate Professor of Social Work at the School of Social Welfare, University of Wisconsin-Milwaukee, USA.

Carissa van den Berk-Clark is Assistant Professor at the Department of Family and Community Medicine, Saint Louis University, USA.

Julie Vannerson is Associate Professor of Clinical Medicine at Indiana University School of Medicine, USA.

Maureen A. Walton is Professor in the Department of Psychiatry, University of Michigan Medical School, USA.

Fiona Weeks is a Wisconsin Population Health Service Fellow with dual placements at the Institute for Child and Family Well-Being, University of Wisconsin-Milwaukee, USA, and the City of Milwaukee Health Department in the Family and Community Health Division.

Sha-Lai Williams is Assistant Professor at the Department of Social Work, University of Missouri, USA. Her research interests include cultural competence among social work and helping professionals and racial/ethnic disparities in access to and utilization of quality mental health services, with an emphasis on African Americans and emerging adults.

Susan Woodruff is Professor at the School of Social Work, San Diego State University, USA. Her work looks at tobacco and drug use research, particularly with high-risk and underserved populations, health disparity research, research methodology, and statistics.

Introduction
Implementing the Grand Challenge of Reducing and Preventing Alcohol Misuse and Its Consequences

AUDREY L. BEGUN, MSW, PhD ⓘ

DIANA M. DiNITTO, PhD

The Grand Challenges for Social Work initiative, launched by the American Academy of Social Work and Social Welfare (AASWSW) in 2012, identified a series of 12 broad social work challenges. Each challenge addressed a "deeply significant problem widely recognized by the public whose solution is within our grasp in the next decade, given concentrated scientific and practical attention" (AASWSW, 2016). This special double issue of the *Journal of Social Work Practice in the Addictions* addresses the Social Work Grand Challenge called *Reducing and Preventing Alcohol Misuse and Its Consequences* (Begun, Clapp, & The Alcohol Misuse Grand Challenge Collective, 2016).[1] The AASWSW Grand Challenges initiative leadership situated the alcohol misuse challenge under the umbrella of "Close the Health Gap." Solutions under this health-related umbrella are expected to "lead to broad gains in the health of our entire society" and promote greater health equity across the population.[2] Reducing and preventing the consequences of alcohol misuse would make major contributions by addressing one of America's major health gaps.

---

[1]   The original Alcohol Misuse Grand Challenge paper can be found at http://aaswsw.org/wp-content/uploads/2015/12/WP14-with-cover.pdf. It has been reprinted with minor changes as Begun, Clapp, and The Alcohol Misuse Grand Challenge Collective (2016).
[2]   More information on Close the Health Gap Grand Challenge can be found at http://aaswsw.org/grand-challenges-initiative/12-challenges/close-the-health-gap/.

Since the AASWSW posted the alcohol misuse grand challenge paper on alcohol misuse, members of the Alcohol Misuse Grand Challenge Collective have initiated several efforts to respond to this challenge. These have included disseminating the challenge itself to an interdisciplinary audience, organizing conference sessions that bring together scholars in the area, and producing this special issue of the *Journal of Social Work Practice in the Addictions* for scholars, practitioners, and other audiences. These efforts are intended to showcase what social work is doing to address the alcohol misuse grand challenge and to provide direction for the future.

WHY IT MATTERS

The *Reducing and Preventing Alcohol Misuse and Its Consequences* Grand Challenge effort is particularly meaningful because alcohol misuse is a large, significant, and compelling national and global problem related to many health and social concerns. Authors of the challenge paper elected to define alcohol misuse as involving "drinking in greater quantities or more frequently than is advisable, and may involve drinking in risky situations or circumstances" (Begun et al., 2016, p. 73). The U.S. Surgeon General defined it as use of the substance in such a manner that it causes harm to users or those around them (U.S. Department of Health and Human Services, Office of the Surgeon General, 2016). In terms of health consequences, the World Health Organization (WHO) identified alcohol use as responsible for almost 6% of deaths globally (3.3 million annually) and just over 5% of the global disease burden (WHO, 2014). During 2011, the United Nations General Assembly adopted a resolution concerning the prevention and control of four leading noncommunicable diseases—all of which are exacerbated by alcohol misuse (United Nations, 2011). The WHO has published a goal of effecting a 10% decrease in harmful use of alcohol between 2015 and 2020 (WHO, 2015). In the United States, an average of just under 88,000 deaths annually are associated with alcohol misuse, making it the fourth leading cause of preventable deaths (Stahre, Roeber, Kanny, Brewer, & Zhang, 2014).

Alcohol misuse is a contributing factor in risk for injury, addiction, and dangerous drug interactions. Furthermore, it causes or contributes to health problems, such as lifelong, irreversible developmental complications from fetal exposure; significant damage to multiple organ systems in the body (e.g., brain, heart, liver, immune system); and the development of major disease conditions (e.g., some forms of cancer, Type II diabetes, liver and heart disease, as well as multiple types of psychiatric and mental health disorders). In addition to these physical health concerns, alcohol misuse is a frequent concomitant or prelude to many serious social, behavioral, economic, and legal problems affecting individuals, families, communities, and social institutions. These include family and other forms of interpersonal violence (e.g., intimate partner violence, child maltreatment, and sexual assault), driving under the influence (including mass transit drivers), suicidality, problem gambling, human trafficking, housing insecurity, legal and criminal justice system involvement, job loss or poor work performance, sexual risk taking, unintended pregnancy, and more.

Social workers play vital roles in addressing all these problems in the many settings in which they work. With concerted effort, social workers, along with allied professionals and the public's support, can make significant progress toward reducing and preventing alcohol misuse and its consequences. The recent release of the U.S. Surgeon General's (U.S. Department of Health and Human Services, Office of the Surgeon General, 2016) first report on alcohol, drugs, and health is further reminder of the need to redouble efforts to reduce alcohol misuse. The report was produced in recognition of the health and social problems associated with substance misuse, including alcohol, and the need for a comprehensive approach to address the problems in the United States (pp. 1–3).

THIS SPECIAL ISSUE

Our initial call for manuscripts was broad. We wanted to elicit a response from a variety of social work scholars engaged in work related to the aims described in the Grand Challenge paper. The result is presented here as 10 articles submitted by individuals and teams of scholars. The articles fall into two groups. One group addresses a more general set of issues, including articles that focus on specific populations that are critical to meeting the grand challenge. Indicative of social work, we were pleased to see that these articles address micro, mezzo, and macro level issues and solutions. The second group addresses a social work workforce development agenda, in particular, implementation of Screening, Brief Intervention, and Referral to Treatment (SBIRT). In addition, we conducted interviews on two topics not specifically addressed in the 10 articles that we also thought warranted inclusion—fetal alcohol spectrum disorders and the federal government's role in meeting the grand challenge.

The General Papers

The general papers address several topics. With national attention focused on reducing health disparities (U.S. Department of Health and Human Services, n.d.), it is not surprising that two of the articles focus on this topic. One of these articles (Manuel) addresses whether treatment utilization for alcohol misuse and alcohol use disorders has increased, especially among Black, Hispanic, and Asian men and women, since passage of the

Patient Protection and Affordable Care Act, also known as the Affordable Care Act (ACA) and "Obamacare." Under the ACA, 20 million more Americans now have health insurance (U.S. Department of Health and Human Services, 2016). The ACA added new requirements for health insurance plans to include treatment for alcohol and drug problems. However, rather than increased utilization of services for alcohol use misuse and use disorders for all groups as hoped, Manuel found that treatment utilization increased for some racial and gender groups and decreased for others. The results must be viewed cautiously, because factors other than the ACA (e.g., patient preferences, stigma, provider biases, cultural attitudes, or other factors) might continue to inhibit more optimal levels of treatment use. We join the authors in calling for approaches such as culturally relevant services and greater use of models such as integrated behavioral health care as means of remedying inequities in treatment for alcohol misuse and use disorders. With uncertainly in the national health care environment given the new administration's desire to take a different course than that mandated by the ACA, those involved in preventing and treating substance misuse and substance use disorders will be carefully monitoring the health insurance environment and advocating to ensure a continued focus on increasing access to treatment.

The second article on racial disparities examines whether government-funded substance use treatment programs in counties with majority and minority Black populations differed in their provision of evidence-supported treatments (ESTs) from 2008 to 2010 (van den Berk-Clark, Patterson Silver Wolf [Adelv Unegv Waya], and Williams). After controlling for a variety of agency or organization and community factors, findings suggest that although programs in majority Black communities might provide somewhat fewer ESTs than those in minority Black communities, programs in both community types embrace EST use. Although the authors recommend viewing the findings cautiously due to limitations in the variables available for inclusion and the self-report data of treatment personnel, the findings tend to contradict other studies and popular beliefs that Blacks receive inferior treatment. With the scientific community focused on the need to promote the use of ESTs and interventions, more research like this is needed to determine whether, how, and where ESTs are being used.

Two articles turn our attention to programs addressing alcohol misuse among adolescents and emerging adults. One describes programmatic features relevant to the growing Recovery School movement (Holleran Steiker and McElrath). This article is a useful introduction and primer for those interested in high school settings specifically designed for young people who are in recovery from alcohol and drug problems. The article emphasizes the need for such programs because many students in typical high school environments face significant pressure to use alcohol (as well as other drugs). Students in recovery high schools generally have access to a variety of supportive services that help them sustain recovery while earning their high school degree, a necessary credential for engaging in the workforce and moving toward a productive life as an adult. Another article related to youth in this special issue explores the organizational characteristics that empower staff and volunteers in community coalitions that target underage drinking (Powell, Gold, Peterson, Borys, and Hallcom). It is not surprising that empowerment coalitions like these received attention in the U.S. Surgeon General's recent report. Mobilizing community members is key to solving problems such as underage drinking, and keeping staff and volunteers engaged is a necessary condition for effective coalitions. The study found that although there was some overlap, different factors affected staff and volunteers' sense of empowerment and views of coalition effectiveness. For example, among staff members, the opportunity to engage in specific roles was particularly important, while fostering leadership and a sense of community was critical for volunteers. With knowledge such as this, more emphasis can be placed on training and developing staff and volunteers to increase coalition involvement and effectiveness.

The Hohman, Barker, and Woodruff team studied the intersection between trauma and posttraumatic stress disorder (PTSD), which are often related to alcohol misuse. Their focus was clients in programs designed for individuals arrested for driving under the influence (DUI). The likelihood of experiencing particular traumatic events differed for men and women in this treatment population, but clients with higher blood alcohol concentrations were more likely to screen positive for PTSD. As a means of preventing future DUI incidents and improving client overall well-being, the authors implore those working in DUI programs to identify trauma, help clients see the relationship between trauma and alcohol use, and refer clients to services that can help address trauma when needed.

The last of our general topic articles discusses the Grand Challenge implications of three technology-based interventions for reducing alcohol misuse and its consequences (Resko, Brown, Lister, Ondersma, Cunningham, and Walton). With the growing emphasis on teletherapy and applications accessed via smartphones and other electronic devices to provide physical and mental health services, it is no wonder that interest in using technology to deliver interventions to reduce substance misuse is growing. These interventions are particularly attractive for their ease of access, availability, privacy considerations (and challenges), and cost effectiveness. They seem destined to grow in popularity among people of all age groups. In the quest to reduce alcohol misuse and its consequences, we must experiment with a variety of tools to expand our reach and attract more individuals to use them. We also need to remain mindful of their limitations.

The Workforce Development Papers

Responding to the alcohol misuse grand challenge requires a workforce dedicated to reducing and preventing alcohol misuse and its consequences. Four of our special issue articles focus on workforce development. To reduce alcohol misuse and its consequences, the Substance Abuse and Mental Health Services Administration (SAMHSA) has provided substantial funding to see that health and allied health professionals are prepared to engage in the evidence-based practice called SBIRT. These four articles describe initiatives to prepare social work professionals to provide SBIRT. Although there will continue to be a need for specialized alcohol treatment services, the alcohol misuse grand challenge cannot be met without interventions that tap into the problems much earlier in their development and present motivating opportunities and access to a wider audience. Thus, these training projects are responsive to calls for bringing alcohol misuse interventions into general practice arenas and mainstream social work practice across setting types.

In the first of these articles, the team of Carlson, Agley, Gassman, McNelis, Schwindt, Vannerson, Crabb, and Khaja found that following SBIRT training, master's of social work (MSW) students at a large, urban, public university made gains in perceived competence, comfort making alcohol-related statements, and positive attitudes toward working with patients who drink at risky levels. The training included Microsoft PowerPoint presentations, online educational modules, and face-to-face training that included simulated role-playing. A second of these articles (Sacco, Ting, Crouch, Emery, Moreland, Bright, Frey, and DiClemente) reports on an SBIRT course that included didactic sessions, role-playing, and videotaped standardized patient interactions for MSW students. Sacco and colleagues also report that SBIRT behaviors, confidence, skills, and knowledge increased following the course. In a third article, Putney, O'Brien, Collin, and Levine prepared MSW as well as a smaller number of bachelor's of social work students and a group of field instructors to use SBIRT. The students' training was based on existing SBIRT curricula adapted for social workers and was embedded in the social work foundation curriculum. Training was online and in class and included skills practice. Field instructors were trained in a 3-hr seminar that also included information on mentoring students in SBIRT use. Similar to the other studies, Putney and colleagues found evidence of SBIRT training's feasibility and acceptability and preliminary evidence of its effectiveness.

In addition to SBIRT training, and as noted in discussing the Hohman et al. article earlier, trauma-informed care has gained social workers' attention (SAMHSA, 2015). The fourth workforce development article (Topitzes, Berger, Otto-Salaj, Mersky, Weeks, and Ford) reports on efforts to combine trauma services with SBIRT (they call it T-SBIRT) with a sample comprised largely of low-income African American and Latino clients served by community health clinics. The investigators found T-SBIRT to be feasible and acceptable with the potential to increase treatment referrals for substance misuse or substance use disorder and trauma. They also point to the need for integrating behavioral services in primary health care services. Those of us dedicated to preparing the next generations of social workers hope that SBIRT for alcohol misuse and related problems will become part of the education of all students in social work, as well as other physical and behavioral health disciplines.

The Interviews

Finally, we invited two scholars to participate in interviews about topics we thought were important to include, but were not covered in the manuscripts we received. In the first interview, Dr. Peggy Murray, a senior official with the National Institute on Alcohol Abuse and Alcoholism (NIAAA), spoke with us about NIAAA's research mission, research agenda, and the global challenge of reducing and preventing alcohol misuse and its consequences. Murray empha-sizes opportunities for social workers to obtain research funding and to use data sets from other studies. She describes major NIAAA-funded studies on the adolescent brain and cognitive development, the genetics of alcoholism, medication-assisted treatment, fetal alcohol spectrum disorders (FASD), and college drinking. Murray underscores the importance of screening and brief intervention and efforts of the World Health Organization, the Organization for Economic Cooperation and Development, and the United Nations to reduce and prevent alcohol misuse and use disorders and their consequences. She encourages social workers to become part of research teams tackling the big issues in alcohol misuse because the social work perspective is always needed. For the second interview, we asked Dr. Shauna Acquavita, whose work has been in physical and behavioral health, including addressing substance use disorders among pregnant women, to talk with us about fetal alcohol exposure. Preventing fetal alcohol exposure is critical in meeting the grand challenge of reducing and preventing alcohol misuse and its consequences. Acquavita defines FASD, updates us on efforts to prevent it, and discusses social work's roles in the process, especially collaboration with members of other disciplines in concerted efforts to prevent drinking during pregnancy and to help those with the range of FASD achieve their full potential.

MOVING FORWARD WITH THE CHALLENGE

Social work is not alone in recognizing the significance of alcohol misuse as a major contributor to physical health, mental health, and social problems. Members of the Alcohol Misuse Grand Challenge Collective believe that demonstrable progress can be made toward reducing alcohol misuse and preventing its consequences in the next decade. Doing so requires new approaches to collaboration—multidisciplinary, interdisciplinary, and transdisciplinary—as well as multisectorial approaches that transcend traditional lines between systems and levels of study or intervention. Social workers often use the term *biopsychosocial* to refer to this comprehensive approach. Sustainable solutions will require significant, transformative, and innovative strategies (Begun et al., 2016).

In conclusion, this special issue of the *Journal of Social Work Practice in the Addictions* presents important contributions for responding to the Social Work Grand Challenge of Reducing and Preventing Alcohol Misuse and Its Consequences. We hope that the journal readership, practitioners, scholars, policymakers, educators, and the public are inspired to join us in addressing the alcohol misuse grand challenge because much remains to be done. By joining together, we can develop and invest in additional initiatives for responding to the challenge. Each of us can also find innovative ways to become engaged in the effort and assume leadership roles in organizing responses to the challenge. With concerted efforts, the cumulative effect can be significant reductions in alcohol misuse and its consequences.

ORCID

Audrey L. Begun ⓘ http://orcid.org/0000-0002-1672-0315

REFERENCES

American Academy of Social Work and Social Welfare (AASWSW). (2016). *Grand challenges of social work initiative: Impact model. Scope, products, impacts, and timeframe.* Retrieved from http://aaswsw.org/wp-content/uploads/2016/01/Oct24_GC-ImpactModel-Statement-and-Model-REV.pdf

Begun, A. L., Clapp, J. D., & The Alcohol Misuse Grand Challenge Collective. (2016). Reducing and preventing alcohol misuse and its consequences. *International Journal of Alcohol and Drug Research, 5*(2), 73–83. doi:10.7895/ijadr.v5i2.223

Stahre, M., Roeber, J., Kanny, D., Brewer, R. D., & Zhang, X. (2014). Contribution of excessive alcohol consumption to deaths and years of potential life lost in the United States. *Centers for Disease Control and Prevention: Preventing Chronic Disease, 11.* Retrieved from https://www.cdc.gov/pcd/issues/2014/13_0293.htm

Substance Abuse and Mental Health Services Administration. (2015). *Trauma informed approach and trauma-specific interventions.* Retrieved from https://www.samhsa.gov/trauma

U.S. Department of Health and Human Services. (n.d.). *HHS action plan to reduce racial and ethnic health disparities: A nation free of disparities in health and health care.* Washington, DC: Author. Retrieved from https://minorityhealth.hhs.gov/assets/pdf/hhs/HHS_Plan_complete.pdf

U.S. Department of Health and Human Services. (2016, March 3). *20 million have gained health insurance coverage because of the Affordable Care Act, new estimates show* (DHHS press release). Retrieved from https://www.hhs.gov/about/news/2016/03/03/20-million-people-have-gained-health-insurance-coverage-because-affordable-care-act-new-estimates

U.S. Department of Health and Human Services, Office of the Surgeon General. (2016, November). *Facing addiction in America: The Surgeon General's report on alcohol, drugs, and health*. Retrieved from https://addiction.surgeongeneral.gov

United Nations. (2011). *2011 high level meeting on prevention and control of non-communicable diseases*. Retrieved from http://www.un.org/en/ga/ncdmeeting2011/

World Health Organization. (2014). *Global status report on alcohol and health*. Geneva, Switzerland: Author. Retrieved from http://apps.who.int/iris/bitstream/10665/112736/1/9789240692763_eng.pdf?ua=1

World Health Organization. (2015). *Target 2: Reduce harmful use of alcohol. Global Monitoring Framework for NCDs (non-communicable diseases)*. Retrieved from http://www.who.int/nmh/ncd-tools/target2/en/

The Grand Challenge of Reducing Gender and Racial/Ethnic Disparities in Service Access and Needs Among Adults with Alcohol Misuse

JENNIFER I. MANUEL, PhD

This study examined the impact of the Affordable Care Act (ACA) on gender and racial and ethnic disparities in accessing and using behavioral health services among a national sample of adults who reported heavy or binge alcohol use (n = 52,496) and those with alcohol use disorder (AUD; n = 22,966). Difference-in-differences models estimated service-related disparities before (2008–2009) and after (2011–2014) health care reform. A subanalysis was conducted before (2011–2013) and after (2014) full implementation of the ACA. Asian subgroups among respondents with heavy or binge drinking were excluded from substance use disorder (SUD) treatment and unmet need outcome models due to insufficient cell size. Among heavy or binge drinkers, unmet SUD treatment need decreased among Black women and increased among Black men. Mental health (MH) treatment decreased among Asian men, whereas unmet MH treatment need decreased among Hispanic men. MH treatment increased among Hispanic women with AUD. Although there were improvements in service use and access among Black and Hispanic women and Hispanic men, there were setbacks among Black and Asian men. Implications for social workers are discussed.

Alcohol misuse is a major public health problem, affecting almost a quarter of the population aged 12 years and older in the United States (Center for Behavioral Health Statistics and Quality, [CBHSQ] 2015b). Alcohol misuse, defined as excessive drinking beyond the recommended amounts, includes a continuum of alcohol problems, ranging from binge drinking (i.e., five or more drinks on the same occasion on at least 1 day or more in the past 30 days) and heavy episodic drinking (i.e., five or more drinks on the same occasion on at least 5 days or more in the past 30 days) to alcohol use disorder (AUD). In 2014, approximately 60.9 million (23%) adults aged 12 years and older reported binge alcohol use, and 16.3 million (6.2%) reported heavy alcohol use in the past year (CBHSQ, 2015b). Of the 21.5 million (8.1%) people aged 12 years and older who had a substance use disorder (SUD) in 2014, the majority (~17 million) had an AUD (CBHSQ, 2015b). Of those with an AUD, the majority were adults aged 18 years and older (~16.3 million), of whom 65% were men and 35% were women (CBHSQ, 2015b). Although Whites (13.8%) are more likely to have a life-time AUD than Blacks (8.4%) and Hispanics (9.5%), recurrent or persistent AUD is more prevalent among Blacks and Hispanics once AUD occurs (Chartier & Caetano, 2010; Dawson et al., 2005; Hasin, Stinson, Ogburn, & Grant, 2007). Asian Americans have an estimated lifetime AUD prevalence of 3.6%, however, significant variation exists among Asian subgroups (Chartier & Caetano, 2010).

The health, social, and economic impacts of alcohol misuse are substantial, especially among vulnerable and marginalized groups, and represent an immense challenge for health and behavioral health providers, including social workers. Globally, alcohol misuse makes up about 5.1% of the burden of disease and injury and is a leading risk factor for early death and disability (World Health Organization [WHO], 2014). In the United States, the economic burden of alcohol misuse is more than $200 billion annually, of which three-quarters is related to binge drinking (Research Society on Alcoholism, 2015; Sacks, Gonzales, Bouchery, Tomedi, & Brewer, 2015). Alcohol misuse is a leading risk factor for numerous health- and injury-related conditions, most notably liver disease, cancers, and injury due to traffic crashes and falls (O'Brien et al., 2006; WHO, 2014), as well as social and legal problems (Begun, Clapp, & The Alcohol Misuse Grand Challenge Collective, 2016). The prevalence of alcohol misuse among persons with mental health (MH) disorders is also high, ranging from 45% to 60% in national studies (Grant et al., 2004; Hasin et al., 2007; Kessler et al., 1996). Despite the prevalence and adverse consequences of alcohol misuse, the vast majority of risky drinkers and people with AUD do not receive treatment (Han et al., 2015; Harris & Edlund, 2005; Ilgen et al., 2011; McLellan & Woodworth, 2014; Mojtabai, 2005).

GENDER AND RACIAL/ETHNIC DISPARITIES
IN SERVICE USE AND ACCESS

Existing research on gender disparities in SUD treatment is well established. However, little attention has been paid to understanding the intersection of gender and race and ethnicity with respect to service disparities. Women have consistently been underrepresented groups in SUD treatment programs (Chartier & Caetano, 2010; Dawson et al., 2005; Greenfield, Trucco, McHugh, Lincoln, & Gallop, 2007; Ilgen et al., 2011; Marsh, Cao, & D'Aunno, 2004; Tuchman, 2010; Zemore, Mulia, Yu, Borges, & Greenfield, 2009). Historically, women have been less likely to enter treatment than men (Greenfield et al., 2007). Differences in treatment entry could reflect gaps in income and health care coverage. Compared to men, women typically earn less, on average, leading to greater challenges in paying for and accessing services over their lifetime (Fitzgerald, Cohen, Hyams, Sullivan, & Johnson, 2014). Women are also less likely to be covered by insurance because they have frequent job transitions and work part time (Henry J. Kaiser Family Foundation, 2012). Women are more likely to be insured as a dependent on their spouse's or partner's health insurance policy than through their own job, which places them at risk of losing their benefits if their spouse or partner loses their job or if they become divorced or widowed (Henry J. Kaiser Family Foundation, 2012). Other research suggests that gender disparities in service use might reflect differences in medical, MH, and other psychosocial problems between women and men (Marsh et al., 2004; Tuchman, 2010). For example, Weinberger, Mazure, Morlett, and McKee (2013) found that depression, which is more prevalent among women than men (Kessler, McGonagle, Swartz, Blazer, & Nelson, 1993; Wolk & Weissman, 1995), negatively affected women's SUD treatment outcomes.

Studies also point to disparities in SUD treatment among racial and ethnic minority groups (Chartier & Caetano, 2011; Mulia, Tam, & Schmidt, 2014; Mulvaney-Day, DeAngelo, Chen, Cook, & Alegria, 2012; Schmidt, Ye, Greenfield, & Bond, 2007; Weisner, Matzger, Tam, & Schmidt, 2002; Wells, Klap, Koike, & Sherbourne, 2001; Witbrodt, Mulia, Zemore, & Kerr, 2014), although research findings are less consistent due to differences in sample populations and methodology. Mulvaney-Day and colleagues (2012) compared two national surveys of community samples with SUDs and found that both surveys showed a lower likelihood of perceived unmet need for SUD treatment among Black respondents and a greater likelihood among Hispanic respondents than non-Hispanic White respondents (Mulvaney-Day et al., 2012). Earlier data show a different pattern of unmet need for alcohol treatment. Specifically, Asian and Hispanic respondents who reported a need for alcohol treatment had a lower likelihood of using alcohol specialty services compared to non-Hispanic White and Black respondents (Chartier & Caetano, 2010). Other research suggests racial and ethnic variation in service use by differences in access to resources. For example, Weisner and colleagues (2002) surveyed a probability sample of adult problem and dependent drinkers and found a greater likelihood of SUD treatment among Black compared to White respondents, even after adjusting for health insurance. However, Hispanic respondents were associated with a lower likelihood of SUD treatment. Differences in service use could also depend on alcohol severity. Schmidt and colleagues (2007) found that both Black and Hispanic respondents with more severe alcohol problems were less likely to receive any treatment services compared to White respondents with similar alcohol problem severity.

HEALTH CARE POLICIES TO IMPROVE ACCESS TO CARE

The 2008 Mental Health Parity and Addiction Equity Act (MHPAEA) and 2010 Affordable Care Act (ACA) offer new provisions to reduce gender and race and ethnic disparities in accessing behavioral health services and improve the overall quality of care (Clemans-Cope, Kenney, Buettgens, Carroll, & Blavin, 2012; Gettens, Henry, & Himmelstein, 2012). For example, the ACA considers SUD and MH treatment as essential benefits that new health plans must offer, extending federal parity under the MHPAEA. Under the ACA, access to health insurance exchanges in all states and Medicaid expansion in most states serve as mechanisms for increased coverage and affordable options for low-income populations. In addition, women now have expanded coverage for preventive services and comparable insurance premium rates as men for the same plan. Health care providers are receiving new opportunities for training in cultural competence (Andrulis, 2010; Salganicoff, Ranji, Beamesderfer, & Kurani, 2014). Other initiatives, such as health homes and accountable care organizations, aim to better facilitate the delivery of integrated care to improve the efficiency, quality, and coordination of health and behavioral health services.

Under the ACA, 30 million people are expected to gain coverage (Beronio, Glied, & Frank, 2014), including more than 5 million in need of behavioral health services (Ali, Mutter, & Teich, 2015). An increase in access to behavioral health services is expected to increase the demand for and use of services and presumably reduce unmet needs for such services. However, concerns exist about whether these new policies will translate to better access, especially for vulnerable populations. For example, the ACA is expected to have an impact on SUD treatment more than any other health care legislation. It is unclear, however, whether SUD treatment programs will have the capacity to meet the increased demands that might arise due to increased coverage (Humphreys & Frank, 2014). In addition, the 2012 ruling of the U.S. Supreme Court made Medicaid expansion voluntary for state governments, which will likely affect low-income and racial and ethnic minority groups. The Congressional Budget Office (2012) estimated that, without Medicaid expansion, approximately 3 million fewer people will have health insurance. As such, low-income individuals (i.e., income at or below 133% of the federal poverty level) will struggle in purchasing health insurance coverage. This includes Hispanic immigrants who have been in the United States fewer than 5 years. In states without Medicaid expansion, individuals might be expected to pay for coverage or pay a tax penalty.

THE CURRENT STUDY

Research on health care reform remains limited with respect to ACA's impact on gender and racial and ethnic disparities in behavioral health service use and access. To date, preliminary research on the ACA's impact suggests significant increases in insurance coverage overall and evidence of some reduction in racial and ethnic disparities (Chen, Vargas-Bustamante, Mortensen, & Ortega, 2016; McMorrow, Long, Kenney, & Anderson, 2015; Sommers, Musco, Finegold, Gunja, Burke, & McDowell, 2014). Other research has extended this work to investigate changes in treatment utilization by race and ethnicity before and after ACA implementation and found an overall increase in MH service use, particularly among Hispanics and Asians (Creedon & Cook, 2016). However, no significant changes in substance abuse treatment were found post-ACA reform, despite significant gains in insurance coverage (Creedon & Cook, 2016). The lack of significant changes might reflect other prominent barriers, such as stigma or negative attitudes about treatment (Kaufmann, Chen, Crum, & Mojtabai, 2014; Mojtabai, Chen, Kaufmann, & Crum, 2014).

In addition, given advances in gender-specific and culturally congruent services over the past decade, there might be important subgroup differences in service use and access by gender and race and ethnicity (Amaro, Arevalo, Gonzalez, Szapocznik, & Iguchi, 2006; Polak, Haug, Drachenberg, & Svikis, 2015). To date, however, limited research has investigated the intersection of gender and race and ethnicity with service use and access. Specific to alcohol misuse, a literature search produced one recent study that examined the intersection of gender and race and ethnicity and found lower service use among Black and Hispanic women versus White women and lower utilization among Hispanic versus White men with a lifetime AUD (Zemore, Mulia, Yu, Borges, & Greenfield, 2014). However, this research precedes the ACA and does not differentiate among different alcohol risk groups.

The primary objective of this study is to evaluate the impact of the ACA on reducing gender and race and ethnic disparities in behavioral health service use (i.e., SUD and MH treatment utilization) and access (i.e., perceived unmet needs for SUD and MH treatment) in a national sample of adults with alcohol misuse. In light of recent evidence (Creedon & Cook, 2016), the study hypothesizes that there will be improvement in MH service use and access and limited changes in SUD service use and access in combined gender and racial and ethnic minority groups after health care reform. Because alcohol misuse includes a continuum of risky drinking patterns that might require different types of services to meet needs, analyses were stratified by alcohol risk group (i.e., heavy or binge alcohol use vs. AUD). Given the negative consequences of alcohol misuse, understanding the impact of health care reform on gender and racial and ethnic disparities in service use and access among alcohol risk groups is critical for effective policy and practice planning. The social work profession is well positioned to take leadership in addressing this challenge given its commitment to social justice, advocacy for oppressed groups, and a person-in-environment perspective. Results from this study will equip social workers and other health care providers with important information about the intersection of gender and race and ethnicity with service use and access to inform gender- and culturally grounded approaches to improve access to and engagement in treatment and ultimately reduce the negative impact of alcohol misuse. Findings from this study will inform interventions and policies to improve the efficiency and equity of the health care system.

METHODS

Study Design and Sampling

The study used 2008–2009 and 2011–2014 data from the National Survey on Drug Use and Health (NSDUH), a national representative survey of the civilian, non-institutionalized population in the United States. Conducted annually, the NSDUH uses a multistage stratified sampling design to generate national estimates of alcohol and drug use, MH and SUDs, and use of and access to behavioral health treatment services. The NSDUH interview response rates ranged from 71% to 76% over the study period. The NSDUH data are weighted to account for the survey's complex design. More detailed information on the NSDUH survey design and methodology can be found elsewhere (CBHSQ, 2015a). The New York University Institutional Review Board deemed the study exempt.

Participants

The analysis included adult respondents aged 18 years and older and classified as either having reported heavy or binge drinking use in the past year but did not meet diagnostic criteria for AUD (unweighted $N = 52,496$; weighted $N = 37,698,482$), or having met diagnostic criteria for past-year AUD (unweighted $N = 22,966$; weighted $N = 13,991,980$).

Measures

SERVICE USE AND ACCESS

Four sets of dichotomous outcomes were assessed: SUD treatment, MH treatment, perceived unmet need for SUD treatment, and perceived unmet need for MH treatment. SUD treatment was defined as using any substance abuse treatment services in the past year. This variable categorizes those who receive formal outpatient and inpatient SUD services, including treatment received in primary care and emergency room visits, and excludes informal services such as self-help groups, which are typically free and do not require insurance coverage. MH treatment was defined as the use of one or more of the following services: outpatient treatment, inpatient treatment, and psychotropic medication. Respondents who endorsed having a perceived unmet need for SUD treatment reported not receiving SUD treatment in the past year but perceiving a need for such treatment or perceiving a need for additional treatment if they used SUD treatment in the past year. Respondents who reported a perceived unmet need for MH treatment indicated that they perceived a need for MH treatment or counseling in the past 12 months but did not receive it. Use of MH treatment and perceived unmet need for MH treatment were included as outcomes given the high cooccurrence of MH conditions among people with or at risk for AUD, and based on evidence that people with SUD might seek MH treatment instead of SUD treatment (Edlund, Booth, & Han, 2012; Mojtabai, 2005).

GENDER AND RACE AND ETHNICITY

Respondents self-reported their gender as either female or male. Self-reported race and ethnicity were measured based on the U.S. Census categories: non-Hispanic White, non-Hispanic Black, Hispanic, and Asian, based on self-reports. Other racial and ethnic groups were excluded because they were either unknown or comprised small sample sizes.

ALCOHOL RISK GROUPS: HEAVY OR BINGE ALCOHOL USE AND ALCOHOL USE DISORDER

Binge alcohol use was defined as drinking five or more drinks on the same occasion on at least 1 day or more in the past 30 days, and heavy alcohol use was defined as drinking five or more drinks on the same occasion on at least 5 days or more in the past 30 days. To increase the power to detect low incidence of service use and unmet treatment needs, respondents who reported either heavy or binge alcohol use in the past 30 days were combined into one group. Respondents in this group did not meet diagnostic criteria for AUD. Heavy or binge alcohol use was defined as a dichotomous (yes–no) variable.

Respondents were defined as having an AUD if they met abuse or dependence criteria according to the *Diagnostic and Statistical Manual of Mental Disorders* (4th ed. [*DSM–IV*; American Psychiatric Association, 1994). Respondents were asked a series of questions that assessed alcohol abuse and dependence in the past year. Abuse-related questions evaluated alcohol-related problems with respect to home, work, and school functioning; health-related risks; legal trouble; and difficulties in relationships with family and friends. Dependence-related questions assessed alcohol problems associated with tolerance, withdrawal, drinking larger amounts or for longer periods, inability to cut down, time spent using alcohol, giving up activities, and continued drinking despite problems. AUD was defined as a dichotomous (yes–no) variable.

PREDISPOSING, NEED, AND ENABLING COVARIATES

The Andersen–Newman behavioral model of health service use guided the selection of covariates that are relevant to service use and access, as well as alcohol-related problems (Andersen, 1995). This model assumes that service use and access are a function of predisposing factors, such as gender, age, race and ethnicity, education level, marital status, and arrest history; need factors, including physical health problems; and enabling factors that facilitate or hinder service use and access, including employment, income, and health insurance.

In addition to gender and race and ethnicity, predisposing variables included in this analysis were age (18–20, 21–29, 30–49, and ≥ 50 years), education level (less than high school, high school, some college, and college graduate), marital status (married, separated, divorced or widowed, and single), and lifetime arrest history (yes–no). The analysis controlled for lifetime arrest history as a predisposing variable for past-year service use and unmet need given the high prevalence of SUD and mental illness among persons in the criminal justice system (James & Glaze, 2006; Teitelbaum & Hoffman, 2013). Although imperfect, arrest history could provide insight into persons who are at risk for unaddressed SUD needs, MH needs, or both, and for being mandated to or not engaged in services.

The enabling variables included employment (currently employed full-time or part-time, unemployed, and not working due to other reasons), family income (US$ < 20,000, 20,000–49,999, 50,000–74,999, > 75,000), and health insurance (private, Medicaid, Medicare, other insurance, and uninsured).

Self-reported physical health need was measured from poor to excellent on a 5-point scale. For the purposes of this analysis, physical health was dichotomized into fair to poor (*fair* and *poor*) and good to excellent (*excellent, very good*, and *good*).

Drug use disorder and mental illness were included in the analysis as covariates given their common cooccurrence with alcohol misuse (Grant et al., 2015). Similar to AUD, drug use disorder was derived from a series of questions based on *DSM–IV* criteria for abuse and dependence for the following drugs: marijuana, crack or cocaine, heroin, hallucinogens, inhalants, pain relievers, tranquilizers, stimulants, and sedatives. Drug use disorder was defined as a dichotomous (yes–no) variable.

Estimates of mental illness were generated using data from a subsample of NSDUH participants who completed diagnostic clinical interviews, which were combined with other NSDUH data based on questions from Kessler's screening for psychological distress (Kessler et al., 2003), the WHO Disability Assessment Schedule (WHODAS; Novak, Colpe, Barker, & Gfroerer, 2010), suicidal ideation, major depressive episode, and age (Aldworth et al., 2010; Liao et al., 2012). NSDUH statisticians used these data to generate a prediction model for mental illness. Predicted probability estimates from the prediction model were then used to create three indicators of mental illness, including mild, moderate, and severe. For the purposes of this study, an indicator for any mental illness (yes–no) was created from the mental illness severity measure. A more detailed description of the methodology used to create mental illness indicators can be found elsewhere (Aldworth et al., 2010).

Analysis

Stata/MP version 14.0 was used for all statistical analyses. Survey weights were used in the analyses to produce nationally representative estimates of the target population. A weight adjustment procedure recommended by the Substance Abuse and Mental Health Services Administration (SAMHSA) corrected for combining data by dividing the sampling weights by the number of years of pooled data (CBHSQ, 2015a). All percentages reported in the results section are weighted. Chi-square tests were conducted to compare predisposing, need, and enabling characteristics for each alcohol risk group and gender and race and ethnicity subgroup before (2008–2009) and after (2011–2014) the ACA was implemented. In addition, linear probability models were used to test the significance of changes in the unadjusted probability of SUD and MH treatment and unmet treatment needs before and after the ACA by gender and race and ethnicity for each alcohol risk group.

To address the primary study objective, a difference-in-differences method was used to estimate the differential change in behavioral health service use and perceived unmet treatment needs among adults with heavy or binge alcohol use or an AUD before and after the ACA. A difference-in-differences approach is often used to examine the impact of policy changes (Angrist & Pischke, 2008; Imbens & Wooldridge, 2009). In this study, racial and ethnic differences were estimated postreform (2011–2014) compared to prereform (2008–2009) by gender and alcohol risk group. The year 2010 was excluded given that the ACA was signed into law midyear on March 23, 2010. In addition to the pre–post analysis, a subanalysis of data from 2011 to 2014 was examined given the uncertainty and evolving health care environment since the enactments of these policies in 2010 and full implementation of ACA's fundamental provisions as of January 1, 2014 (McDonough & Adashi, 2014). This analysis will provide important information about the short-term progress of health care reform on reducing gender and racial and ethnic disparities since these policies went into effect. The subanalysis of data from 2011 to 2014 estimated changes in gender and racial and ethnic differences among the alcohol risk groups in 2014 compared to 2011 to 2013.

The dependent variables included in the difference-in-differences models were SUD treatment use, MH treatment use, perceived unmet need for SUD treatment, and perceived unmet need for MH treatment. The independent variables of principal interest were interaction terms between the variables postreform period (coded as 1 for 2011–2014, and 0 for 2008–2009 in the main analysis, or coded as 1 for 2014, and 0 for 2011–2013 in the subanalysis) and race and ethnicity, with White respondents serving as the reference category. The interaction terms, which are the difference-in-differences estimates, are interpreted as the difference between each of the racial and ethnic groups (i.e., Black, Hispanic, Asian) included in the model and the White reference group in the average change in the outcome (i.e., service use and perceived unmet treatment needs) from the prereform period to the postreform period. All models were stratified by gender and alcohol risk group and controlled for the predisposing, enabling, and need variables described earlier.

Linear probability models were used for the difference-in-differences analysis because of the dichotomous outcome variables and the difficulty in interpreting interaction terms in nonlinear difference-in-differences models. When a nonlinear model is used, such as logit or probit regression, the difference-in-differences interpretation of the modeled interaction term is lost and might not be a reliable indicator of the policy effect (Athey & Imbens, 2002). Linear probability models lead to heteroskedastic estimates of standard errors, which could result in incorrect statistical inferences. To address this limitation, linear probability models were estimated using heteroskedastically robust jackknife standard errors. In a sensitivity analysis, logistic regression models yielded similar results.

To reduce the risk of Type I error due to multiple testing, a conservative alpha value of $p < .01$ was used to assess statistical significance. Adjusting for Type I error also increases the chance of Type II errors (Feise, 2002). As such, the included tables indicate those findings that are significant at the $p < .05$ level. These findings are discussed with caution given that they are statistically provisional. In addition, based on model fit statistics, the Asian subgroups among respondents with heavy or binge drinking were excluded from SUD treatment and unmet need outcome models due to insufficient cell size. With these adjustments, model fit statistics revealed significant overall F tests for the SUD-related (excluding Asian subgroups) and MH-related outcome models, suggesting that the cell sizes for other subgroups were of sufficient size.

RESULTS

Sample Characteristics

Approximately 72.7% of the sample population met criteria for heavy or binge alcohol use, and 27.3% met criteria for an AUD. Tables 1 and 2 show the predisposing, enabling, and need characteristics of respondents with heavy or binge drinking and AUD, respectively, by gender and race and ethnicity pre- and postreform. Due to the large sample size, most between-group comparisons were statistically significant ($p < .01$). Notably, a greater percentage of Black and Hispanic respondents across the gender and alcohol risk groups reported having less than a high school education and being unemployed compared to White and Asian groups. Most racial and ethnic minority groups, regardless of gender and alcohol risk group, reported having a household income less than $20,000 in the past year and were uninsured. Having a lifetime arrest was more prevalent among Black men than other racial and ethnic groups regardless of alcohol risk group.

Unadjusted Rates of Service Use and Unmet Needs

Figures 1 and 2 show the unadjusted probability of behavioral health service use and perceived unmet needs before and after the ACA was implemented. Notably, there was a significant reduction in the use of MH treatment postreform compared to prereform among Asian men identified as heavy or binge drinking users ($p < .01$). The rate of unmet need for SUD treatment decreased from pre- to postreform for Black men in this same group ($p < .05$). Among respondents with AUD, there was a significant increase in receiving any MH treatment postreform compared to prereform for Hispanic women ($p < .01$).

Difference-in-Differences Estimates of Service Use and Unmet Needs

The adjusted models show the differential changes in service use and perceived unmet needs postreform for both alcohol risk groups (see Tables 3 and 4). For heavy or binge drinkers, perceived unmet need for SUD treatment increased by 1 percentage point in 2011 to 2014 compared to 2008 to 2009 among Black women ($p < .05$), whereas this type of unmet need decreased by 1.65 percentage points among Black men ($p < .05$). However, the subanalysis shows a decrease by 1.32 percentage points in perceived unmet SUD treatment need among Black women ($p < .05$), whereas this type of unmet need increased by 1.12 percentage points among Black men ($p < .05$). Among Asian men, use of any MH treatment decreased by 7.1 percentage points in 2011 to 2014 compared to 2008 to 2009 ($p < .01$). Similarly, the subanalysis indicates a significant decrease by 5.08 percentage points in using any MH treatment among Asian men ($p < .01$).

TABLE 1 Sample Characteristics Among Adults with Heavy or Binge Drinking by Gender and Race and Ethnic Subgroups: National Survey on Drug Use and Health 2008–2009 and 2011–2014

	Women (N = 22,078)								Men (N = 30,418)							
	Pre-ACA: 2008–2009 (n = 7,190)				Post-ACA: 2011–2014 (n = 14,888)				Pre-ACA: 2008–2009 (n = 9,951)				Post-ACA: 2011–2014 (n = 20,4□)			
	White (73.2%)	Black (11.6%)	Hispanic (12.8%)	Asian (2.5%)	White (67.9%)	Black (13.3%)	Hispanic (15.3%)	Asian (3.6%)	White (71.2%)	Black (9.4%)	Hispanic (16.6%)	Asian (2.8%)	White (69.6%)	Black (10.0%)	Hispanic (17.0%)	Asian (_.4%)
Age in years[b]***, c***, d***																
18–25	26.1%	24.0%	28.8%	28.6%	24.3%	22.5%	27.0%	30.0%	18.3%	19.3%	19.9%	23.1%	18.0%	19.2%	22.7%	23.3%
26–34	21.2%	24.0%	30.9%	19.5%	22.3%	19.7%	26.9%	26.0%	20.9%	19.9%	27.8%	30.8%	20.7%	23.0%	27.2%	2□.6%
35–49	29.8%	32.7%	26.7%	32.9%	28.0%	32.2%	30.0%	20.7%	29.8%	30.8%	36.9%	28.1%	28.2%	28.5%	32.6%	2□.7%
50 years+	22.9%	19.3%	13.7%	19.1%	25.4%	25.7%	16.1%	23.7%	31.0%	30.0%	15.4%	18.0%	33.2%	29.2%	17.6%	2□.5%
Marital status[a]***, b***, c***, d***																
Married	48.3%	20.3%	43.8%	49.1%	45.4%	19.5%	38.2%	37.2%	54.8%	35.1%	50.4%	52.2%	50.7%	31.6%	49.6%	4□.4%
Separated, divorced or widowed	17.3%	24.4%	16.1%	7.0%	18.5%	24.1%	19.0%	16.2%	13.1%	18.2%	10.8%	3.1%	15.8%	17.7%	11.1%	□1%
Never married	34.4%	55.4%	40.1%	43.9%	36.0%	56.5%	42.8%	46.6%	32.1%	46.7%	38.8%	□4.7%	33.5%	50.7%	39.3%	4□5%
< High school education[a]**, b***, c**, d**	8.8%	15.6%	26.1%	4.9%	7.1%	13.2%	22.3%	6.2%	10.0%	22.4%	32.0%	3.7%	9.1%	19.1%	28.3%	8□5%
Ever arrested[a]**, b***, c***, d***	14.9%	17.8%	12.0%	3.2%	14.5%	16.7%	13.2%	4.7%	32.6%	41.6%	29.0%	18.2%	34.7%	42.7%	25.8%	1□4%
Unemployed[a]**, b***, c**, d**	5.4%	12.6%	7.6%	7.5%	4.5%	12.4%	7.3%	6.3%	5.1%	11.1%	7.7%	4.6%	5.1%	13.2%	8.0%	□0%
Household income < $20,000[a]**, b***, c**, d**	15.1%	36.7%	25.2%	14.1%	17.3%	41.0%	25.4%	22.3%	11.3%	26.8%	17.2%	16.5%	12.9%	32.9%	19.1%	1□5%
Uninsured[a]**, b***, c**, d**	16.3%	20.8%	32.0%	17.6%	13.3%	18.2%	28.5%	17.8%	15.3%	25.6%	35.9%	15.0%	14.2%	27.7%	36.5%	1□7%
Drug use disorder[c]*, d*	3.2%	4.0%	2.5%	0.5%	2.7%	3.0%	1.9%	1.1%	3.1%	5.6%	3.4%	2.5%	3.5%	5.5%	3.6%	□0%
Any mental illness[b]*, d**	24.0%	19.2%	25.0%	20.5%	23.3%	20.6%	18.8%	18.7%	11.2%	10.0%	10.4%	14.8%	12.0%	10.2%	9.2%	1□1%
Fair or poor health[a]***, b***, c*, d***	6.4%	13.5%	13.3%	3.5%	6.8%	16.9%	13.3%	10.9%	8.3%	12.7%	10.2%	13.8%	8.7%	13.4%	13.5%	5□%

Note: ACA = Affordable Care Act. [a]Significant between-group comparison for women pre-ACA. [b]Significant between-group comparison for women post-ACA. [c]Significant between-group comparison for men pre-ACA. [d]Significant between-group comparison for men post-ACA. *p < .05. **p < .01. ***p < .001.

TABLE 2 Sample Characteristics Among Adults with Alcohol Use Disorder by Gender and Race and Ethnic Subgroups, National Survey of Drug Use and Health 2008–2009 and 2011–2014

	Women (N = 8,987)								Men (N = 13,979)							
	Pre-ACA: 2008–2009 (n = 3,325)				Post-ACA: 2011–2014 (n = 5,662)				Pre-ACA: 2008–2009 (n = 5,270)				Post-ACA: 2011–2014 (n = 8,709)			
	White (76.6%)	Black (9.6%)	Hispanic (11.4%)	Asian (2.5%)	White (71.3%)	Black (10.8%)	Hispanic (15.1%)	Asian (2.8%)	White (67.7%)	Black (12.6%)	Hispanic (17.6%)	Asian (2.2%)	White (68.4%)	Black (10.8%)	Hispanic (18.0%)	Asian (2.8%)
Age in years[b**, c**, d**]																
18–25	34.4%	35.6%	44.3%	54.3%	29.6%	31.6%	44.0%	45.9%	31.3%	22.4%	27.9%	43.4%	25.3%	23.9%	31.5%	40.1%
26–34	21.2%	31.3%	25.7%	24.3%	21.9%	28.8%	28.5%	35.4%	21.6%	24.4%	35.3%	23.3%	22.6%	24.5%	29.3%	27.2%
35–49	26.7%	24.9%	22.2%	21.4%	25.4%	22.5%	20.7%	16.0%	27.4%	30.6%	25.3%	18.2%	26.0%	29.8%	29.2%	22.5%
50 years+	17.6%	8.3%	7.8%	0.0%	23.1%	17.2%	6.9%	2.7%	19.7%	22.7%	11.5%	15.2%	26.1%	21.8%	10.0%	10.2%
Marital status[a*, b**, d***]																
Married	35.6%	13.8%	25.7%	23.9%	33.4%	14.2%	24.6%	23.2%	36.0%	31.4%	36.4%	40.0%	37.5%	25.7%	36.5%	27.5%
Separated, divorced or widowed	16.8%	16.5%	17.7%	5.1%	21.6%	18.2%	15.1%	3.8%	16.5%	17.3%	12.4%	3.6%	16.2%	14.1%	12.8%	7.8%
Never married	47.6%	69.8%	56.6%	71.1%	45.1%	67.6%	60.3%	73.0%	47.5%	51.4%	51.2%	56.8%	46.3%	60.2%	50.7%	64.8%
High school education[a**, b**, c*, d**]	9.0%	19.0%	28.4%	7.6%	6.2%	19.4%	21.0%	6.0%	13.0%	20.4%	34.8%	7.6%	11.2%	23.2%	28.9%	4.4%
Ever arrested[a**, b**, c*, d**]	27.1%	37.9%	21.8%	11.1%	26.2%	35.2%	27.4%	15.2%	51.2%	57.8%	45.8%	28.4%	46.3%	60.8%	43.0%	28.5%
Unemployed[b***, c, d***]	6.7%	12.2%	10.1%	4.5%	7.1%	13.1%	8.4%	17.9%	8.8%	15.5%	11.9%	1.8%	7.6%	17.6%	8.8%	8.9%
Household income $20,000[a**, b**, c**, d**]	18.7%	42.4%	24.2%	23.5%	20.7%	45.4%	36.1%	39.0%	17.2%	31.8%	22.0%	21.9%	18.7%	33.2%	24.1%	19.0%
Uninsured[a*, b**, c**, d**]	16.1%	27.6%	28.2%	30.6%	15.2%	24.4%	30.8%	21.3%	22.7%	29.7%	43.6%	15.7%	19.6%	37.7%	39.5%	24.5%
Drug use disorder[b**, c, d*]	14.4%	16.0%	16.5%	9.3%	11.8%	22.2%	15.6%	15.2%	15.0%	20.9%	15.9%	6.7%	13.5%	22.6%	15.4%	9.0%
Any mental illness	49.3%	51.4%	41.8%	60.4%	49.1%	50.5%	51.4%	39.9%	29.7%	27.3%	25.6%	30.1%	31.4%	32.5%	26.9%	26.1%
Fair or poor health[a*, b**, c*, d**]	7.6%	19.8%	14.1%	7.1%	11.7%	25.8%	12.2%	10.2%	11.4%	10.1%	17.7%	12.0%	12.6%	18.4%	15.0%	9.1%

Note: ACA = Affordable Care Act.

[a] Significant between-group comparison for women pre-ACA. [b] Significant between-group comparison for women post-ACA. [c] Significant between-group comparison for men pre-ACA. [d] Significant between-group comparison for men post-ACA. *p < .05. **p < .01. ***p < .001.

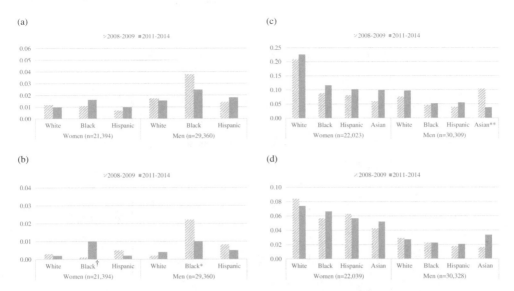

FIGURE 1 Proportion of service use and unmet needs among adults with heavy or binge alcohol use, by gender and race and ethnicity. (a) Proportion of any substance use disorder (SUD) treatment. (b) Proportion of any unmet need for SUD treatment (c) Proportion of any mental health (MH) treatment. (d) Proportion of any unmet need for MH treatment. $^{\dagger}p < .10$. $^{*}p < .05$. $^{**}p < .01$. $^{***}p < .001$.

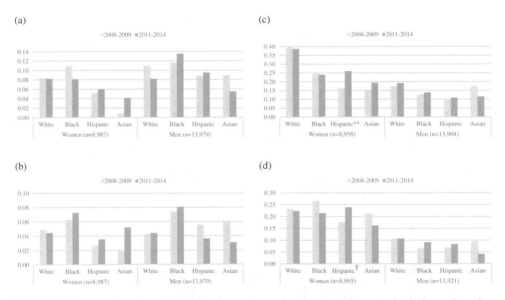

FIGURE 2 Proportion of service use and unmet needs among adults with alcohol use disorder, by gender and race and ethnicity. (a) Proportion of any substance use disorder (SUD) treatment. (b) Proportion of any unmet need for SUD treatment (c) Proportion of any mental health (MH) treatment. (d) Proportion of any unmet need for MH treatment. $^{\dagger}p < .10$. $^{*}p < .05$. $^{**}p < .01$. $^{***}p < .001$.

TABLE 3 Difference-in-Differences Estimates of Service Use and Perceived Unmet Need for Black, Hispanic, and Asian Adults with Heavy or Binge Drinking, by Gender

| | Post-ACA: 2011–2014 (vs. 2008–2009) | | | | | | | Subanalysis, Post-ACA: 2014 (vs. 2011–2013) | | | | | |
| | Black (vs. White) | | Hispanic (vs. White) | | Asian (vs. White) | | Black (vs. White) | | Hispanic (vs. White) | | Asian (vs. White) | |
Outcome	DiD Estimate[a] (%)	95% CI	DiD Estimate[a] (%)	95% CI	DiD Estimate[a] (%)	95% CI	DiD Estimate[a] (%)	95% CI	DiD Estimate[a] (%)	95% CI	DiD Estimate[a] (%)	95% CI
Women												
SUD treatment	0.72	-0.64 2.09	0.48	-0.64 1.44	—	— —	1.19	-0.78 3.18	-0.03	-1.19 1.11	—	— —
MH treatment	0.35	-3.92 4.61	1.95	-2.42 6.39	2.94	-4.13 10.02	-1.23	-6.66 4.19	-2.60	-7.78 2.57	-3.79	-13.66 6.09
Unmet need, SUD treatment	1.02*	0.14 1.91	-0.26	-1.12 0.60	—	— —	-1.32*	-2.52 -0.13	-0.15	-0.53 0.23	—	— —
Unmet need, MH treatment	1.76	-1.16 4.67	1.45	-1.27 4.17	1.23	-3.46 5.91	-3.42	-7.40 0.55	-0.35	-3.55 2.85	-2.36	-6.68 1.97
Men												
SUD treatment	-1.19	-3.62 1.25	0.76	-0.41 1.93	—	— —	1.45	-0.94 0.038	-0.66	-1.97 0.70	—	— —
MH treatment	-1.48	-4.71 1.75	-0.04	-2.45 2.37	-7.10**	-12.40 -1.78	-2.40	-6.15 1.34	1.05	-2.40 4.53	-5.08**	-9.32 -0.83
Unmet need, SUD treatment	-1.65*	-3.30 -0.001	-0.45	-1.23 0.33	—	— —	1.12*	0.07 0.02	0.85	-0.27 1.98	—	— —
Unmet need, MH treatment	0.44	-1.05 1.93	0.80	-0.38 1.97	3.01	-0.35 6.37	0.45	-1.43 2.32	-2.06**	-3.67 -0.45	2.09	-3.56 7.73

Note: All models controlled for predisposing, enabling, and need variables. The models estimating unmet needs for substance use disorder (SUD) treatment and mental health (MH) treatment also controlled for past-year SUD treatment and past-year MH treatment, respectively. ACA = Affordable Care Act.[a]The Difference-in-Differences (DiD) estimates are derived from the b coefficients (i.e., probabilities) from the regression models and presented as percentage points.*p < .05. **p < .01. ***p < .001.

TABLE 4 Difference-in-Differences Estimates of Service Use and Perceived Unmet Need for Black, Hispanic, and Asian Adults with Alcohol Use Disorder, by Gender

| | Post-ACA: 2011–2014 (vs. 2008–2009) | | | | | | Subanalysis, Post-ACA: 2014 (vs. 2011–2013) | | | | | |
| | Black (vs. White) | | Hispanic (vs. White) | | Asian (vs. White) | | Black (vs. White) | | Hispanic (vs. White) | | Asian (vs. White) | |
Outcome	DiD Estimate[a] (%)	95% CI	DiD Estimate[a] (%)	95% CI	DiD Estimate[a] (%)	95% CI	DiD Estimate[a] (%)	95% CI	DiD Estimate[a] (%)	95% CI	DiD Estimate[a] (%)	95% CI
Women												
SUD treatment	−4.11	−11.88 3.67	−0.82	−5.02 3.38	2.70	−3.09 8.49	−0.43	−7.94 7.09	−3.56	−8.8 1.69	4.58	−5.71 14.87
MH treatment	−1.03	−11.60 9.54	7.44*	0.67 14.20	0.09	−0.08 0.26	0.45	−12.12 13.01	−5.84	−17.53 5.84	5.14	−17.58 27.86
Unmet need, SUD treatment	0.52	−4.11 5.15	1.09	−2.11 4.29	4.47	−2.05 11.00	4.86	−3.66 13.38	−0.96	−5.41 3.49	−2.36	−13.50 8.78
Unmet need, MH treatment	−4.79	−13.50 3.92	2.67	−4.96 10.30	−1.61	−18.25 15.01	3.72	−7.21 14.65	−0.78	−8.94 7.38	−1.56	−22.49 19.38
Men												
SUD treatment	3.57	−1.71 8.85	3.07	−2.06 8.20	−1.46	−13.16 10.25	1.89	−5.66 9.44	1.69	−4.94 8.33	2.84	−4.46 10.14
MH treatment	−0.67	−7.75 6.42	−0.15	−5.39 5.09	−6.61	−19.91 6.69	1.42	−6.79 9.63	1.15	−4.88 7.17	−1.57	−10.98 7.84
Unmet need, SUD treatment	−0.31	−5.55 4.92	−1.86	−4.77 1.06	−3.45	−13.66 6.76	−0.97	−7.15 5.22	−1.90	−4.37 0.57	−1.28	−6.43 −3.88
Unmet need, MH treatment	0.99	−2.56 4.55	1.31	−2.92 5.53	−3.46	−13.00 6.08	3.90	−2.34 10.17	−3.75	−8.57 1.07	1.10	−6.11 8.31

Note: All models controlled for predisposing, enabling, and need variables. The models estimating unmet needs for substance use disorder (SUD) treatment and mental health (MH) treatment also controlled for past-year SUD treatment and past-year MH treatment, respectively. ACA = Affordable Care Act. [a]The Difference-in-Differences (DiD) estimates are derived from the *b* coefficients (i.e., probabilities) from the regression models and presented as percentage points.*p ≤ .05. **p ≤ .01. ***p < .001.

In 2014, Hispanic men had a 2.06 percentage point decrease in perceived unmet MH treatment need ($p < .01$).

Adjusted models estimating the probability of service use and perceived unmet needs among respondents with AUD suggested few changes postreform. Notably, use of any MH treatment increased by 7.44 percentage points for Hispanic women postreform (2011–2014) compared to prereform rates ($p < .05$). No significant changes were found in the subanalysis between 2011 and 2014 among respondents with an AUD.

DISCUSSION

Gender and racial and ethnic disparities in SUD treatment have been well established in the literature. The ACA is recent legislation that is expected to reduce these disparities and increase access to services. This study found mixed results in examining the impact of the ACA on reducing gender and racial and ethnic disparities in behavioral health service use and access among adults who misuse alcohol.

Most of the pre–post reform changes found in this study occurred among heavy or binge alcohol users. Notably, although unmet need for SUD treatment increased postreform (2011–2014) for Black (vs. White) women, the subanalysis showed a decrease in 2014 compared to 2011 to 2013, suggesting that the rate of unmet need in this population might be improving now that full implementation of the ACA is underway. In contrast, changes in unmet need for SUD treatment among Black (vs. White) men showed the opposite pattern, suggesting a worsening of treatment access in 2014 compared to 2011 to 2013. The descriptive analysis indicated higher uninsured rates among Black men compared to Black women, which could help explain these differences. Black men also had higher rates of cooccurring drug use disorder than Black women, suggesting the potential role of gender differences in the type of substances used or SUD severity. It is important to note, however, that these results are statistically provisional and should be viewed with caution. Whether these changes are the result of the ACA warrants continued monitoring as the provisions are more fully integrated into the health care system or if any of the ACA provisions are dismantled.

Both the main and subanalyses found a decrease in using any MH treatment among Asian men who are heavy or binge drinkers. The declining trend is concerning given that the descriptive analysis showed a higher rate of mental illness among Asian men but the lowest rate of any past-year MH treatment compared to men of other racial and ethnic groups. These rates are consistent with past research, suggesting a lower rate of MH treatment among Asians compared to other racial and ethnic groups (Sue, Yan Cheng, Saad, & Chu, 2012). Previous research also suggests that immigration status and limited English proficiency are barriers to accessing services among Asian Americans

(Chen, Vargas-Bustamante, & Ortega, 2013). Studies on help-seeking behaviors report that Asian Americans often seek help from nonprofessional sources or general medical providers (Chu, Hsieh, & Tokars, 2011). Given the emphasis on integrated care, the declines in MH treatment might reflect increases in other sources of informal or formal care, such as primary care, a topic worth exploring in future research.

After full ACA implementation in 2014, there was a significant decrease in unmet MH treatment need among Hispanic men compared to the initial years in 2011 to 2013. Although Hispanic men have the highest uninsured rates compared to other groups in this sample, a descriptive analysis revealed a decrease in the uninsured rate among Hispanic men after full implementation of the ACA. In 2014, the uninsured rate among Hispanic men was about 31% compared to 39% in 2011 to 2013. Indeed, recent research indicates a decline in the uninsured rates among Hispanics (Chen et al., 2016; Creedon & Cook, 2016). Similarly, a statistically provisional improvement was also found in using any MH treatment among Hispanic women with AUD. A recent study found that Hispanic respondents, regardless of gender, were more likely to be screened for depression, which could reflect improvements in access to bilingual care (Hahm, Le Cook, Ault-Brutus, & Alegra, 2015).

Although these findings are promising, it is worth noting that Hispanic women and men, as well as other racial and ethnic minority groups, continue to lag behind their White counterparts in using and accessing services (Creedon & Cook, 2016). Between 40% and 50% of Hispanic women with AUD in this study reported a cooccurring mental illness, yet less than a quarter used MH treatment in any given year, and they had among the lowest use rates of all groups of women. Whether these MH service disparities can be explained by differences in patient preferences, attitudes toward care, or provider bias and stereotyping (Ashton et al., 2003; Fiscella, Franks, Doescher, & Saver, 2002; McGuire & Miranda, 2008) are important factors to consider in future research.

Limitations

This study has several limitations. First, past drinking and service use behaviors are based on self-reported data and are subject to recall bias; however, a strength of NSDUH is the use of computer-assisted software to facilitate interview administration, which is associated with lower rates of recall and social desirability biases (Breslin, Borsoi, Cunningham, & Koski-Jannes, 2001; Killeen, Brady, Gold, Tyson, & Simpson, 2004). Second, people who reported binge and heavy drinking were combined and analyzed together given that the small frequency of heavy drinkers was not sufficient to analyze separately. It could be that binge and heavy drinkers have different service use patterns and needs, although based on a descriptive analysis, the two groups had similar rates of SUD and MH treatment and unmet treatment needs compared to the AUD group. Nevertheless, the conclusions regarding gender and racial and ethnic disparities among heavy or binge drinkers should be examined in future research. Third, the study was underpowered to examine differences in SUD treatment-related outcomes of Asian respondents. Fourth, the large confidence intervals in analyses estimating the impact of SUD-related outcomes and in analyses that included Asian subgroups prompt caution regarding the interpretation of the actual magnitude or value of the estimates in the multivariate models. Fifth, there is likely variation in service use and unmet needs within racial and ethnic subgroups that are not accounted for in this analysis. Sixth, the subanalysis examining service-related outcomes in 2014 compared to 2011 to 2013 provides limited time to investigate the full impact of the health care reform. Finally, although a difference-in-differences design was used to estimate the impact of the ACA on service use and access, caution is needed to infer causal associations between these policies and the outcomes given the cross-sectional, observational design of NSDUH. Prospective, longitudinal studies are needed to better establish temporal ordering of these relationships and to monitor service use and access trends among the same cohort of respondents over time.

Implications for Social Work Practice

This study produced mixed findings on the ACA's impact in reducing gender and racial and ethnic disparities in behavioral health service use and access among alcohol risk groups. Although there was limited progress overall, service use and access improved among Black and Hispanic women and Hispanic men. However, there were setbacks among Black and Asian men. These findings have broad implications for social work practitioners and policymakers in addressing the challenge of reducing service-related disparities in alcohol misuse and related problems. First, gender- and culturally grounded engagement, assessment, and intervention approaches are needed in direct practice settings, especially non-substance-abuse treatment settings where social workers often encounter individuals and families affected by alcohol misuse. Service disparities will likely continue without focusing on unique barriers of gender and racial and ethnic minority groups, such as stigma, attitudes toward treatment, provider bias, and language. Additionally, evidence-based practices, such as Screening, Brief Intervention, and Referral to Treatment (SBIRT) (SAMHSA, 2012), are critical to implement in non-substance-abuse treatment settings.

Second, social workers approach practice from a biopsychosocial perspective, which is often overlooked but important to understanding and addressing the complexity of alcohol misuse and its associated problems.

Social workers view problems from a broader perspective than other health professions, considering not only the MH challenges that often lead to substance abuse, but also the struggles in a person's social environment (e.g., poverty, unstable housing, low levels of education, unemployment, partner and community violence, and poor access to resources and services) that negatively affect the individual's well-being. Through this vantage point, social workers can help individuals understand how their alcohol misuse and internal and external struggles are interconnected.

Third, engaging and intervening with individuals and families affected by alcohol misuse requires effective training and supervision. However, few health care providers, including social workers, consistently provide alcohol and illicit drug screening or intervention in practice (Pringle et al., 2012). Research specific to social work education suggests few MSW programs require or offer elective courses in substance abuse. In a survey of 58 MSW programs, representing all 50 states in the United States, Russett and Williams (2015) found that only one program required a course in substance abuse and 37 offered at least one substance abuse elective course. Notably, about one third of MSW programs sampled did not have a designated course in substance abuse (Russett & Williams, 2015). Yet, experts in the SUD treatment field emphasize the importance of training all social workers in evidence-based practices, such as SBIRT, given the high prevalence of alcohol and other drug misuse and abuse in non-substance-abuse treatment settings (Straussner & Senreich, 2002).

Finally, at a policy level, expanded coverage offered by the ACA is likely not sufficient to reduce long-standing and entrenched gender and racial and ethnic disparities found in behavioral health service use and unmet needs. The higher rates of MH treatment compared to SUD treatment also suggest the importance of integrated models of care, which are now a priority of health homes and accountable care organizations under the ACA. Social workers have made significant contributions to increasing access to services and resources and improving the social conditions of individuals and families (Popple & Leighninger, 2005). The ACA provides social work with an opportunity to take a leadership role in implementing community-based interventions that are culturally grounded and tailored to the specific needs of individuals and communities, as well as providing workforce training opportunities in these approaches. Interventions and policies that target barriers specific to the service experiences of racial and ethnic minority groups are important to consider in future research. Ongoing monitoring and tracking of our evolving health care system and its impact on behavioral health service use and access among gender and racial and ethnic subgroups will be critical in the years ahead. Future research is also needed to examine changes in the health quality and experiences in care, as well as treatment outcomes.

FUNDING

This article was supported by Grant K01DA035330 from the National Institute on Drug Abuse.

REFERENCES

Aldworth, J., Colpe, L. J., Gfroerer, J. C., Novak, S. P., Chromy, J. R., Barker, P. R., … Spagnola, K. (2010). The National Survey on Drug Use and Health Mental Health Surveillance Study: Calibration analysis. *International Journal of Methods in Psychiatric Research, 19*, 61–87. doi:10.1002/mpr.312

Ali, M. M., Mutter, R., & Teich, J. L. (2015). *The CBHSQ report: State participation in the Medicaid expansion provision of the Affordable Care Act: Implications for uninsured individuals with a behavioral health condition*. Rockville, MD: Substance Abuse and Mental Health Services Administration, Center for Behavioral Health Statistics and Quality.

Amaro, H., Arevalo, S., Gonzalez, G., Szapocznik, J., & Iguchi, M. Y. (2006). Needs and scientific opportunities for research on substance abuse treatment among Hispanic adults. *Drug and Alcohol Dependence, 84*, S64–S75. doi:10.1016/j.drugalcdep.2006.05.008

American Psychiatric Association. (1994). *Diagnostic and statistical manual of mental disorders* (4th ed.). Washington, DC: Author.

Andersen, R. M. (1995). Revisiting the behavioral model and access to medical care: Does it matter? *Journal of Health and Social Behavior, 36*(1), 1–10.

Andrulis, D. P. (2010). *Patient Protection and Affordable Care Act of 2010 advancing health equity for racially and ethnically diverse populations*. Washington, DC: Joint Center for Political and Economic Studies.

Angrist, J. D., & Pischke, J.-S. (2008). *Mostly harmless econometrics: An empiricist's companion*. Princeton, NJ: Princeton University Press.

Ashton, C. M., Haidet, P., Paterniti, D. A., Collins, T. C., Gordon, H. S., O'Malley, K., … Street, R. L., Jr. (2003). Racial and ethnic disparities in the use of health services: Bias, preferences, or poor communication? *Journal of General Internal Medicine, 18*, 146–152.

Athey, S., & Imbens, G. W. (2002). *Identification and inference in nonlinear difference-in-differences models*. Stanford, CA: Stanford Institute for Economic Policy Research.

Begun, A. L., Clapp, J. D., & The Alcohol Misuse Grand Challenge Collective. (2016). Reducing and preventing alcohol misuse and its consequences: A Grand Challenge for social work. *The International Journal of Alcohol and Drug Research, 5*(2), 73–83. doi:10.7895/ijadr.v5i2.223

Beronio, K., Glied, S., & Frank, R. (2014). How the Affordable Care Act and Mental Health Parity and Addiction Equity Act greatly expand coverage of behavioral health care. *Journal of Behavioral Health Services & Research, 41*(4), 410–428. doi:10.1007/s11414-014-9412-0

Breslin, F. C., Borsoi, D., Cunningham, J. A., & Koski-Jannes, A. (2001). Help-seeking timeline followback for problem drinkers: Preliminary comparison with agency records of treatment contacts. *Journal of Studies on Alcohol, 62,* 262–267.

Center for Behavioral Health Statistics and Quality. (2015a). *2014 National Survey on Drug Use and Health: Methodological summary and definitions.* Retrieved from http://www.samhsa.gov/data/sites/default/files/NSDUH-MethodSumm-Defs2014/NSDUH-MethodSummDefs2014.htm

Center for Behavioral Health Statistics and Quality. (2015b). *Behavioral health trends in the United States: Results from the 2014 National Survey on Drug Use and Health* (HHS Publication No. SMA 15-4927, NSDUH Series H-50). Retrieved from https://www.samhsa.gov/data/sites/default/files/NSDUH-FRR1-2014/NSDUH-FRR1-2014.pdf

Chartier, K. G., & Caetano, R. (2010). Ethnicity and health disparities in alcohol research. *Alcohol Research and Health, 33*(1–2), 152–160.

Chartier, K. G., & Caetano, R. (2011). Trends in alcohol services utilization from 1991–1992 to 2001–2002: Ethnic group differences in the U.S. population. *Alcoholism: Clinical and Experimental Research, 35,* 1485–1497. doi:10.1111/j.1530-0277.2011.01485.x

Chen, J., Vargas-Bustamante, A., Mortensen, K., & Ortega, A. N. (2016). Racial and ethnic disparities in health care access and utilization under the Affordable Care Act. *Medical Care, 54,* 140–146. doi:10.1097/MLR.0000000000000467

Chen, J., Vargas-Bustamante, A., & Ortega, A. N. (2013). Health care expenditures among Asian American subgroups. *Medical Care Research and Review, 70,* 310–329. doi:10.1177/1077558712465773

Chu, J. P., Hsieh, K. Y., & Tokars, D. A. (2011). Help-seeking tendencies in Asian Americans with suicidal ideation and attempts. *Asian American Journal of Psychology, 2*(1), 25–38. doi:10.1037/a0023326

Clemans-Cope, L., Kenney, G. M., Buettgens, M., Carroll, C., & Blavin, F. (2012). The Affordable Care Act's coverage expansions will reduce differences in uninsurance rates by race and ethnicity. *Health Affairs, 31,* 920–930. doi:10.1377/hlthaff.2011.1086

Congressional Budget Office. (2012). *Estimates for the insurance coverage provisions of the Affordable Care Act updated for the recent Supreme Court decision.* Washington, DC: Author.

Creedon, T. B., & Cook, B. L. (2016). Access to mental health care increased but not for substance use, while disparities remain. *Health Affairs, 35,* 1017–1021. doi:10.1377/hlthaff.2016.0098

Dawson, D. A., Grant, B. F., Stinson, F. S., Chou, P. S., Huang, B., & Ruan, W. J. (2005). Recovery from DSM–IV alcohol dependence: United States, 2001–2002. *Addiction, 100,* 281–292. doi:10.1111/j.1360-0443.2004.00964.x

Edlund, M. J., Booth, B. M., & Han, X. (2012). Who seeks care where? Utilization of mental health and substance use disorder treatment in two national samples of individuals with alcohol use disorders. *Journal of Studies on Alcohol and Drugs, 73,* 635–646.

Feise, R. J. (2002). Do multiple outcome measures require p-value adjustment? *BMC Medical Research Methodology, 2,* 8.

Fiscella, K., Franks, P., Doescher, M. P., & Saver, B. G. (2002). Disparities in health care by race, ethnicity, and language among the insured: Findings from a national sample. *Medical Care, 40*(1), 52–59.

Fitzgerald, T., Cohen, L., Hyams, T., Sullivan, K. M., & Johnson, P. A. (2014). Women and health reform: How national health care can enhance coverage, affordability, and access for women (examples from Massachusetts). *Women's Health Issues, 24*(1), e5–e10. doi:10.1016/j.whi.2013.11.006

Gettens, J., Henry, A. D., & Himmelstein, J. (2012). Assessing health care reform: Potential effects on insurance coverage among persons with disabilities. *Journal of Disability Policy Studies, 23*(1), 3–13. doi:10.1177/1044207311416584

Grant, B. F., Goldstein, R. B., Saha, T. D., Chou, S. P., Jung, J., Zhang, H., ... Hasin, D. S. (2015). Epidemiology of DSM–5 alcohol use disorder: Results from the National Epidemiologic Survey on Alcohol and Related Conditions III. *JAMA Psychiatry, 72*, 757–766. doi:10.1001/jamapsychiatry.2015.0584

Grant, B. F., Stinson, F. S., Dawson, D. A., Chou, S. P., Dufour, M. C., Compton, ... Kaplan, K. (2004). Prevalence and co-occurrence of substance use disorders and independent mood and anxiety disorders: Results from the National Epidemiologic Survey on Alcohol and Related Conditions. *Archives of General Psychiatry, 61*, 807–816. doi:10.1001/archpsyc.61.8.807

Greenfield, S. F., Trucco, E. M., McHugh, R. K., Lincoln, M., & Gallop, R. J. (2007). The Women's Recovery Group Study: A Stage I trial of women-focused group therapy for substance use disorders versus mixed-gender group drug counseling. *Drug and Alcohol Dependence, 90*(1), 39–47. doi:10.1016/j.drugalcdep.2007.02.009

Hahm, H. C., Le Cook, B., Ault-Brutus, A., & Alegra, M. (2015). Intersection of race-ethnicity and gender in depression care: Screening, access, and minimally adequate treatment. *Psychiatric Services, 66*, 258–264. doi:10.1176/appi.ps.201400116

Han, S. Y., Cho, M. J., Won, S., Hong, J. P., Bae, J. N., Cho, S. J., ... Chang, S. M. (2015). Sociodemographic factors and comorbidities associated with remission from alcohol dependence: Results from a nationwide General Population Survey in Korea. *Psychiatry Investigation, 12*, 316–323. doi:10.4306/pi.2015.12.3.316

Harris, K. M., & Edlund, M. J. (2005). Use of mental health care and substance abuse treatment among adults with co-occurring disorders. *Psychiatric Services, 56*, 954–959. doi:10.1176/appi.ps.56.8.954

Hasin, D. S., Stinson, F. S., Ogburn, E., & Grant, B. F. (2007). Prevalence, correlates, disability, and comorbidity of DSM–IV alcohol abuse and dependence in the United States—Results from the National Epidemiologic Survey on Alcohol and Related Conditions. *Archives of General Psychiatry, 64*, 830–842. doi:10.1001/archpsyc.64.7.830

Henry J. Kaiser Family Foundation. (2012). *Women's health insurance coverage: Fact sheet*. Menlo Park, CA: Author. Retrieved from http://kff.org/womens-health-policy/fact-sheet/womens-health-insurance-coverage-fact-sheet/

Humphreys, K., & Frank, R. G. (2014). The Affordable Care Act will revolutionize care for substance use disorders in the United States. *Addiction, 109*(12), 1957–1958. doi:10.1111/add.12606

Ilgen, M. A., Price, A. M., Burnett-Zeigler, I., Perron, B., Islam, K., Bohnert, A. S., & Zivin, K. (2011). Longitudinal predictors of addictions treatment utilization in treatment-naive adults with alcohol use disorders. *Drug and Alcohol Dependence, 113,* 215–221. doi:10.1016/j.drugalcdep.2010.08.006

Imbens, G. W., & Wooldridge, J. M. (2009). Recent developments in the econometrics of program evaluation. *Journal of Economic Literature, 47*(1), 5–86. doi:10.1257/jel.47.1.5

James, D. J., & Glaze, L. E. (2006). *Mental health problems of prison and jail inmates.* Washington, DC: Bureau of Justice Statistics. Retrieved from www.bjs.gov/content/pub/pdf/mhppji.pdf

Kaufmann, C. N., Chen, L. Y., Crum, R. M., & Mojtabai, R. (2014). Treatment seeking and barriers to treatment for alcohol use in persons with alcohol use disorders and comorbid mood or anxiety disorders. *Social Psychiatry and Psychiatric Epidemiology, 49,* 1489–1499. doi:10.1007/s00127-013-0740-9

Kessler, R. C., Barker, P. R., Colpe, L. J., Epstein, J. F., Gfroerer, J. C., Hiripi, E., … Zaslavsky, A. M. (2003). Screening for serious mental illness in the general population. *Archives of General Psychiatry, 60*(2), 184–189. doi:10.1001/archpsyc.60.2.184

Kessler, R. C., McGonagle, K. A., Swartz, M., Blazer, D. G., & Nelson, C. B. (1993). Sex and depression in the National Comorbidity Survey, I: Lifetime prevalence, chronicity and recurrence. *Journal of Affective Disorder, 29*(2–3), 85–96.

Kessler, R. C., Nelson, C. B., McGonagle, K. A., Edlund, M. J., Frank, R. G., & Leaf, P. J. (1996). The epidemiology of co-occurring addictive and mental disorders: Implications for prevention and service utilization. *American Journal of Orthopsychiatry, 66*(1), 17–31.

Killeen, T. K., Brady, K. T., Gold, P. B., Tyson, C., & Simpson, K. N. (2004). Comparison of self-report versus agency records of service utilization in a community sample of individuals with alcohol use disorders. *Drug and Alcohol Dependence, 73,* 141–147.

Liao, D., Kott, P., Aldworth, J., Yu, F., Karg, R., Shook-Sa, B., & Davis, T. (2012). *2011 Mental Health Surveillance Study: Design and estimation report.* Research Triangle Park, NC: RTI International.

Marsh, J. C., Cao, D., & D'Aunno, T. (2004). Gender differences in the impact of comprehensive services in substance abuse treatment. *Journal of Substance Abuse Treatment, 27,* 289–300. doi:10.1016/j.jsat.2004.08.004

McDonough, J. E., & Adashi, E. Y. (2014). Realizing the promise of the Affordable Care Act–January 1, 2014. *Journal of the American Medical Association, 311,* 569–570. doi:10.1001/jama.2013.286067

McGuire, T. G., & Miranda, J. (2008). New evidence regarding racial and ethnic disparities in mental health: Policy implications. *Health Affairs, 27,* 393–403. doi:10.1377/hlthaff.27.2.393

McLellan, A. T., & Woodworth, A. M. (2014). The Affordable Care Act and treatment for "substance use disorders": Implications of ending segregated behavioral healthcare. *Journal of Substance Abuse Treatment, 46*(5), 541–545. doi:10.1016/j.jsat.2014.02.001

McMorrow, S., Long, S. K., Kenney, G. M., & Anderson, N. (2015). Uninsurance disparities have narrowed for black and Hispanic adults under the Affordable Care Act. *Health Affairs, 34*(10), 1774–1778. doi:10.1377/hlthaff.2015.0757

Mojtabai, R. (2005). Use of specialty substance abuse and mental health services in adults with substance use disorders in the community. *Drug and Alcohol Dependence, 78*, 345–354. doi:10.1016/j.drugalcdep.2004.12.003

Mojtabai, R., Chen, L. Y., Kaufmann, C. N., & Crum, R. M. (2014). Comparing barriers to mental health treatment and substance use disorder treatment among individuals with comorbid major depression and substance use disorders. *Journal of Substance Abuse Treatment, 46*, 268–273. doi:10.1016/j.jsat.2013.07.012

Mulia, N., Tam, T. W., & Schmidt, L. A. (2014). Disparities in the use and quality of alcohol treatment services and some proposed solutions to narrow the gap. *Psychiatric Services, 65*, 626–633. doi:10.1176/appi.ps.201300188

Mulvaney-Day, N., DeAngelo, D., Chen, C. N., Cook, B. L., & Alegria, M. (2012). Unmet need for treatment for substance use disorders across race and ethnicity. *Drug and Alcohol Dependence, 125*(Suppl. 1), S44–S50. doi:10.1016/j.drugalcdep.2012.05.005

Novak, S. P., Colpe, L. J., Barker, P. R., & Gfroerer, J. C. (2010). Development of a brief mental health impairment scale using a nationally representative sample in the USA. *International Journal of Methods in Psychiatric Research, 19*(Suppl. 1), 49–60. doi:10.1002/mpr.313

O'Brien, M. C., McCoy, T. P., Champion, H., Mitra, A., Robbins, A., Teuschlser, H., … DuRant, R. H. (2006). Single question about drunkenness to detect college students at risk for injury. *Academic Emergency Medicine, 13*, 629–636. doi:10.1197/j.aem.2005.12.023

Polak, K., Haug, N. A., Drachenberg, H. E., & Svikis, D. S. (2015). Gender considerations in addiction: Implications for treatment. *Current Treatment Options in Psychiatry, 2*, 326–338.

Popple, P. R., & Leighninger, L. (2005). *Social work, social welfare, and American society* (6th ed.). Boston, MA: Allyn & Bacon.

Pringle, J. L., Melczak, M., Johnjulio, W., Campopiano, M., Gordon, A. J., & Costlow, M. (2012). Pennsylvania SBIRT medical and residency training: Developing, implementing, and evaluating an evidenced-based program. *Substance Abuse, 33*, 292–297. doi:10.1080/08897077.2011.640091

Research Society on Alcoholism. (2015). *White paper: Impact of alcoholism and alcohol induced disease and disorders on America*. Retrieved from http://rsoa.org/RSA-2014WhitePaperFinalVersionVH.pdf

Russett, J. L., & Williams, A. (2015). An exploration of substance abuse course offerings for students in counseling and social work programs. *Substance Abuse, 36*(1), 51–58. doi:10.1080/08897077.2014.933153

Sacks, J. J., Gonzales, K. R., Bouchery, E. E., Tomedi, L. E., & Brewer, R. D. (2015). 2010 national and state costs of excessive alcohol consumption. *American Journal of Preventive Medicine, 49*(5), e73–79. doi:10.1016/j.amepre.2015.05.031

Salganicoff, A., Ranji, U., Beamesderfer, A., & Kurani, N. (2014). *Women and health care in the early years of the Affordable Care Act*. Menlo Park, CA: Henry J. Kaiser Family Foundation.

Schmidt, L. A., Ye, Y., Greenfield, T. K., & Bond, J. (2007). Ethnic disparities in clinical severity and services for alcohol problems: Results from the National Alcohol Survey. *Alcoholism: Clinical and Experimental Research, 31*(1), 48–56. doi:10.1111/j.1530-0277.2006.00263.x

Sommers, B. D., Musco, T., Finegold, K., Gunja, M. Z., Burke, A., & McDowell, A. M. (2014). Health reform and changes in health insurance coverage in 2014. *New England Journal of Medicine, 371*(9), 867–874. doi:10.1056/NEJMsr1406753

Straussner, S. L., & Senreich, E. (2002). Educating social workers to work with individuals affected by substance use disorders. *Substance Abuse, 23*(Suppl. 3), 319–340.

Substance Abuse and Mental Health Services Administration. (2012). *State of SBIRT 2003–2012: Review and discussion of SAMHSA funded SBIRT initiatives*. Rockville, MD: Department of Health and Human Services, Substance Abuse and Mental Health Services Administration, Center for Substance Abuse Treatment.

Sue, S., Yan Cheng, J. K., Saad, C. S., & Chu, J. P. (2012). Asian American mental health: A call to action. *American Psychologist, 67*, 532–544. doi:10.1037/a0028900

Teitelbaum, J. B., & Hoffman, L. G. (2013). Health reform and correctional health care: How the Affordable Care Act can improve the health of ex-offenders and their communities. *Fordham Urban Law Journal, 40*, 1323–1356.

Tuchman, E. (2010). Women and addiction: The importance of gender issues in substance abuse research. *Journal of Addictive Diseases, 29*, 127–138. doi:10.1080/10550881003684582

Weinberger, A. H., Mazure, C. M., Morlett, A., & McKee, S. A. (2013). Two decades of smoking cessation treatment research on smokers with depression: 1990-2010. *Nicotine and Tobacco Research, 15*(6), 1014–1031. doi:10.1093/ntr/nts213

Weisner, C., Matzger, H., Tam, T., & Schmidt, L. (2002). Who goes to alcohol and drug treatment? Understanding utilization within the context of insurance. *Journal of Studies on Alcohol and Drugs, 63*, 673–682.

Wells, K., Klap, R., Koike, A., & Sherbourne, C. (2001). Ethnic disparities in unmet need for alcoholism, drug abuse, and mental health care. *American Journal of Psychiatry, 158*, 2027–2032. doi:10.1176/appi.ajp.158.12.2027

Witbrodt, J., Mulia, N., Zemore, S. E., & Kerr, W. C. (2014). Racial/ethnic disparities in alcohol-related problems: Differences by gender and level of heavy drinking. *Alcoholism: Clinical and Experimental Research, 38*, 1662–1670. doi:10.1111/acer.12398

Wolk, S. I., & Weissman, M. M. (1995). Women and depression: An update. In J. M. Oldham & M. B. Riba (Eds.), *Review of psychiatry* (Vol. 14, p. 227–259). Washington, DC: American Psychiatric Press.

World Health Organization. (2014). *Global status report on alcohol and health*. Retrieved from http://www.who.int/substance_abuse/publications/global_alcohol_report/msb_gsr_2014_1.pdf?ua=1

Zemore, S. E., Mulia, N., Yu, Y., Borges, G., & Greenfield, T. K. (2009). Gender, acculturation, and other barriers to alcohol treatment utilization among Latinos in three national alcohol surveys. *Journal of Substance Abuse Treatment, 36*, 446–456. doi:10.1016/j.jsat.2008.09.005

Impact of Race on the Implementation of Empirically Supported Treatments in Substance Abuse Treatment

CARISSA VAN DEN BERK-CLARK, PhD, MSW

DAVID A. PATTERSON SILVER WOLF (ADELV UNEGV WAYA), PhD

SHA-LAI WILLIAMS, PhD, LCSW

The effort to address the gap between research and practice in substance abuse treatment has largely neglected the role of local resources and political trends. This study seeks to clarify the role of the local environment in implementing empirically supported treatments (ESTs). The study consisted of secondary data analysis of substance abuse treatment centers (N = 13,079) and U.S. Census data to determine the likelihood of using EST by substance abuse treatment centers in counties with 50% or more Black residents. Bivariate and multivariate models were employed. After controlling for various factors, results indicate that substance use disorder treatment agencies that accept federal funding are less likely to use ESTs if they are located in counties with predominantly (> 50%) Black residents. Implementation of ESTs could be influenced by community racial distribution (% Black), but environmental constraints and events might shift implementation patterns.

Untreated substance use disorders (SUDs) continue to be a major health issue in the United States (National Drug Intelligence Center, 2011). Tens of thousands of Americans die prematurely each year and the financial cost to the nation's economy extends beyond $200 billion annually (Bouchery, Harwood, Sacks, Simon, & Brewer, 2011). In 2007, approximately 20 million Americans needed SUD treatment and the amount of people seeking treatment could double as a result of the Affordable Care Act (Johnson, 2013). Yet, most people who seek professional services are not treated with services that are empirically tested or empirically supported treatments (ESTs) (Aarons, 2004). ESTs are defined as "clearly specified psychological treatments shown to be efficacious in controlled research with a delineated population" (Chambless & Hollon, 1998, p. 7). Because the gold standard of quality care is providing clients with ESTs, there is a great need to understand the barriers and pathways to implementing ESTs in standard clinical health services.

Meanwhile, the National Institute on Drug Abuse's (NIDA) report, *Adoption of NIDA's Evidence-Based Treatments in Real World Settings* (NIDA, 2012), indicates that developing and adding new interventions to the list of ESTs is not sufficient. The field must also investigate ways to implement and sustain ESTs in real-world agencies. Scientifically addressing the chasm between identifying effective ESTs and their efficient delivery process is a stated priority for the National Institutes of Health (Institute of Medicine, 2000, 2006; USDHHS, 2006). The chasm has been connected with various factors and a combination of individual, organizational, and system-level conditions (Patterson, 2015).

This article focuses specifically on how this research–practice chasm affects Black communities. Blacks often come to treatment with comorbid conditions that complicate the course of treatment (e.g., untreated psychiatric disorders, lower income, criminal justice problems) and often have reduced access to SUD treatment (Jacobson, Robinson, & Bluthenthal, 2007; Nahra, Alexander, & Pollack, 2009) or experience stigma from family and friends when utilizing mental health treatment (Thornicroft, 2008). Additional evidence suggests that they usually access SUD treatment centers that are of considerably lower quality (e.g., where clinicians have less education, there are fewer training opportunities available, and there are fewer licensures; Wheeler & Nahra, 2000) and studies have shown that these quality indicators affect EST implementation (Aarons, 2005; Proctor et al., 2011). As a result of these barriers, the retention rates of Blacks are often much lower compared to those of Whites or other racial groups (Saloner & Lê Cook, 2013). This study examines the possible existence of systematic barriers experienced by Blacks, by examining whether or not county-level racial distribution (percentage of Black population) affects the degree to which SUD treatment agencies use ESTs.

INDIVIDUAL AND ORGANIZATIONAL BARRIERS TO USING ESTs

There have been extensive discussions regarding the many reasons why ESTs are not sufficiently implemented. In the next two sections, we discuss numerous barriers to the implementation process, including individual barriers such as worker characteristics (McGovern et al., 2004; Nelson, Steele, & Mize, 2006) and organizational barriers like poor organizational context (Aarons, 2005; Glisson et al., 2008; Hoagwood & Burns, 2005; Patterson, Dulmus, & Maguin, 2013; Patterson & Dulmus, 2012). Studies of implementation tend to focus primarily on factors in both of these broad domains.

Individual Barriers

There is a new branch of literature emerging that focuses on worker attitudes toward ESTs. According to these studies, providers' attitudes toward new clinical practices could hamper or facilitate the implementation of ESTs in practice settings (Patterson et al., 2013). A measure of workers' attitudes toward implementing ESTs—the Evidence-Based Practice Attitudinal Scale (EBPAS)—has been developed and validated, and attitudes have been investigated in relation to a set of individual differences (Aarons, 2004; Aarons & Sawitzky, 2006; Garland, Kruse, & Aarons, 2003; Stahmer & Aarons, 2009). The studies that reported educational attainment (Aarons, 2004; Ogborne et al., 1998) found that more highly educated workers conveyed more positive attitudes compared to those with less education (Stahmer & Aarons, 2009). Other studies found attitudinal differences between workers with different educational, race, and gender backgrounds (Patterson, Maguin, Ramsey, & Stringfellow, 2014).

Many frontline workers at SUD treatment centers identify themselves as "recovering addicts." This professional identity typically encompasses a consistent combination of attributes, beliefs, values, motives, preferences, and experiences that workers will use to define themselves in their professional role (see Watkins-Hayes, 2009). This professional identity could either strengthen or weaken EST implementation through its ability to influence attitudes and openness toward new interventions. Among recovering addicts, there might be less openness toward interventions that do not utilize 12-step models, like cognitive behavior therapy or different types of trauma therapies (Miller, Sorensen, Selzer, & Brigham, 2006).

Public-sector organizations such as community mental health organizations and SUD treatment agencies also often employ Black practitioners, especially in areas with large Black populations (Greene & Rogers, 1994; Hewitt, 2004). Studies show that Black workers also have a professional identity whereas they often position race as a source of solidarity and support for same-race Black clients (Watkins-Hayes, 2011). In other words, their race and other aspects of their personal experiences are part of their identity and affect their decisions in the workplace. A major weakness of studies focused on individual barriers to utilization, however, is that they are commonly conducted using only a few organizations in one specific location, which might not be representative of SUD treatment organizations generally and they tend to ignore both organizational and structural barriers (van den Berk-Clark et al., 2015).

Organizational Barriers

Unlike their professional identity, which individual workers establish through life experience, organizations assign professional roles to workers that are dictated by a combination of organizational leadership and professional identities (Watkins-Hayes, 2009). Literature that focuses on EST implementation barriers generally uses measures of organizational culture and climate to characterize this environment (Hemmelgarn et al., 2006). Although characterizing the culture and climate of a specific organization is often difficult (Schneider, Ehrhart, & Macey, 2011; Verbeke, Volgering, & Hessels, 1998), organizational culture is generally described as the "way things are done around here." Workers within an organization communicate shared norms, beliefs, and behavioral expectations that are valued by the organization (Hasenfeld & Powell, 2004), and these values determine training availability, the value of different types of accreditation, and even the value of worker education. Most important of all, these organizational norms and values affect worker attitudes toward ESTs (Patterson, Ramsey, & van den Berk-Clark, 2015).

Sometimes these values can be affected by the organizational structures. For example, nonprofit organizations will prioritize a number of different missions related to client well-being, along with sustainability, whereas for-profit organizations' main mission is profit (Anheier, 2005). However, one limitation to this approach is that there is no broad theoretical framework to explain how organizations, by means of workers and leadership, interpret institutional, economic, and political cues and how this has the potential to affect EST implementation.

THE GAP IN IMPLEMENTATION KNOWLEDGE AT THE COUNTY LEVEL RELATED TO RACE

EST implementation in SUD treatment is largely affected by state and local governments (D'Aunno, 2006) and requires sufficient financial and human resources, including stakeholder collaboration, capacity building, quality improvement practices, service delivery training, and infrastructure building (Aarons, 2005). In a highly decentralized system, with no federal policies for governing systems to measure health disparities, states have enormous discretion regarding the provision of incentives for the implementation of ESTs (Kerwin, Walker-Smith, & Kirby, 2006). States can determine whether to draft administrative rules and regulations, and whether to assume the cost of providing financial incentives, initial training, and initiatives related to measuring fidelity (Knudsen & Abraham, 2012).

Studies have shown that this policy environment is heavily influenced by nonminority attitudes toward Blacks and the size of a state's minority population. According to the racial threat paradigm (Blalock, 1967; Key, 1949; Percival, 2009), nonminority groups perceive growing minority populations, especially Black populations (Percival, 2010), as threatening to their economic and political interests and therefore become hostile toward them and attempt to repress their interests. This has been reflected by policy shifts in states and counties with a higher proportion of Blacks. For instance, higher Black census rates increase the likelihood of electing politicians who might be considered racist (Giles & Buckner, 1993). These politicians might in turn enact laws and policies that will negatively affect minority populations, such as antiminority ballot initiatives (Hero & Tolbert, 2004), decreased education funding in minority districts (Hartney & Flavin, 2013; Hero & Tolbert, 1996), lower levels of welfare benefits (Barrilleaux & Bernick, 2003; Fellowes & Rowe, 2004; Hero & Tolbert, 2004; Tolbert, Mossberger, & McNeal, 2008), and increased incarceration or other types of punitive policies (Percival, 2010).

The racial threat paradigm could also affect the allocation of sufficient resources for full-EST implementation throughout SUD treatment agencies. According to the adaption theory of organizations (Pfeffer & Salancik, 1978), decisions about implementation by organizational stakeholders are usually made within the context of social networks and funding constraints that change over time. For example, an organization that is part of a federal department (e.g., Veterans Affairs) will likely have differing funding constraints and will thus conduct itself differently than an organization that takes funding from private insurance companies (Arfken & Kubiak, 2009; Hasenfeld & Powell, 2004). If there is a significant change to health policy at the federal level, like for instance when the Affordable Care Act passed (Buck, 2011), both organizations would likely need to make changes to their organizational processes, but these changes will likely vary by their specific relation with the federal government (Hasenfeld & Powell, 2004).

Currently, SUD treatment is primarily funded through single state agencies (SSAs). Since 2008, federal grants have represented a mere 24% of funding for SUD treatment at the county level, and this funding mechanism has been further reduced by 11% (Buck, 2011). Although the total addiction costs in the United States will increase from $24.3 billion in 2009 to $42.0 billion by 2020, expansions in Medicaid standards require implementation of new types of costly medical technology, including electronic health record systems, that might not be supported by SSAs (Andrews et al., 2015).

Moreover, since the passing of the Affordable Care Act in 2008, both private and public insurers are required to cover services for SUDs (White House, 2008). This could lead to a better substance abuse treatment in counties with high Black populations, thereby reducing the imbalance with counties with low Black populations (Banks, 2014). However, many states with larger Black populations have refused to expand Medicaid, and a larger proportion of Blacks remain underinsured compared to their White counterparts (Henry J. Kaiser Family Foundation, 2016).

Thus, it is possible that such policies might not improve access to SUD treatment for Blacks, much less ensure high-quality SUD treatment services. Furthermore, research by Buck (2011) indicates that fee-for-service funding is more likely to go to larger, better operated SUD treatment centers (over less established ones), favoring medical services under the supervision of physicians (over psychosocial services). Meanwhile, Blacks generally have lower mean incomes compared to nonminorities, might delay psychiatric care, and often enter treatment through court involvement or coercion (Wells, Klap, Koike, & Sherbourne, 2001). Given these financial deficits, many Blacks are likely to access second-tier treatment centers that use fragmented treatment systems of inferior quality (i.e., less licensure, less skilled staff, etc.; Archibald & Rankin, 2013; Arfken & Kubiak, 2009) and that have lower EST take up and fidelity (Aarons et al., 2012; Aarons, Zagursky, & Palinkas, 2006).

In this study, we use a combination of racial threat and adaption theory to assess whether there is a link between the ethnic composition of a county (in particular with regard to Blacks) and the likelihood of utilizing ESTs by SUD treatment providers. The primary questions for this study are:

1. What is the proportion of SUD treatment organizations that report utilization of ESTs?
2. Does county-level racial composition affect the proportion of utilization of ESTs among these organizations?
3. Does this stay consistent over time?

Because government-subsidized organizations will be more affected by resources available in the environment (Fording, Soss, & Schram, 2007; Pfeffer & Salancik, 1978), we stratify by government subsidization. We hypothesize that different ESTs will be used by SUD treatment providers that are located in communities with higher percentages of Blacks (Hypothesis 1) and that, overall, these communities will implement fewer EST treatments (Hypothesis 2). However, given the significant changes occurring in the United States from 2008 to 2010 (including the "great recession" and Affordable Care Act), other environmental forces might shift implementation patterns (Hypothesis 3).

METHOD

Data Sets

To understand utilization of ESTs related to counseling in SUD treatment, we used the National Survey of Substance Abuse Treatment Services (N-SSATS; Substance Abuse and Mental Health Services Administration [SAMHSA], 2013). The N-SSATS was derived from SAMHSA's Behavioral Health Information System (BHSIS), which quantifies the dynamic atmosphere of the U.S. substance abuse delivery system. BHSIS collects information on SUD treatment providers in the United States, such as ownership, services available, primary focus, size, and funding. It is essentially an annual census of all treatment facilities listed in the Inventory of Substance Abuse Treatment Services, an electronic master list of all SUD treatment providers known to SAMHSA. SUD treatment facility representatives complete either a Web-based questionnaire, a paper questionnaire, or a telephone interview (94% response rate; SAMHSA, 2013). As a "point-prevalence" survey, it provides cross-sectional snapshots of SUD treatment agencies on specific reference dates. The N-SSATS also provides county-level data and, for the purposes of this study, includes all 50 states. A total of 40,058 substance abuse treatment organizations that offered counseling services in 2008 (n = 13,688), 2009 (n = 13,513), and 2010 (n = 13,339) were included in the study.

Measures

UTILIZATION OF ESTS

The frequency of utilizing EST practices related to education and psychosocial support were recorded using a scale ranging from 1 (*never*) to 4 (*always or often*) and included 11 items: 12-step facilitation, brief intervention, cognitive-behavioral therapy, contingency management, motivational interviewing, trauma-related counseling, anger management, Matrix model, community reinforcement plus vouchers, rational emotive behavioral therapy (REBT), and relapse prevention. The score for all 11 EST items was summed to create a total EST score for each treatment organization that ranged from 11 (*lowest*) to 44 (*highest*).

RACIAL THREAT AND RESOURCE DEPENDENCE

Two variables were used to assess the role of racial threat and resource dependence: (a) the percentage of Blacks within the particular county, and (b) whether the substance abuse treatment facility received federal, state, or local funding. The percentage of Blacks in a particular county was derived from census data and dichotomized with a cutoff of 50% to reflect demographic variation of counties, because this cutoff score has been found to be associated with increasing racial tension (Tolbert & Hero, 2001). That is, counties with 50% Blacks or more will be referred to as majority Black counties, whereas those with less than 50% Blacks will be labeled minority Black counties. Organizations were considered to be receiving government funding if they provided the following responses to corresponding questions: (a) "Does this facility receive any funding or grants from the federal government, or state, county, or local governments, to support its substance abuse treatment programs?" (response = "yes"), and (b) "Which of the following types of client payments or insurance are accepted by this facility for substance abuse treatment?" (response = "Medicaid").

ORGANIZATIONAL CONTEXT

To elucidate the organizational context of each SUD treatment organization, standard practices and organizational characteristics were measured. We used the following five standard practice items to assess quality: (a) provide continuing education to staff, (b) perform drug tests on clients, (c) engage in quality case review, (d) utilization review, and (e) assess client satisfaction (Archibald & Rankin, 2013). Organization characteristics such as size (number of annual clients), funding and payment mechanisms, ownership status (nonprofit, federal agency, hospital-operated agency), and licensure status (through state substance abuse agency, state mental health department) were also used to assess access to resources.

AREA DEMOGRAPHICS

To better understand the interacting role of population density and gender, when it comes to community racial distribution and EST implementation, a continuous measure of population density (total population size) and male population (0–100) were used.

Data Analysis

To assess Hypothesis 1, initial bivariate analysis compared organizations that received government funding to organizations that did not receive government funding. We compared county racial distribution (majority Black vs. minority Black), types of EST utilization, organizational quality standards, and other organizational characteristics (see Table 1 for more details) using 2008, 2009, and 2010 data. As Table 1 shows, we made comparisons between 2008 and 2010 to evaluate the adaption of SUD agencies over time (Hypothesis 3), especially when it comes to their use of ESTs, standards, or organizational structure.

To assess Hypotheses 2 and 3, we implemented a multilevel mixed effects regression model to identify the characteristics that independently predicted the level of EST utilization and controlled for randomness in inter-annual variability between different surveys (year was categorical with 2010 as reference). This was done to determine whether significant turbulence occur-ring in both social services and among SUD treatment agencies during this time period might have affected EST utilization (see D'Aunno, 2006; Hasen-feld, Kil, Chen, Parent, & Guihama, 2013; Miller & Moulton, 2014). A stepwise multivariate analysis included an unadjusted model (Step 1) and an adjusted model for demographics (total population, % male; Step 2), standards of practice (continuing education of staff, drug tested clients, case review through quality review committee, periodic utilization review, periodic client satisfaction survey; Step 3), organizational characteristics (nonprofit status, organizational integration with hospital status, federal agency status, whether organization provided services at no charge, whether organization accepted private insurance, whether organization accepted Medicaid, whether 50% or more clients at agency had a psychiatric disorder, whether organization was accredited by state substance abuse agency, whether organization was accre-dited by state mental health department, and total admissions; Step 4), and the full model (Step 5). All variables included in the multivariate analysis were tested for multicollinearity by assessing the size of variance inflation factors using the 'vif' command in Stata version 13.0, and variables that were highly correlated with other covariates were excluded from the analysis. Around 5% of the data were discovered to be missing at random using the Stata version 13 'misstable patterns' command. Auxiliary variables were chosen and tested using a Pearson's correlation test. We then used the 'mi impute' command to impute missing variables (Royston, 2004).

RESULTS

In 2010, there were 609 fewer SUD treatment centers than in 2008 and this loss was concentrated among SUD agencies that received government funding (see Supplemental Material for tables reflecting 2008 and 2009 characteristics; Table 1 reflects 2010 characteristics). In 2008, SUD agencies that received federal funding were more likely to always or often implement 12-step facil-itation (58% vs. 48%), $\chi^2 = 15.54$, $p < .001$; cognitive-behavior therapy (67% vs. 57%), $\chi^2 = 19.86$, $p < .001$; motivational interviewing (56% vs. 47%), $\chi^2 = 14.71$, $p < .001$; trauma-related counseling (23% vs. 18%), $\chi^2 = 4.67$, $p < .03$; anger management (40.5% vs. 34.7%), $\chi^2 = 6.00$, $p < .014$; and the matrix model (17.1% vs. 10.5%), $\chi^2 = 13.24$, $p < .001$, if they were located in Black counties (see Hypothesis 1). However, contrary to Hypothesis 1, differences between majority and minority Black counties seemed to diminish over time. The supplemental tables show that SUD agencies in minority Black counties seemed to reduce the amount of implementation of ESTs and SUD agencies in majority Black counties seemed to increase the amount of implementation

TABLE 1 Characteristics of Substance Abuse Treatment Centers That Receive and Do Not Receive Government Funding by County Racial Distribution in 2010

| Characteristic | All Centers N (%) N = 13,079[a] | Receive Government Funding (n = 10,267[a]) | | Do Not Receive Government Funding (n = 2,812[b]) | |
		AA– Counties (n = 9,837[a])	AA+ Counties (n = 430[a])	AA– Counties (n = 2,786[b])	AA+ Counties (n = 87[c])
Evidence-based counseling practices (always/often)					
12-step facilitation	7,193 (53.9)[a]	5,428 (54.1)[a]	**213 (48.7)**[b]	1,513 (54.3)[b]	118 (59.9)[b]
Brief intervention	4,636 (34.8)[a]	3,505 (35.0)[a]	**194 (44.4)**[b]	**898 (32.2)**[a]	**39 (44.8)**[b]
Cognitive-behavioral therapy	8,628 (64.7)[a]	6,550 (65.3)[a]	284 (64.9)[b]	1736 (62.3)[b]	58 (66.7)[b]
Contingency management	3,385 (25.4)[a]	**2,502 (25.0)**[a]	**153 (35.0)**[b]	**696 (25.0)**[a]	**34 (39.1)**[b]
Motivational interviewing	7,332 (55.0)[a]	5,789 (57.7)[a]	256 (58.6)[b]	**1236 (44.4)**[b]	**51 (58.6)**[b]
Trauma-related counseling	2,864 (21.5)[a]	2,295 (22.9)[a]	92 (21.1)[b]	463 (16.6)[a]	14 (16.1)[a]
Anger management	4,762 (35.7)[a]	**3,656 (36.5)**[a]	**203 (46.5)**[b]	876 (31.4)[a]	27 (31.0)[a]
Matrix model	2,261 (16.6)[a]	1,838 (18.3)[a]	80 (18.3)[b]	285 (10.2)[a]	13 (14.9)[a]
Community reinforcement/voucher	604 (4.5)[b]	**474 (4.7)**[a]	**50 (11.4)**[b]	**71 (2.6)**[a]	**9 (10.3)**[b]
Relational emotive behavior therapy	2,135 (16.0)[a]	**1,492 (14.9)**[a]	**99 (22.7)**[b]	**250 (18.7)**[a]	**24 (27.6)**[b]
Relapse prevention	11,434 (85.7)[a]	**8,681 (86.6)**[a]	**358 (81.9)**[b]	2322 (83.4)[a]	73 (83.9)[a]
Standard practices					
Continuing education, staff	12,910 (96.8)[b]	9,765 (97.4)[b]	420 (96.1)[b]	2647 (95.0)[b]	**78 (89.7)**[b]
Drug testing	11,410 (85.5)[b]	**8,573 (85.5)**[b]	**402 (92.0)**[b]	2359 (84.7)[b]	76 (87.4)[b]
Quality case review	9475 (71.0)[a]	**7,442 (74.2)**[b]	**351 (80.3)**[b]	1626 (58.4)[a]	56 (64.4)[a]
Utilization review	11,313 (84.8)[b]	8,821 (88.0)[a]	374 (85.6)[b]	2053 (73.7)[a]	65 (74.7)[b]
Client satisfaction surveys	12,205 (91.5)[b]	9,416 (93.9)[b]	383 (87.6)[b]	2333 (83.7)[b]	73 (83.9)[b]
Organizational characteristics					
Nonprofit status	7,683 (57.6)[a]	6,655 (66.4)[a]	291 (66.6)[a]	**702 (25.2)**[a]	**35 (40.2)**[b]
Located in/operated by hospital	1,490 (11.2)[a]	1,222 (12.2)[a]	48 (11.0)[a]	212 (7.6)[a]	8 (9.2)[a]
Federal government agency	348 (2.6)[b]	277 (2.8)[a]	10 (2.3)[b]	—	—
Payment: Treatment at no charge	6,676 (50.1)[b]	**5,724 (57.1)**[a]	**307 (70.3)**[b]	**618 (22.2)**[b]	**27 (31.0)**[a]
Payment: Medicaid	7,478 (56.1)[b]	**7,222 (72.0)**[b]	**237 (54.2)**[b]	—	—
Payment: Private health insurance	8,648 (64.8)[b]	**6,860 (68.4)**[b]	**214 (49.0)**[a]	**1,541 (55.3)**[b]	33 (37.9)[b]
Over 50% psychiatric diagnosis	4,528 (34.0)[b]	**3,717 (37.1)**[b]	**123 (28.2)**[a]	670 (24.1)[b]	13 (20.7)[b]
Over 500 annual clients	1,761 (13.2)[a]	1,449 (14.5)[a]	52 (11.9)[c]	245 (9.1)[c]	6 (6.9)[b]
Licensed state substance abuse agency	10,924 (81.9)[b]	8,356 (83.3)[b]	365 (83.5)[b]	2,130 (76.5)[b]	73 (83.9)[b]
Licensed mental health department	4,712 (35.3)[a]	**3,719 (37.1)**[a]	**243 (55.6)**[b]	**712 (25.6)**[a]	**38 (43.7)**[b]

Note: AA = African American. Values shown in bold have a significant difference between AA+ and AA– at *p* < .05. [a]Percentage decreases since 2008. [b]Percentage increases since 2008 and 2010. [c]No difference between 2008 and 2010.

of ESTs (see Hypothesis 3). By 2010, agencies that received government funding in majority Black counties were more likely to always or often implement brief intervention (44% vs. 35%), $\chi^2 = 16.35$, $p < .001$; contingency management (25% vs. 35%), $\chi^2 = 22.4$, $p < .001$; anger management (47% vs. 37%), $\chi^2 = 17.99$, $p < .001$; community reinforcement (11% vs. 5%), $\chi^2 = 39.71$, $p < .001$; and relational emotive therapy (23% vs. 15%), $\chi^2 = 19.65$, $p < .001$. By 2010, agencies in minority Black counties were only more likely to implement 12-step facilitation (54% vs. 49%), $\chi^2 = 4.88$, $p < .03$; and relapse prevention (87% vs. 82%), $\chi^2 = 7.65$, $p < .01$ (data not shown).

There were steady increases in the use of standard practices for all agencies from 2008 to 2010 and the pattern of utilization remained about the same. That is, SUD agencies with government funding located in majority Black counties were more likely to use drug testing (92% vs. 86%), $\chi^2 = 14.52$, $p < .001$; and quality case review (80% vs. 74%), $\chi^2 = 8.24$, $p < .004$; and SUD agencies with government funding located in minority Black counties were more likely to use client satisfaction surveys (94% vs. 88%), $\chi^2 = 27.37$, $p < .001$. Although there were 143 fewer nonprofit and 59 fewer hospital-based SUD agencies in 2010 compared to 2008, many of the organizational characteristics stayed consistent over time. That is, SUD agencies with government funding located in majority Black counties were consistently more likely to offer treatment at no charge (70% vs. 57%), $\chi^2 = 29.78$, $p < .001$; and to be licensed by the state mental health department (56% vs. 37%), $\chi^2 = 61.08$, $p < .001$. SUD agencies receiving government funding located in majority Black counties were consistently more likely to take Medicaid (72% vs. 54%), $\chi^2 = 64.63$, $p < .001$; or private health insurance (68% vs. 49%), $\chi^2 = 72.18$, $p < .001$ (see Table 1, results reflect 2010).

Table 2 shows the effect of a county's racial composition (percent Black, specifically) on the utilization of ESTs based on unadjusted (Step 1) and adjusted models for demographics (Step 2), standards of care (Step 3), organizational characteristics (Step 4), and all variables (Step 5; see Hypothesis 2 and 3). The interannual variability between 2010 and other years was tested for random effects that were found to be significant at $p < .0001$ in all models, confirming that the multilevel test was appropriate. In Step 1 of Model 1 (SUD agencies with government funding), $\chi^2(1) = 6.14$, $p < .01$, the level of EST utilization was reduced by 35% when SUD agencies were located in a majority Black county ($z = -2.93$, $p < .003$). When the total population and the percentage of males (Step 2) were added to the model, the Wald increased to $\chi^2(3) = 17.29$, $p < .001$, and EST remained steady at $\beta = -0.39$ ($z = -2.79$, $p < .005$). When standards of care—including whether agencies continually educated staff, provided drug testing, engaged in quality case or utilization review, and routinely assessed client satisfaction—were added to Model 1 (Step 3), Wald increased to χ^2 (7) = 1723.09, $p < .001$, and the effect of a county's Black population size increased to $\beta = -0.44$ ($z = -3.77$, $p < .001$). After organizational characteristics (nonprofit, hospital, and federal government), payment status (no charge,

TABLE 2 Association (β; 95% CI) Between County Racial Distribution Residential Distribution (Cutoff at 50% Distribution of AA), Government Funding (Federal Grants and Medicaid), and Utilization of Evidence-Based Practices (EBPs) in Local Substance Abuse Treatment Facilities

AA+ Counties vs. AA− Counties	β EBPs[a]	β EBPs (Demographics)[b]	β EBPs (Standards)[c]	β EBPs (Organizational)[d]	β EBPs (Full model)
(1) AA+ with funding	−0.35 [−0.59, −0.12]	−0.39 [−0.66,−0.12]	−0.44 [−0.67, −0.21]	−0.32 [−0.55, −0.09]	−0.41 [−0.67, −0.15]
(2) AA+ without funding	0.70 [0.15, 1.24]	0.43 [−0.21, 1.06]	0.59 [0.07, 1.12]	0.78 [0.25, 1.31]	0.57 [−0.02, 1.16]

Note: AA = African American. Values shown in bold are significant at $p < .05$. Model 1 exposure variable is agencies located in counties with a 50% or more AA population that receive government funding. Model 2 exposure variable is agencies located in counties with a 50% or more AA population that do not receive government funding. To improve parsimony, variables in Table 1 and **2** were dropped from the model when significance fellow below $p < .01$. β are adjusted for random effects of year of the survey (2008–2010, 2010 reference) and was significant at $p < .001$ for all models.

[a]Total population was significant in Model 1 at $p < .004$ and percentage male was significant in Model 2 at $p < .032$. [b]All standards variables were significantly associated with EBP utilization at $p < .001$. [c]All organizational variables significant at $p < .001$ accept for nonprofit status in Models 1 and 2 and total admissions in Model 2. [d]All variables were significant at $p < .05$ except percentage male in Model 1 and total population, nonprofit status, and substance abuse license in Model 2.

Medicaid, or private), client size (total admissions and total number of clients with mental health diagnosis), and licensure status (SSA and state mental health agency) were added to Model 1 in Step 4, Wald decreased to $\chi^2(11) = 1449.55$, $p < .001$, and county majority Black population status remained significant ($\beta = -0.32$, $z = -2.32$, $p < .02$. County majority Black population also remained significant ($\beta = -0.41$, $z = -3.09$, $p < .002$) in the full model: Step 5, $\chi^2(19) = 3158.76$, $p < .001$.

Model 2 (SUD agencies without federal funding) was significant in Steps 1, 3, and 4. It appeared that county total population and percentage males, which were both significant in Step 2, might have moderated the effect of county racial distribution. Standards also reduced the level of effect from the exposure variable (majority Black counties) in Step 3 ($\beta = 0.59$, $z = 2.20$, $p < .03$), whereas organizational factors seemed to increase the level of effect in Step 4 ($\beta = 0.78$, $z = 2.90$, $p < .004$). In the final model controlling for all variables, county racial distribution was no longer significant.

DISCUSSION AND IMPLICATIONS FOR PRACTICE

The purpose of this study was to examine whether the racial composition of a county, with particular regard to Black residents, affected the likelihood of utilizing ESTs among SUD treatment agencies. We found that a larger percentage of government-funded SUD treatment agencies were in majority Black counties and that SUD treatment agencies that received government funding implemented ESTs more comprehensively. However, in majority Black counties, we found several significant differences in SUD agencies receiving government funding compared to minority Black counties, but these differences appeared to disappear over time. First, EST practices were less fully implemented among SUD agencies receiving government aid that were located in majority Black counties in 2008 and 2009, but not in 2010. Second, bivariate results showed that more SUD agencies in majority Black counties used drug testing, provided services at no charge, and had state mental health licensure. Fewer SUD agencies in majority Black communities employed reviews for client satisfaction surveys, or took Medicaid or private insurance.

One plausible explanation for these findings is that SUD agencies receiving government aid that were in majority Black counties might have faced different constraints due to their reliance on Medicaid and private insurance payers that caused them to shift toward supporting less medical and more behavioral interventions from 2008 to 2010 (see Andrews et al., 2015; Miller & Moulton, 2014). SUD agencies in majority Black counties might have relied on a behavioral health organizational "niche" to ensure survival in this environment (Pfeffer & Salancik, 1978; Popielarz & Neal, 2007). This niche likely provides the agency with a significant amount of legitimacy and appeal, along with an already existing set of organizations and social networks on which to rely. A behavioral health niche might be why these agencies were more likely to have state mhntal Health licensure and to more fully implement a range of different behavioral health interventions over time.

SUD agencies in majority Black counties might also have a criminal justice niche and thus specialize in providing services to incarcerated populations or populations transitioning from jail or prison. The increased use of drug testing in these facilities might be an obvious response to these constraints of drug courts and probation officers, not to mention the fact that geographic areas with higher Black populations tend to focus more on punitive criminal justice policies (Percival, 2010), which leads to larger corrections budgets, which thereby provide incentives for more drug testing in treatment (Kubiak, Arfken, & Gibson, 2009). Alexander (2012) referred to this as the "new Jim Crow"; that is, communities that feel that there is a racial threat will be more inclined to devise strategies by which to reduce Black citizen rights. Mass incarceration and supervision through SUD treatment centers is one such strategy.

Findings related to quality improvement practices and licensure in this study are different from studies showing that Blacks tend to use second-tier SUD agencies that often hire less qualified staff and have lower levels of accreditation (Archibald & Rankin, 2013; Arfken & Kubiak, 2009; Kubiak et al., 2009; Wheeler & Nahra, 2000). Although N-SSATS did not provide information on staff education levels, it did show that by 2010, SUD agencies located in majority Black counties used similar levels of continuing education as SUD agencies located in minority Black counties. A similar rate of utilization review and higher levels of quality case review between SUD agencies that received government funding located in majority Black and minority Black counties was also observed by 2010.

Limitations

Although this study used a relatively large sample, it should be interpreted with caution because N-SSATS only provided a selection of available EST items, which means that the full extent to which ESTs are used in different agencies remains unclear. N-SSATS does not include worker-level variables that reflect whether implementation of ESTs at those organizations are universal or variable. There are also no data on worker demographics, training, and attitudes toward ESTs. To assess the willingness to use ESTs, worker attitude scales would have to be measured along with rates of EST implementation. The reason that N-SSATS lacks such data is because organizational-level responses reflect the bias of the individual who participates in the survey. The data set also lacks actual address data, so there could be significant within-county variance when it comes to race. We also are comparing different types of ESTs that have a range of different levels of efficacy. For this reason, results from this study only hint at the implementation of ESTs according to community racial distribution. Future studies should used individual worker-level responses, and also use measures of state-level funding for SUD agencies and substance use, political makeup of state legislative body, and utilization of regulations or incentives for EST utilization.

CONCLUSION

Despite these limitations, this study provides valuable insight, as it is the first to analyze county-level data in relation to how factors such as race and funding sources can impact SUD treatment frontline clinical activities. In the absence of any guidance regarding the investigation of barriers to using ESTs from current disciplines, such as implementation science, the best route for discussing potential implications for practice would be Blalock's (1967) theory of racial threat and adaption theory. Blalock hinted at the existence of repressive state control mechanisms in regard to the size of a minority population. When nonminorities perceive the potential loss of economic and political powers, specific practices are encouraged to protect their power and privileges (Hughey, 2015; Tolbert & Hero, 2001). This usually translates into reduced funding for social services, higher levels of incarceration of minority populations, and reduced Medicaid access. SUD treatment facility management and viability, to a large extent, rely on these factors (Buck, 2011; Wheeler & Nahra, 2000). In this study, racial threat theorists would likely point out the lack of ESTs encouraged in 2008 and 2009. However, changes occurring in 2010 might be the result of these agencies adapting to constraints posed by new funding streams for SUD treatment (Buck, 2011), and shifting economic forces that led to tougher competition and increasing numbers of SUD treatment closures (Miller & Moulton, 2014).

It is important to understand the dynamics involved in EST implementation because treatment for SUDs is a well-planned, goal-based process that is specifically targeted at achieving abstinence and improving overall health and wellness outcomes (Walker, 2009). Failure to provide or receive adequate SUD treatment has negative implications both for the individual and the community as a whole, including financial difficulties, poor health, increased rates of HIV, and increased burden on loved ones (Alterman, McKay, Mulvaney, & McLellan, 1996; United Nations, 2012). Majority Black counties appear to be fully embracing SUD behavioral health treatments supported by evidence to produce the best health and wellness outcomes; however, their progress lagged behind minority Black communities. ESTs are used in practice due to a considerable amount of scientific evidence indicating that client outcomes are improved with ESTs (Corrigan, 2005; Institute of Medicine, 2000, 2006). Furthermore, scientifically verified services have a higher level of legitimacy with the public as well as with funders (Brown et al., 2006;

Institute of Medicine, 2006; USDHHS, 2006). Given the benefits of using ESTs, research exploring the impact of organizational characteristics and client population on the use of ESTs remains crucial.

SUPPLEMENTARY MATERIAL

Supplemental data for this article can be accessed on the publisher's website: http://dx.doi.org/10.1080/1533256X.2017.1302883

REFERENCES

Aarons, G. A. (2004). Mental health provider attitudes toward adoption of evidence-based practice: The Evidence-Based Practice Attitude Scale (EBPAS). *Mental Health Services Research, 6*(2), 61–74. doi:10.1023/B:MHSR.0000024351.12294.65

Aarons, G. A. (2005). Measuring provider attitudes toward evidence-based practice: Consideration of organizational context and individual differences. *Child and Adolescent Psychiatric Clinics of North America, 14,* 255–271. doi:10.1016/j.chc.2004.04.008

Aarons, G. A., Glisson, C., Green, P. D., Hoagwood, K., Kelleher, K. J., Landsverk, J. A., & Health, R. N. O. Y. M. (2012). The organizational social context of mental health services and clinician attitudes toward evidence-based practice: A United States national study. *Implementation Science, 7*(1), 56. doi:10.1186/1748-5908-7-56

Aarons, G. A., & Sawitzky, A. C. (2006). Organizational culture and climate and mental health provider attitude toward evidence-based practices. *Psychological Services, 3,* 61–72.

Aarons, G. A., Zagursky, K., & Palinkas, L. (2006, February). *Multiple stakeholder perspectives on evidence-based practice implementation.* Paper presented at the Annual Research Conference of the University of South Florida, Tampa, FL.

Alexander, M. (2012). *The new Jim Crow: Mass incarceration in the age of color-blindness.* New York, NY: The New Press.

Alterman, A. I., McKay, J. R., Mulvaney, F. D., & McLellan, A. (1996). Prediction of attrition from day hospital treatment in lower socioeconomic cocaine-dependent men. *Drug and Alcohol Dependence, 40,* 227–233. doi:10.1016/0376-8716(95)01212-5

Andrews, C., Abraham, A., Grogan, C. M., Pollack, H. A., Bersamira, C., Humphreys, K., & Friedmann, P. (2015). Despite resources from the ACA, most states do little to help addiction treatment programs implement health care reform. *Health Affairs, 34,* 828–835. doi:10.1377/hlthaff.2014.1330

Anheier, H. (2005). *Nonprofit organizations: Approaches, management, policy.* New York, NY: Routledge.

Archibald, M. E., & Rankin, C. P. (2013). Community context and healthcare quality: The impact of community resources on licensing and accreditation of substance abuse treatment agencies. *The Journal of Behavioral Health Services & Research, 40,* 442–456. doi:10.1007/s11414-013-9340-4

Arfken, C. L., & Kubiak, S. P. (2009). Substance abuse treatment and services by criminal justice and other funding sources. *Addictive Behaviors, 34*, 613–615. doi:10.1016/j.addbeh.2009.03.015

Banks, A. J. (2014). The public's anger: White racial attitudes and opinions toward health care reform. *Political Behavior, 36*, 493–514. doi:10.1007/s11109-013-9251-3

Barrilleaux, C., & Bernick, E. (2003). Deservingness, discretion, and the state politics of welfare spending, 1990–96. *State Politics & Policy Quarterly, 3*(1), 1–22. doi:10.1177/153244000300300101

Blalock, H. M. (1967). *Toward a theory of minority-group relations.* New York, NY: Wiley.

Bouchery, E. E., Harwood, H. J., Sacks, J. J., Simon, C. J., & Brewer, R. D. (2011). Economic costs of excessive alcohol consumption in the US, 2006. *American Journal of Preventive Medicine, 41*, 516–524. doi:10.1016/j.amepre.2011.06.045

Brown, L. S., Jr, Kritz, S. A., Goldsmith, R. J., Bini, E. J., Rotrosen, J., Baker, S., … McAuliffe, P. (2006). Characteristics of substance abuse treatment programs providing services for HIV/AIDS, hepatitis C virus infection, and sexually transmitted infections: The national drug abuse treatment clinical trials network. *Journal of Substance Abuse Treatment, 30*, 315–321. doi:10.1016/j.jsat.2006.02.006

Buck, J. A. (2011). The looming expansion and transformation of public substance abuse treatment under the Affordable Care Act. *Health Affairs, 30*, 1402–1410. doi:10.1377/hlthaff.2011.0480

Chambless, D. L., & Hollon, S. (1998). Defining empirically supported therapies. *Journal of Consulting and Clinical Psychology, 66*(1), 7–18. doi:10.1037/0022-006X.66.1.7

Corrigan, J. M. (2005). Crossing the quality chasm. In P. P. Reid, W. D. Compton, J. H. Grossman, & G. Fanjang (Eds.), *Building a better delivery system: A new engineering/health care partnership* (pp. 95–98). Washington, DC: The National Academies Press.

D'Aunno, T. (2006). The role of organization and management in substance abuse treatment: Review and roadmap. *Journal of Substance Abuse Treatment, 31*, 221–233. doi:http://dx.doi.org/10.1016/j.jsat.2006.06.016

Fellowes, M. C., & Rowe, G. (2004). Politics and the new American welfare states. *American Journal of Political Science, 48*, 362–373. doi:10.1111/j.0092-5853.2004.00075.x

Fording, R. C., Soss, J., & Schram, S. F. (2007). Devolution, discretion, and the effect of local political values on TANF sanctioning. *Social Service Review, 81*, 285–316. doi:10.1086/517974

Garland, A. F., Kruse, M., & Aarons, G. A. (2003). Clinicians and outcome measurement: What's the use? *Journal of Behavioral Health Services and Research, 30*, 393–405.

Giles, M. W., & Buckner, M. A. (1993). David Duke and black threat: An old hypothesis revisited. *The Journal of Politics, 55*, 702–713. doi:10.2307/2131995

Glisson, C., Landsverk, J., Schoenwald, S., Kelleher, K., Hoagwood, K. E., Mayberg, S., … Health, R. N. O. Y. M. (2008). Assessing the organizational social context (OSC) of mental health services: Implications for research and practice. *Administration and Policy in Mental Health and Mental Health Services Research, 35* (1–2), 98–113. doi:10.1007/s10488-007-0148-5

Greene, M., & Rogers, J. E. (1994). Education and the earnings disparities between Black and White men: A comparison of professionals in the public and private sectors. *The Journal of Socio-Economics*, *23*(1), 113–130. doi:10.1016/1053 5357 (94)90023-X

Hartney, M. T., & Flavin, P. (2013). The political foundations of the black–white education achievement gap. *American Politics Research*, *42*, 3–33. doi:10.1177/ 1532673x13482967

Hasenfeld, Y., & Powell, L. (2004). The role of non-profit agencies in the provision of welfare-to-work services. *Administration in Social Work*, *28*(3), 91–110. doi:10.1300/J147v28n03_05

Hasenfeld, Z., Kil, H. K., Chen, M., Parent, B., & Guihama, J. (2013). *Stressed and stretched: The recession, poverty, and human services nonprofits in Los Angeles. Annual state of the sector report 2002–2012*. Los Angeles, CA: UCLA Center for Civil Society.

Hemmelgarn, A. L., Glisson, C., & James, L. R. (2006). Organizational culture and climate: Implications for services and interventions research. *Clinical Psychology: Science and Practice*, *13*, 73–89.

Henry J. Kaiser Family Foundation. (2016). *Status of state action on Medicaid expansion decision*. Washington, DC: Author.

Hero, R. E., & Tolbert, C. J. (1996). A racial/ethnic diversity interpretation of politics and policy in the states of the U.S. *American Journal of Political Science*, *40*, 851–871. doi:10.2307/2111798

Hero, R. E., & Tolbert, C. J. (2004). Minority voices and citizen attitudes about government responsiveness in the American states: Do social and institutional context matter? *British Journal of Political Science*, *34*, 109–121. doi:10.1017/ S0007123403000371

Hewitt, C. M. (2004). African-American concentration in jobs the political economy of job segregation and contestation in Atlanta. *Urban Affairs Review*, *39*, 318–341. doi:10.1177/1078087403253416

Hoagwood, K. E., & Burns, B. J. (2005). Evidence-based practice: Part II. Effecting change. *Child and Adolescent Psychiatric Clinics of North America*, *14*(2), xv–xvii. doi:10.1016/j.chc.2004.11.001

Hughey, M. W. (2015) The five I's of five-O: Racial ideologies, institutions, interests, identities, and interactions of police violence. *Critical Sociology 41*(6): 857–871.

Institute of Medicine. (2000). *To err is human: Building a safer health system*. Washington, DC: National Academy Press.

Institute of Medicine. (2006). *Improving the quality of health care for mental and substance-use conditions*. Washington, DC: National Academy Press.

Jacobson, J. O., Robinson, P., & Bluthenthal, R. N. (2007). A multilevel decomposition approach to estimate the role of program location and neighborhood disadvantage in racial disparities in alcohol treatment completion. *Social Science & Medicine*, *64*, 462–476. doi:10.1016/j.socscimed.2006.08.032

Johnson, C. K. (2013, April 27). Obamacare could overwhelm addiction services. *The Mercury*. Retrieved from http://www.pottsmerc.com/article/20130427/NEWS04/ 130429295/obamacare-could-overwhelm-addiction-services#full_story

Kerwin, M. E., Walker-Smith, K., & Kirby, K. C. (2006). Comparative analysis of state requirements for the training of substance abuse and mental health counselors.

Journal of Substance Abuse Treatment, 30, 173–181. doi:10.1016/j. jsat.2005.11.004

Key, V. (1949). *Southern politics in state and nation.* New York, NY: Knopf.

Knudsen, H. K., & Abraham, A. J. (2012). Perceptions of the state policy environment and adoption of medications in the treatment of substance use disorders. *Psychiatric Services, 63*(1), 19–25. doi:10.1176/appi.ps.201100034

Kubiak, S. P., Arfken, C. L., & Gibson, E. S. (2009). Departments of corrections as purchasers of community-based treatment: A national study. *Journal of Substance Abuse Treatment, 36,* 420–427. doi:10.1016/j.jsat.2008.08.009

McGovern, M. P., Fox, T. S., Xie, H., & Drake, R. E. (2004). A survey of clinical practices and readiness to adopt evidence-based practices: Dissemination research in an addiction treatment system. *Journal of Substance Abuse Treatment, 26,* 305–312.

Miller, S. M., & Moulton, S. (2014). Publicness in policy environments: A multilevel analysis of substance abuse treatment services. *Journal of Public Administration Research and Theory, 24,* 553–589. doi:10.1093/jopart/mus065

Miller, W. R., Sorensen, J. L., Selzer, J. A., & Brigham, G. S. (2006). Disseminating evidence-based practices in substance abuse treatment: A review with suggestions. *Journal of Substance Abuse Treatment, 31,* 25–39. doi:10.1016/j.jsat.2006.03.005

Nahra, T. A., Alexander, J., & Pollack, H. (2009). Influence of ownership on access in outpatient substance abuse treatment. *Journal of Substance Abuse Treatment, 36,* 355–365. doi:10.1016/j.jsat.2008.06.009

National Drug Intelligence Center. (2011). *The economic impact of illicit drug use on American society.* Washington, DC: U.S. Department of Justice.

National Institute on Drug Abuse. (2012). *Adoption of NIDA's evidence-based treatments in real world settings: A National Advisory Council on Drug Abuse workgroup report.* Washington, DC: Author.

Nelson, T. D., Steele, R. G., & Mize, J. A. (2006). Practitioner attitudes toward evidence based practice: Themes and challenges. *Administration and Policy in Mental Health, 33,* 398–409.

Ogborne, A. C., Wild, T. C., Braun, K., & Newton-Taylor, B. (1998). Measuring treatment process beliefs among staff of specialized addiction treatment services. *Journal of Substance Abuse Treatment, 15,* 301–312.

Patterson, D. A. (2015). Factors influencing the implementation of a brief alcohol screening and educational intervention in social settings not specializing in addiction services. *Social Work in Health Care, 54,* 345–364. doi:10.1080/00981389.2015.1005270

Patterson, D. A., & Dulmus, C. N. (2012). Organizational barriers to adopting an alcohol screening and brief intervention in community-based mental health organizations. *Best Practices in Mental Health, 8*(1), 16–28.

Patterson, D. A., Dulmus, C. N., & Maguin, E. (2013). Is openness to using empirically supported treatments related to organizational culture and climate? *Journal of Social Service Research, 39,* 562–571. doi:10.1080/01488376.2013.804023

Patterson, D. A., Maguin, E., Ramsey, A. L., & Stringfellow, E. (2014). Measuring attitudes towards empirically supported treatment in real world addiction services. *Journal of Social Work Practice in the Addictions, 14,* 141–154. doi:10.1080/1533256X.2014.902717

Patterson, D. A., Ramsey, A. T., & van den Berk-Clark, C. (2015). Implementing outside the box: Community-based social service provider experiences with using an alcohol screening and intervention. *Journal of Social Service Research*, *41*, 233–245. doi:10.1080/01488376.2014.980963

Percival, G. L. (2009). Testing the impact of racial attitudes and racial diversity on prisoner reentry policies in the U.S. states. *State Politics & Policy Quarterly*, *9*, 176–203. doi:10.1177/153244000900900203

Percival, G. L. (2010). Ideology, diversity, and imprisonment: Considering the influence of local politics on racial and ethnic minority incarceration rates. *Social Science Quarterly*, *91*, 1063–1082. doi:10.1111/ssqu.2010.91.issue-4

Pfeffer, J., & Salancik, G. (1978). *The external control of organizations: A resource dependence perspective*. Palo Alto, CA: Stanford University Press.

Popielarz, P. A., & Neal, Z. P. (2007). The niche as a theoretical tool. *Sociology*, *33*(1), 65–84. doi:10.1146/annurev.soc.32.061604.123118

Proctor, E., Silmere, H., Raghavan, R., Hovmand, P., Aarons, G., Bunger, A., … Hensley, M. (2011). Outcomes for implementation research: Conceptual distinctions, measurement challenges, and research agenda. *Administration and Policy in Mental Health and Mental Health Services Research*, *38*(2), 65–76. doi:10.1007/s10488-010-0319-7

Royston, P. (2004). Multiple imputation of missing values. *The Stata Journal*, *4*, 227–241.

Saloner, B., & Lê Cook, B. (2013). Blacks and Hispanics are less likely than Whites to complete addiction treatment, largely due to socioeconomic factors. *Health Affairs*, *32*, 135–145. doi:10.1377/hlthaff.2011.0983

Schneider, B., Ehrhart, M. G., & Macey, W. H. (2011). Perspectives on organizational climate and culture. In S. Zedeck (Ed.), *APA Handbook of Industrial and Organizational Psychology: Vol. 1. Building and Developing the Organization* (pp. 373–414). Washington, DC: American Psychological Association.

Stahmer, A. C., & Aarons, G. A. (2009). Attitudes toward adoption of evidence-based practices: A comparison of autism early intervention teachers and children's mental health providers. *Psychological Services*, *6*, 223–234.

Substance Abuse and Mental Health Services Administration. (2013). *National Survey of Substance Abuse Treatment Services (N-SSATS): 2013*. Washington, DC: Author.

Thornicroft, G. (2008). Stigma and discrimination limit access to mental health care. *Epidemiologia e Psichiatria Sociale*, *17*(1), 14–19. doi:10.1017/S1121189X00002621

Tolbert, C. J., & Hero, R. E. (2001). Dealing with diversity: Racial/ethnic context and social policy change. *Political Research Quarterly*, *54*, 571–604. doi:10.1177/106591290105400305

Tolbert, C. J., Mossberger, K., & McNeal, R. (2008). Institutions, policy innovation, and E-government in the American states. *Public Administration Review*, *68*, 549–563. doi:10.1111/j.154h210.2008.00890.x

United Nations. (2012). *World drug report 2012*. New York, NY: Author.

U.S. Department of Health & Human Services. (2006). *The road ahead: Research partnerships to transform services: A report by the National Advisory Mental Health Council's Workgroup on Services and Clinical Epidemiology Research*. Bethesda, MD: National Institutes of Health, National Institute of Mental Health.

van den Berk-Clark, C. (2015) The dilemmas of frontline staff working with the homeless: Discretion and the task environment. *Housing Policy Debate, 26*(1), 105–122.

Verbeke, W., Volgering, M., & Hessels, M. (1998). Exploring the conceptual expansion within the field of organizational behavior: Organizational climate and organizational culture. *Journal of Management Studies, 35,* 303–329.

Walker, R. (2009). Retention in treatment—Indicator or illusion: An essay. *Substance Use & Misuse, 44*(1), 18–27. doi:10.1080/10826080802525967

Watkins-Hayes, C. (2009). Race-ing the bootstrap climb: Black and Latino bureaucrats in post-reform welfare offices. *Social Problems, 56,* 285–310. doi:10.1525/sp.2009.56.2.285

Watkins-Hayes, C. (2011). Race, respect, and red tape: Inside the black box of racially representative bureaucracies. *Journal of Public Administration Research and Theory, 21*(Suppl. 2), i233–i251. doi:10.1093/jopart/muq096

Wells, K., Klap, R., Koike, A., & Sherbourne, C. (2001). Ethnic disparities in unmet need for alcoholism, drug abuse, and mental health care. *American Journal of Psychiatry, 158,* 2027–2032. doi:10.1176/appi.ajp.158.12.2027

Wheeler, J. R., & Nahra, T. A. (2000). Private and public ownership in outpatient substance abuse treatment: Do we have a two-tiered system? *Administration and Policy in Mental Health and Mental Health Services Research, 27,* 197–209. doi:10.1023/A:1021357318246

White House. (2008). *Substance abuse and the Affordable Care Act.* Retrieved from https://www.whitehouse.gov/ondcp/healthcare

Recovery Schools Rise to the Challenge: Shifting Alcohol Norms and Behaviors in Youth and Emerging Adults

LORI HOLLERAN STEIKER, PhD

JULIE McELRATH, LMSW

Alcohol is a huge challenge for youth and therefore for the field of social work. The confluence of biopsychosocial factors place youth at risk. Early initiation to alcohol use is a serious risk factor for depression, anxiety, and suicide. The focus of this article is on the collaborative use of resources and evidence-based practices and innovative mechanisms for shifting youth mores around alcohol and providing alternative peer groups, especially in abstinence-hostile settings, such as high schools and college campuses. Recovery schools are drawing national attention and becoming a part of the fabric of the advancing recovery movement for youth. This article discusses the Recovery School movement; its impact on youth, families, and communities; and the impact it can have on the Social Work Grand Challenges. It culminates with a case study of a university community that demonstrates how lives and norms around alcohol can shift for youth and young adults.

"Reducing and Preventing Alcohol Misuse and Its Consequences" is a critical and formidable Grand Challenge for the social work profession. Alcohol is the most commonly used drug among youth. For example, 2012 data from the

Monitoring the Future Survey indicate that 72% percent of 12th graders (nearly three out of four) have tried alcohol, and 39% of 8th graders have reported some alcohol use in their lifetime (Johnston, O'Malley, Bachman, & Schulenberg, 2014). Of greater concern is the widespread occurrence of episodes of drunkenness and binge drinking. The rates of self-reported drunkenness in the past 30 days were 55%, 14%, and 25%, respectively, for Grades 8, 10, and 12, and the prevalence rates of binge drinking (occasions of consuming five or more drinks in a row in the previous 2 weeks) were 8%, 16%, and 25% for the three grades, respectively. Over half (52%) of 12th graders and one eighth (12%) of 8th graders in 2013 reported having been drunk at least once in their life (Johnston et al., 2014). One in four Americans who began using any addictive substance including alcohol before age 18 are addicted, compared to 1 in 25 who started using at age 21 or older. The risk of being addicted is much higher among Americans who begin to use at a younger age (National Center on Addiction and Substance Abuse at Columbia University [NCASA], 2011).

According to the Centers for Disease Control and Prevention, every year more than 80,000 U.S. deaths are the result of binge drinking. Only a percentage of these deaths happen to youth and only a small percentage of those are youth who drink compulsively, but in 2014, an estimated 679,000 adolescents 12 to 17 years old had an alcohol use disorder (Substance Abuse and Mental Health Services Administration [SAMHSA], 2014); this number includes 367,000 females and 311,000 males (SAMHSA), 2014). An estimated 55,000 adolescents (18,000 males and 37,000 females) received treatment for an alcohol problem in a specialized facility in 2014 (SAMHSA, 2014). Substances including alcohol are the most prevalent cause of teen morbidity and mortality in the United States (SAMHSA, 2014). Emerging adults (i.e., college-age students) experience high rates of alcohol-related problems stemming from heavy use patterns and drinking in high-risk contexts (Clapp, Johnson, Voas, Lange, Shillington, & Russell, 2005; Johnston et al., 2014). Alcohol poisonings among emerging adults 18 to 24 years old, for instance, have increased more than 190% over the past two decades (Hingson, 2012, cited in Begun, Clapp, & The Alcohol Misuse Grand Challenge Collective, 2016).

Youth alcohol misuse is even more pervasive in the college years. In 2014, 59.8% of full-time college students, ages 18 to 22, drank alcohol in the past month compared with 51.5% of other persons of the same age who were not in college. More than one third of college students in this age range engaged in binge drinking (five or more drinks on an occasion). Approximately 12% of college students 18 to 22 years old engaged in heavy drinking (five or more drinks on an occasion on five or more occasions per month) in the past month compared with 9.5% of other persons of the same age. Roughly 20% of college students meet the criteria for an alcohol use disorder (Blanco, Okuda, & Wright, 2008).

IMPACT OF ALCOHOL USE DURING ADOLESCENCE AND EMERGING ADULTHOOD

The consequences of youth and emerging adults' alcohol misuse are serious. Research indicates that alcohol use during the teenage years often interferes with normal adolescent development. From a neurobiological perspective, the developing adolescent brain and the delay in the development of the frontal cortex and related executive functions place youth at risk for alcohol and other substance misuse. Given youths' proclivities toward impulsivity, sensation seeking, and disregard of future outcomes, they tend to respond more to alcohol's reward stimuli compared to adults (McLoughlin, Gould, & Malone, 2015).

Biological Aspects

There are many factors associated with alcohol use disorders and its etiology. Genetics accounts for 60% of the variance with regard to whether or not a youth winds up with dependence on alcohol (Erickson, 2007). Those who have genetic predisposition are less able to curtail their phenomenon of craving and therefore continue to drink despite physical, mental, developmental, social, and spiritual consequences. This is often referred to as the "hijacked brain" (NIDA, 2007).

Experimentation with alcohol is normative for youth and emerging adults. In this population, the prefrontal cortex is not fully developed. This results in a lack of executive functioning that can prompt poor decision making. In addition, youth with a predisposition to alcohol use disorders due to what Erickson calls "disrupted pleasure pathways" experience alcohol as a "fix" for insecurity, social fears, and low self-esteem. These youth are often able to drink more without showing the effects of the alcohol—referred to as tolerance. Finally, blackouts, or the inability to remember (i.e., alcohol-induced amnesia), further exacerbate the complexity of the consequences.

Psychological Shifts and Related Social Implications

The sudden and rapid physical, mental, cognitive, and emotional changes that adolescents go through make them very self-conscious, sensitive, and worried about their changes. Due to the fact that alcohol is pervasive in society, is minimized as a drug, and is considered part of teenage and young adult culture, it can profoundly affect the ways that youth view themselves and the world around them. Compared to other life stages, the developmental stage of emerging adulthood confers the highest risk for the onset of harmful alcohol use (Kelly, Stout, & Slaymaker, 2013).

Individuation (or identity separation, making themselves distinct from parents), in some families, might manifest in adolescent rebellion, which could lead to conflict as the parents try to keep control. As adolescents pull away from their parents in a search for their own identity, they shift to their peer group as their locus of control. They might make painful comparisons about themselves with their peers. Their peer group might become a safe haven in which adolescents can test new ideas. Or the peer group (depending on the level of risk-based activities of the group) can be a dangerous place disguised as a sanctuary.

As the youth move into midadolescence, the peer group expands to include romantic friendships. In mid- to late adolescence, young people often feel the need to establish their sexual identity by dating and experimenting sexually. Young people who do not experience positive parents or have minimal intimacy with their peers might have more difficulty with relationships when they are adults (Rauer, Pettit, Lansford, Bates, & Dodge, 2013). On the other hand, youth who experiment sexually in the midst of drug and alcohol use could find themselves with consequences that they did not intend or anticipate. Pregnancy, sexually transmitted diseases (STDs), and sexual abuse—all of these risks are more prevalent when alcohol and drugs are in the picture (Eaton et al., 2012).

Social Aspects

In addition to the role of parents, families, and peers, to be discussed at length later in this article, cultural and social norms are an important consideration with regard to factors affecting alcohol decision making. Starting in the late 1990s, research has illuminated social influences and environmental pressures that can affect age of experimentation, frequency, substance choice, and other factors affecting use and misuse patterns (Oostveen, Knibbe, & De Vries, 1996). For some youth seeking recovery, the cultural milieu where social norms are more tolerant of alcohol and other drug consumption can force a choice between recovery protection and a higher education.

Comorbidities and Consequences

Underage drinking contributes to a range of acute consequences, including injuries, sexual assaults, and even deaths—including those from car crashes (NIAAA, 2006). Although some might consider "underaged drinking" a legal term, it is more relevant, for this discussion, to note that the brain continues to develop in terms of neural plasticity until the age of 25. Therefore, any drinking before the completion of that biological process can result in serious consequences: 1,825 college students between the ages of 18 and 24 die from alcohol-related unintentional injuries, including motor vehicle crashes;,

696,000 students between the ages of 18 and 24 are assaulted by another student who has been drinking; and 97,000 students between the ages of 18 and 24 report experiencing alcohol-related sexual assault or date rape (Hingson, Heeren, & Winter, 2005; Hingson, Zha, & Weitzman, 2009). Adolescent alcohol use, especially among preteens, is a serious risk factor for suicidal ideation and suicide attempts in girls and boys; for example, youth who reported an episode of heavy episodic drinking during the past year were significantly more likely to report a suicide attempt than peers who did not (McLoughlin et al., 2015). In addition, the use of alcohol while feeling depressed is correlated with suicidal behavior among adolescents (McLoughlin et al., 2015).

Research suggests a connection between depression and adolescent substance use, including alcohol (Kaplow, Curran, Angold, & Costello, 2001; Stice, Burton, & Shaw, 2004; Windle & Windle, 2001). Unfortunately, as illuminated by Ohannessian and Hesselbrock (2009), due to the variation in measurements from study to study, the findings related to depression are inconclusive.

Anxiety disorders are also concurrent with alcohol use in high numbers of adolescents (Wu et al., 2010). The associations between anxiety disorders and substance use differs according to the particular anxiety disorders and forms of substance use being examined, as well as by gender. Social phobia was associated with cigarette smoking among boys only. For girls, social phobia appeared to be negatively associated with drug use. For the other anxiety disorders, the associations with substance use tended to be stronger among girls. These findings highlight the need to improve clinical recognition of the anxiety disorders and to improve treatment access for afflicted adolescents. In addition, it is common that eating disorders, gaming, and self-harm are also woven into the presentation of youth with alcohol use disorders (Sussman et al., 2011).

Cooccurring complexities can be more a function of environmental factors, trauma, and socioeconomic status (SES) than psychology. In light of the Challenge related to family violence, the effects of exposure to school violence, community violence, child abuse, and parental intimate partner violence (IPV) on youths' subsequent alcohol and marijuana use are undeniable (Wright, Fagan, & Pinchevsky, 2013). Researchers have found that exposure to violence in a 1-year period increased the frequency of substance use 3 years later. The specific relationships between victimization and use varied for alcohol and marijuana use, with alcohol use not having a statistically significant relationship. Community violence and child abuse (but not school violence or exposure to IPV) have been established as predictive of future marijuana use (Wright et al., 2013). However, the accumulation of exposure to violence across "life domains" was detrimental to both future alcohol and marijuana use.

Alcohol and Academics

Alcohol contributes to academic problems for youth: Dropping out tends to coincide with increased delinquency, teen pregnancy among females, and incidents of alcohol misuse (Audas & Wilms, 2001).

Substance use increases with age, and the highest rate of current illicit drug use is among 18- to 20-year-olds (23.8%), whereas the peak age for alcohol misuse is 25 (SAMHSA, 2014). With regard to education, while in high school, those students who are not college-bound (a decreasing proportion of the total youth population) are considerably more likely to be at risk for using illicit drugs, drinking heavily, and smoking cigarettes (Johnston et al., 2014). Once in college, however, students drink at higher rates than their non-college-attending peers and they are more likely to receive a diagnosis of alcohol use disorder than their peers not attending college (Slutske, 2005). In addition, according to a study at Harvard School of Public Health, about one in four college students report academic consequences from drinking, including missing class, falling behind in class, doing poorly on exams or papers, and receiving lower grades overall (Wechsler, Dowdall, Maenner, Gledhill-Hoyt, & Lee, 1998).

In summary, it is challenging for anyone addicted to alcohol or other drugs to achieve and maintain sobriety, but it is especially challenging for adolescents. Research indicates that typical stressors of adolescence, including hormonal changes, incomplete brain development, a belief that they are invincible, and the importance of fitting in with peers (Berk & Asarnow, 2015), present even greater challenges to teens struggling to overcome addiction (Cates & Cummings, 2003). If teenagers who go through treatment return to a public high school, a majority of them relapse in the period immediately following discharge from the protective environment (Finch & Wegman, 2012).

STRATEGIES FOR ADDRESSING THE PROBLEM

Peers can promote both prosocial and antisocial behaviors. Just as the peer group influences the propensity for youth to engage in drug use, alcohol use, cigarette use, church going, and dropping out of high school (Gaviria & Raphael, 2001), positive peer groups can be a powerful vehicle for shifts from precontemplation to later stages of readiness for change. Mutual support groups have the potential to provide a support network for youth with alcohol problems (Passetti, Godley, & Godley, 2012). Affiliation with peer-based recovery mutual aid groups, as well as the shift from high school to college or the work world, mark distinct periods of opportunity and vulnerability for young people in recovery.

A continuum of care model ideally incorporates interventions for youth that extend far beyond the stages of recovery initiation and stabilization to encompass later stages of recovery maintenance and enhanced quality of life and social functioning. Intervention engagement is key; programs must resonate with the youth who receive them (Holleran Steiker, 2008).

Alternative Peer Groups

PEER-TO-PEER SUPPORTS IN HIGH SCHOOL

Over the last decade, adolescent treatment providers have recognized that services must resemble "wrap around services" (Kutash et al., 2013) in mental health. As described by Positive Behavior and Intervention Supports (PBIS, 2017):

> Wraparound is a philosophy of care with defined planning process used to build constructive relationships and support networks among students and youth with emotional or behavioral disabilities (EBD) and their families. It is community based, culturally relevant, individualized, strength based, and family centered. Wraparound plans are comprehensive and address multiple life domains across home, school, and community, including living environment; basic needs; safety; and social, emotional, educational, spiritual, and cultural needs. (Eber et al., n.d.)

Although there is limited research on mentorship for recovery high school students, there is extensive research on the impact of peer groups. The literature supports the idea that youth might be more likely to be successfully socialized in the presence of a positive peer culture (Lynch, Lerner, & Leventhal, 2013). Mejias, Gill, and Shpigelman (2014) found that a peer support group had a positive impact on young women with disabilities, particularly in the area of enhanced sense of belonging, self-confidence, and disability pride. Blair-McEvoy (1997) found that students who participated in peer support groups in schools scored higher on general, social, academic, and parental self-esteem than nonparticipants. This might not be causal, as it is plausible that youth scoring higher on these features are better equipped to participate in peer support groups. Aspects of behavioral peer culture are correlated with individual achievement, whereas components of both relational and behavioral peer culture are related to school engagement (Lynch et al., 2013). For youth with alcohol use disorders, having a peer group with a culture of sobriety can be critical for ongoing recovery (Collier, Hilliker, & Onwuegbuzie, 2014).

SAMHSA (2009), in a meta-analysis of research that derived guiding principles of systems of care from findings, indicated that a network of personal connections with peers is critical to recovery and that poor social support is a major factor in the return to alcohol or other substance use following recovery initiation. Peer support helps a person in recovery see or visualize others in similar circumstances doing well, which increases a belief in his or her own abilities. It also helps individuals in recovery build or rebuild healthy relationships and play constructive roles in their communities.

Alternative peer groups (APGs) originated in Texas in the late 1970s and many, such as the Palmer Drug Abuse Programs (PDAP), have continued to thrive as supportive settings for youth recovery all these years. The APGs emphasize that youth will not stay in recovery if it is not better for them than alcohol and other substance use (Nash & Collier, 2016). Whereas the original APGs provided peer support only, new versions, such as Teen & Family Services (TAFS), add clinical supports such as individual, family, and group therapeutic sessions. In addition, APGs provide a safe and sober space for youth after school, evenings, and weekends. Some of the APGs even offer summer travel programs. Several of the successful recovery high schools in Texas consider it mandatory that their students belong to an APG to strengthen their chances of staying in recovery during the hours that they are not in school.

COLLEGIATE RECOVERY PROGRAMS AND MENTORSHIP

College campuses have long had an association with excessive alcohol and other substance use, often for the first time in a student's life. For students who recognize their own problematic alcohol use and wish to make a change, there might be no examples of a recovery lifestyle, no recognition that college-aged students can and do find recovery at a young age, and no entry point into a community of recovery readily accessible on or near campus. Enter collegiate recovery programs (CRPs), a refuge of recovery embedded in a college or university campus.

CRPs offer support to college students in recovery from alcohol and substance use disorders. That support is typically centered on a community of students in recovery from substance use disorders, recovery-supportive programming, and the creation of a space on campus where recovery is actively celebrated and normalized. There is significant variation in CRP models, but all center around a core community of support. Although the earliest CRPs date back almost 40 years, the field remained very small until recent years, and the recent rapid proliferation of programs across the country has led to a diversity of CRP models and practices that has not yet been well catalogued (Laudet, Harris, Kimball, Winters, & Moberg, 2015; Laudet, Harris, Winters, Moberg, & Kimball, 2014, 2015).

RECOVERY HIGH SCHOOL MOVEMENT

There is a general consensus among classic and contemporary alcohol researchers that providing support services for persons recovering from alcohol use disorders is one of the most effective ways to increase success (Catalano, Berglund, Ryan, Lonczak, & Hawkins, 1999; Godley, Godley, Dennis, Funk, & Passetti, 2002; Kelly, Myers, & Brown, 2005). Despite the importance of support and guidance to a successful recovery, overall research investigating the effects of such support is sparse. The research that does exist suggests that strong recovery support increases the likelihood of continued abstinence and wellness. Similarly, Kelly et al. (2005) examined the relationship between an adolescent's participation in a 12-step program and alcohol and other substance use during the first 6 months after becoming sober and found that meeting attendance was positively associated with higher rates of abstinence.

Before the existence of recovery high schools, alternative school settings were used to sequester youth who misuse alcohol from others at the school, but these were often punitive, temporary, and insufficient. Instead, recovery schools aim at a strengths-based approach and provide supportive accountability and positive identities for those involved. These models fit well with the social work profession due to the strengths base, evidence base, and focus on vulnerable youth as a critical piece of the overall ecosystem for the success of recovery schools.

Recovery high schools all provide recovery supports while offering academic rigor and ways to pave the way for a future in work or college. Most of the successful schools start with a "Check-In" to start the day with recovery consciousness and to allow for accountability. The classes are like regular high schools (some online and some with teachers), but there are additional recovery-centered activities such as service, recreation, 12-step meetings, and recovery policy advocacy. Also, families are involved in a variety of ways and they are considered an important part of the community. Educational and social events include students and their families. Releases are signed to allow adjunct supports (e.g., recovery sponsors and coaches, probation officers, therapists, etc.) to visit the school and be a part of the solutions.

The National Institutes of Health has recently funded a study of all recovery schools in the nation. Investigators Finch, Moberg, and Krupp (2014) found that there are a variety of models for recovery high schools and many form organically to meet the needs of their unique cultures. For example, some are attached to clinical settings, some are part of school districts, some are charter schools, and still others are private schools. Recovery high schools vary in "enrollment, fiscal stability, governance, staffing, and organizational structure" (Finch et al., 2014, p. 116). Particular challenges to recovery schools include enrollment, funding, lack of primary treatment accessibility, academic rigor, and institutional support (Finch et al., 2014). Recovery schools appear to successfully function as the holistic academic and recovery support environment necessary to reinforce and sustain therapeutic benefits gained from treatment (Moberg

& Finch, 2008). Finch et al.'s study found that small size and recovery-related programming provide the elements that traditional schools cannot. There are approximately 36 recovery high schools in 18 different states (5 of which are in Texas), with two or three new schools opening, on average, each year (Association of Recovery Schools, 2016). All of these schools offer their students a safe academic environment in which they can pursue their high school education.

Lanham and Tirado's (2011) primary focus of research was on recovery high school graduation rates. At the time of the study, more than 90% of the 72 alumni who responded to their survey reported enrolling in college and 6 had graduated. However, many reported struggling with their sobriety once they graduated. Most were no longer participating in 12-step programs, 40% had reentered treatment at some point after high school graduation, 40% had remained sober, and 60% were no longer using illegal drugs.

Although more research is needed, the evidence that exists appears to support that recovery high schools are an important component of the continuum of care for teens (Finch et al., 2014). They can create an empowering and sober environment that helps teens develop a positive sense of identity and be proud of who they are, rather than viewing their former substance misuse as a stigma (Holleran Steiker, Grahovac, & White, 2014). They can also teach skills for resisting peer pressure and reduce social acceptability of using alcohol and other drugs (Sussman, Skara, & Ames, 2008). This could serve to build bridges as teens graduate from high school. Efforts need to be made to continue a continuum of care that supports them during their college and early adult years.

UNIVERSITY HIGH SCHOOL

In forming a school to support high school students struggling with alcohol and other substance use disorders, a critical component is the creation of a recovery culture that includes the principles of integrity, honesty, hope, courage, willingness, fellowship, justice, perseverance, and service. The inspiration for this school came from the Association of Recovery Schools (ARS) Conference in 2012. The University High School (UHS) founders in Austin collaborated with a network of substance use treatment programs, other social service agencies, and community supporters to establish the first recovery high school in the Austin area (Holleran Steiker, Nash, Counihan, White, & Harper, 2012).

The school opened in 2014 as a private 501(c)(3) and in its second year, it was adopted by the University of Texas (UT) Charter School system. It admits students in Grades 9 through 12, who are at various stages in their recovery. Students must have some willingness to be in an abstinent environment and not only participate in the academic and recovery support activities during school, but they must attend support and therapeutic services after school and on weekends. The high school accepts enrollments year round. There is a fee for recovery support programming and services, but scholarships and a sliding fee scale are available. In fact, the school has never turned away a student for financial reasons. The school has one Executive Director, a Director of Wellness and Recovery Support, and a Student Engagement Coordinator who also serves as a recovery coach. UT Charter Schools provides the principal, teachers (presently mathematics, science, and English), curriculum and materials. Sustainability is made possible by donations, grants, and program fees.

Recovery programming includes daily peer-to-peer process groups, weekly meetings of 12-step and other roads to recovery, educational and fun off-campus activities, service opportunities, and individualized brief interventions as needed to provide social and emotional wellness and recovery support. Family recovery support is also a critical piece in the programming (Kumpfer & Alvarado, 2003). Random drug testing is part of the culture. Students hold each other accountable to maintain a safe and sober environment.

College Students in Recovery as Mentors

UHS is innovative in that it incorporates a mentorship program with linkage to an adjacent 10-year-old collegiate recovery program, the UT Center for Students in Recovery (UT CSR). The interactions between the high school and collegiate students in recovery are mutually advantageous.

In 2004, the University of Texas at Austin created the UT CSR, a program that provides a support system for students in recovery to help them achieve academic success. A key aspect of CSR is its 12-step programs and other supportive groups and fellowship, which although attended primarily by UT students, are open to anyone in the community. Research demonstrates that students who frequent the UT CSR stay clean and sober and perform academically at levels equal to, and sometimes surpassing, other students at the university (Holleran & Grahovac, 2014; Holleran, Grahovac, & White, 2014). Students reported that UT CSR provides a safe community where they find hope and support for their recovery. Students also reported that UT CSR provides sober activities and other options in the midst of a world that often is not alcohol- and drug-free. The vast majority of students have adopted positive recovery habits such as having a home group, participating in service work, and sponsoring others. The annual evaluation found that 83% of the students indicated that they have been able to stay free from their substance use since joining UT CSR (Kaye, Stuart, Grahovac, Holleran Steiker, & Maison, 2012).

There is an increase in the number of students who are active in a collegiate recovery program such as the UT CSR who previously attended recovery high schools. Due to their established recovery, these students are particularly well suited to serve as sponsors for teens in the Austin area. The leadership team of UHS determined that the formal mentorship of UHS high school students by collegiate students at the UT CSR could be a powerful innovation. This idea was met with enthusiasm, and other key people who would most likely be supportive, such as parents of youth with alcohol and other substance misuse, parents who had lost a loved one to addiction or overdose, clinicians and therapists working with this population, and members of the local 12-step community were quickly identified and included.

In addition to the CSR mentors, the sponsored student group of Drug and Alcohol Peer Advisors has revolved its service work at UHS providing events (e.g., end-of-school-year Field Day), assistance at UHS and UT CSR events (e.g., Sober Tailgate), advocacy (e.g., helping to testify at the Legislature for the Naloxone Bill, which passed unanimously in 2015), and providing and coordinating the UT Tutoring Program.

UHS prompted other new recovery high schools across the nation to consider a formal relationship with a university through its collegiate recovery program, student internships, and student-sponsored organizations. Being able to "walk in the footsteps" of their older collegiate peers builds the bridge between high school and higher education for many of the recovery school students.

Limitations

Resources are key to a successful recovery high school, but clearly, some recovery school settings do not have the luxury of a local collegiate recovery program to serve as mentors. Such schools often need to rely on the support and guidance of the local recovery community and if there is not a vibrant fellowship of young people in recovery, adults might have to step into these roles until the youth community grows.

Recovery schools must keep safety and security in the forefront to protect the vulnerable youth who attend. Volunteers must be carefully vetted and background screens must be utilized. Because most recovery schools are relatively small (the largest being under 100 students), safety can be maintained with well-written policies and procedures, hiring of highly competent staff, and close supervision of the students attending the setting.

It takes money to have a successful recovery school. There are a variety of funding models and it is best to choose the model that best fits the culture and resources of the setting. Creative sustainability usually includes a combination of fundraising and donations, grants, and consideration of state funds or charter schools to provide the educational piece.

Although this model is fairly new (with the first recovery schools organically beginning in the 1980s), assistance with the creation of a school is available from other successful schools as well as the ARS, which serves recovery high schools, and the Association of Recovery in Higher Education (ARHE), which serves collegiate recovery programs. For the high schools, ARS offers an accreditation process to be sure all aspects of academics and recovery services are well provided. It is wise for new schools to use the ARS Accreditation Standards as a blueprint for creating a successful recovery high school.

WHY ALCOHOL IS THE GRANDEST CHALLENGE OF ALL

For social workers immersed in work with youth (i.e., adolescents 14–18 years old) and emerging adults (i.e., 19–25-year-olds) in high school and college settings, this article highlights the importance of addressing alcohol with young people whose brains are continuing to develop and whose behaviors are being established. The inclusion of "Reducing and Preventing Alcohol Misuse and Its Consequences" as a Grand Challenge for the profession was aptly given a home within the "Close the Health Gap" challenge. To rise to this challenge, the social work profession must focus on our youth. Through education, asset-based communities, healthy attachments, a sense of responsibility, and actively combating stigma, we can break the present cycle of denial and alcohol-related consequences and deaths. To this end, the synthesis of this article points toward the following action steps:

1. Educate locally and nationally to reduce stigma and increase awareness about alcohol, alcohol misuse, and alcohol use disorders.
2. Educate interdisciplinary points of contact about recognizing signs, referring, and knowing local resources.
3. Recognize and make explicit the role of youth alcohol misuse as it ties in with all 12 Grand Challenges.

In addition, specific to recovery schools, it must be emphasized that community collaborations are critical; agencies and organizations serving adolescents and their families need to communicate and determine ways that they can work together rather than compete for resources. Although it is important to have creative brainstorming around innovations that would resonate in a particular community, it is important to learn from the recovery school and APG settings that already exist to avoid pitfalls and build on solid foundations. For example, the ARS Accreditation rubric is an excellent checklist and strategic plan for those starting new schools. Launch teams with connections in overlapping communities of interest (e.g., 12-step programs, local universities, children and youth coalitions, and treatment centers) must build solid working relationships prior to the creation of a recovery school network to build an effective mission statement and culturally grounded strategy for a successful launch. It is recommended that staff and recovery coaches who open the school should have at least some experience in recovery school or APG settings.

Although marketing can be important, the first priority should be building the culture of recovery rather than numbers of students. The vision should grow according to the board-determined strategy and not be haphazard. The students (and family members) who are a success are the best advocates and promoters of the model.

Recovery schools, in conjunction with youth recovery communities, are a powerful piece in the puzzle for solving the problem of youth alcohol misuse. Social workers are in excellent positions to create, administer, and support these settings. Ultimately, the most powerful way to rise to the challenge of youth alcohol misuse is to support young people's positive experiences. Social workers are poised to create, augment, and support settings in which young people can find recovery.

REFERENCES

Association of Recovery Schools. (2016). *The state of recovery high schools: 2016 biennial report*. Retrieved from http://nationalrxdrugabusesummit.org/wp-content/uploads/2016/03/State-of-Recovery-Schools_2-24-16.b.pdf

Audas, R., & Wilms, J. D. (2001). *Engagement and dropping out of school: A life-course perspective* (Working Paper of the Applied Research Branch, Strategic Policy Human Resources Development). Retrieved from http://sbisrvntweb.uqac.ca/archivage/15292281.pdf

Begun, A. L., Clapp, J. D., & The Alcohol Misuse Grand Challenge Collective. (2016). Reducing and preventing alcohol misuse and its consequences: A grand challenge for social work. *International Journal of Alcohol and Drug Research, 5*(2), 73–83. doi:10.7895/ijadr.v5i2.223

Berk, M., & Asarnow, J. R. (2015). Assessment of suicidal youth in the emergency department. *Suicide and Life-Threatening Behavior, 45*, 345–359. doi:10.1111/sltb.2015.45.issue-3

Blair-McEvoy, E. A. (1997). *Peer support groups and rural elementary schools*. Minneapolis, MN: Walden University.

Blanco, C., Okuda, M., & Wright, C. (2008). Mental health of college students and their non-college-attending peers: Results from the national epidemiologic study on alcohol and related conditions. *Archives of General Psychiatry, 65*, 1429–1437. doi:10.1001/archpsyc.65.12.1429

Catalano, R., Berglund, M. L., Ryan, J. A. M., Lonczak, H. S., & Hawkins, J. D. (1999). *Positive youth development in the United States: Research findings on evaluations of positive youth development programs*. Washington, DC: U.S. Department of Health and Human Services.

Cates, J., & Cummings, J. (2003). *Recovering our children: A handbook for parents of young people in early recovery*. New York, NY: Writer's Club Press.

Clapp, J. D., Johnson, M., Voas, R. B., Lange, J. E., Shillington, A., & Russell, C. (2005). Reducing DUI among US college students: Results of an environmental prevention trial. *Addiction, 100*, 327–334. doi:10.1111/j.1360 0443.2004.00917.x

Collier, C., Hilliker, R., & Onwuegbuzie, A. (2014). Alternative peer group: A model for youth recovery. *Journal of Groups in Addiction & Recovery, 9*(1), 40–53. doi:10.1080/1556035X.2013.836899

Dennis, M. L., Feeney, T., & Stevens, L. H. (2006). *Global Appraisal of Individual Needs–Short Screener (GAIN–SS): Administration and scoring manual for the GAINSS version 2.0.1*. Retrieved from http://www.chestnut.org/LI/gain/GAIN_SS/index.html

DeWit, D. J., Adlaf, E. M., Offord, D. R., & Ogborne, A. C. (2000). Age at first alcohol use: A risk factor for the development of alcohol disorders. *American Journal of Psychiatry, 157*, 745–750. doi:10.1176/appi.ajp.157.5.745

Eaton, D. K., Kann, L., Kinchen, S., Shanklin, S., Ross, J., Hawkins, J., … Wechsler, H. (2012). Youth risk behavior surveillance—United States, 2009. *Surveillance Summaries, 61*(4): 1–142.

Eber, L., Hyde, K., Rose, J., Breen, K., McDonald, D., & Lewandowski, H. (n.d.). *Wraparound service and positive behavior support*. Retrieved from https://www.pbis.org/school/tier3supports/wraparound

Erickson, C. (2007). *The science of addiction: From neurobiology to treatment*. New York, NY: Norton.

Finch, A. J., Moberg, D. P., & Krupp, A. L. (2014). Continuing care in high schools: A descriptive study of recovery high school programs. *Journal of Child and Adolescent Substance Abuse, 23*, 116–129. doi:10.1080/1067828X.2012.751269

Finch, A., & Wegman, H. (2012). Recovery high schools: Opportunities for support and personal growth for students in recovery. *Prevention Researcher, 19*(5), 12–16.

Gaviria, A., & Raphael, S. (2001). School-based peer effects and juvenile behavior. *The Review of Economics and Statistics, 83*, 257–268. doi:10.1162/00346530151143798

Godley, M. D., Godley, S. H., Dennis, M. L., Funk, R., & Passetti, L. L. (2002). Preliminary outcomes from the assertive continuing care experiment for adolescents discharged from residential treatment. *Journal of Substance Abuse Treatment, 23*(1), 21–32. doi:10.1016/S0740-5472(02)00230-1

Hingson, R., Heeren, T., & Winter, M. (2005). Magnitude of alcohol-related mortality and morbidity among U.S. college students ages 18–24: Changes from 1998 to 2001. *Annual Review of Public Health, 26*, 259–279. doi:10.1146/annurev.publhealth.26.021304.144652

Hingson, R. W., Zha, W., & Weitzman, E. R. (2009). Magnitude of and trends in alcohol-related mortality and morbidity among U.S. college students ages 18–24, 1998–2005. *Journal of Studies on Alcohol and Drugs* (Suppl. 16), 12–20. doi:10.15288/jsads.2009.s16.12

Hogue, A., Liddle, H. A., Dauber, S., & Samuolis, J. (2004). Linking session focus to treatment outcome in evidence-based treatments for adolescent substance abuse. *Psychotherapy: Theory, Research, Practice, Training, 41*, 83–96. doi:10.1037/0033-3204.41.2.83

Holleran Steiker, L. K. (2008). Making drug and alcohol prevention relevant: Adapting evidence-based curricula to unique adolescent cultures. *Family & Community Health, 31*(1S), S52–S60.

Holleran Steiker, L. K., Counihan, C., White, W., & Harper, K. (2015). Transforming Austin: Augmenting the system of care for adolescents in recovery from substance use disorders. *The Journal of Alcoholism and Drug Dependence, 3*, 203–210. doi:10.4172/2329-6488.1000203

Holleran Steiker, L. K., & Grahovac, I. (2014). Introduction to the special issue: Substance use problems and issues in recovery among college students. *Journal of Social Work Practice in the Addictions, 14*, 1–5. doi:10.1080/1533256X.2014.872937

Holleran Steiker, L. K., Grahovac, I., & White, W. (2014). Social work and collegiate recovery communities. *Social Work, 59*, 177–180. doi:10.1093/sw/swu012

Johnston, L. D., O'Malley, P. M., Bachman, J. G., & Schulenberg, J. E. (2014). *Monitoring the Future national survey results on drug use 1975–2012. 2012 overview: Key findings on adolescent drug use.* Ann Arbor, MI: Institute for Social Research, The University of Michigan. Retrieved from http://monitoringthefuture.org/pubs/monographs/mtf-overview2012.pdf

Kaplow, J. B., Curran, P. J., Angold, A., & Costello, E. J. (2001). The prospective relation between dimensions of anxiety and the initiation of adolescent alcohol use. *Journal of Clinical Child Psychology, 30*, 316–326. doi:10.1207/S15374424JCCP3003_4

Kaye, A. D., Stuart, G., Grahovac, I., & Holleran Steiker, L. K. & Maison, T. (2012). *University of Texas at Austin Center for Students in Recovery assessment report.* Austin, TX: University of Texas at Austin.

Kelly, J. F., Myers, M. G., & Brown, S. A. (2005). The effects of age composition of 12-step groups on adolescent 12-step participation and substance use outcome. *Journal of Child and Adolescent Substance Abuse, 15*, 63–72. doi:10.1300/J029v15n01_05

Kelly, J. F., Stout, R. L., & Slaymaker, V. (2013). Emerging adults' treatment outcomes in relation to 12-step mutual-help attendance and active involvement. *Drug and Alcohol Dependence, 129*, 151–157. doi:10.1016/j.drugalcdep.2012.10.005

Kumpfer, K. L., & Alvarado, R. (2003). Family-strengthening approaches for the prevention of youth problem behaviors. *American Psychologist, 58*, 457–465. doi:10.1037/0003-066X.58.6-7.457

Kutash, K., Acri, M. C., Pollock, M., Armusewicz, K., Olin, S. S., & Hoagwood, K. E. (2013). Quality indicators for multidisciplinary team functioning in community-based children's mental health services. *Administration and Policy in Mental Health and Mental Health Services Research, 41*, 55–68. doi:10.1007/s10488-013-0508-2

Lanham, C., & Tirado, J. (2011). Lessons in sobriety: An exploratory study of graduate outcomes at a recovery high school. *Journal of Groups in Addiction & Recovery, 6:* 245–263.

Laudet, A., Harris, K., Kimball, T., Winters, K. C., & Moberg, D. P. (2014). Collegiate recovery communities programs: What do we know and what do we need to know? *Journal of Social Work Practice in the Addictions, 14*(1), 84–100. doi:10.1080/1533256X.2014.872015

Laudet, A. B., Harris, K., Kimball, T., Winters, K. C., & Moberg, D. P. (2015). Characteristics of students participating in collegiate recovery programs: A national study. *Journal of Substance Abuse Treatment, 51*, 38–46. doi:10.1016/j.jsat.2014.11.004

Laudet, A. B., Harris, K., Winters, K. C., Moberg, D. P., & Kimball, T. (2015). Nation-wide survey of collegiate recovery programs: Is there a single model? *Drug & Alcohol Dependence, 140*, e117. doi:10.1016/j.drugalcdep.2014.02.335

Lynch, A. D., Lerner, R. M., & Leventhal, T. (2013). Adolescent academic achievement and school engagement: An examination of the role of school-wide peer culture. *Journal of Youth and Adolescence, 42*(1), 6–19. doi:10.1007/s10964-012-9833-0

McLoughlin, A. B., Gould, M. S., & Malone, K. M. (2015). Global trends in teenage suicide: 2003–2014. *Quarterly Journal of Medicine, 108*, 765–780. doi:10.1093/qjmed/hcv026

Mejias, N. J., Gill, C. J., & Shpigelman, C. N. (2014). Influence of a support group for young women with disabilities on sense of belonging. *Journal of Counseling Psychology 61*(2): 208–220.

Moberg, D. P., & Finch, A. J. (2008). Recovery high schools: A descriptive study of school programs and students. *Journal of Groups in Addiction & Recovery, 2*, 128–161. doi:10.1080/15560350802081314

Nash, A., & Collier, C. (2016). The alternative peer group: A developmentally appropriate recovery support model for adolescents. *Journal of Addictions Nursing, 27*, 109–119. doi:10.1097/JAN.0000000000000122

National Center on Addiction and Substance Abuse at Columbia University (NCASA). (2011). *National survey of American attitudes on substance abuse XVI: Teens and parents* (Report). Retrieved from http://www.centeronaddiction.org/addiction-research/reports/national-survey-american-attitudes-substance-abuse-teens-parents-2011

National Institute of Drug Abuse (NIDA). (2007). The science of addiction: Drugs, brains, and behavior. *NIH Medline Plus, 2*(2), 14–17. Retrieved from https://medlineplus.gov/magazine/issues/spring07/articles/spring07pg14-17.html

National Institute on Alcohol Abuse and Alcoholism (NIAAA). (2006). *Alcohol alert No. 67: Underage drinking*. Retrieved from http://pubs.niaaa.nih.gov/publications/AA67/AA67.htm

Ohannessian, C. M., & Hesselbrock, V. M. (2009). A finer examination of the role that negative affect plays in the relationship between paternal alcoholism and the onset of alcohol and marijuana use. *Journal of Studies on Alcohol and Drugs, 70*, 400–408. doi:10.15288/jsad.2009.70.400

Oostveen, T., Knibbe, R., & De Vries, H. (1996). Social influences on young adults' alcohol consumption: Norms, modeling, pressure, socializing, and conformity. *Addictive Behaviors, 21*(2), 1X7–1Y7. doi:10.1016/0306-4603(95)00052-6

Passetti, L. L., Godley, S. H., & Godley, M. D. (2012). Youth participation in mutual support groups: History, current knowledge, and areas for future research. *Journal of Groups in Addiction and Recovery, 7*, 253–278. doi:10.1080/1556035X.2012.705707

PBIS. (2017). *Positive Behavioral Interventions and Supports*. Retrieved from https://www.pbis.org/

Rauer, A. J., Pettit, G. S., Lansford, J. E., Bates, J. E., & Dodge, K. A. (2013). Romantic relationship patterns in young adulthood and their developmental antecedents. *Developmental Psychology, 49*, 2159–2171. doi: 10.1037/a0031845

Slutske, W. S. (2005). Alcohol use disorders among US college students and their non–college-attending peers. *Archives of General Psychiatry, 62*, 321–327. doi:10.1001/archpsyc.62.3.321

Stice, E., Burton, E. M., & Shaw, H. (2004). Prospective relations between bulimic pathology, depression, and substance abuse: Unpacking comorbidity in adolescent girls. *Journal of Consulting and Clinical Psychology, 72,* 62–71.

Substance Abuse and Mental Health Services Administration. (2009). *Child Mental Health Initiative Evaluation findings: Report to Congress 2009 on Comprehensive Community Mental Health Services for Children and Their Families Program.* Rockville, MD: Author.

Substance Abuse and Mental Health Services Administration. (2014). *Behavioral health trends in the United States: Results from the 2014 National Survey on Drug Use and Health.* Retrieved from https://www.samhsa.gov/data/sites/default/files/NSDUH-FRR1-2014/NSDUH-FRR1-2014.pdf

Sussman, S., Leventhal, A., Bluthenthal, R. N., Frelruth, M., Forster, M., & Ames, S. L. (2011). A framework for the specificity of addictions. *International Journal of Environmental Research and Public Health, 8,* 3399–3415.

Sussman, S., Skara, S., & Ames, S. L. (2008). Substance abuse among adolescents. *Substance Use and Misuse, 43,* 1802–1828.

Wechsler, H., Dowdall, G. W., Maenner, G., Gledhill-Hoyt, J., & Lee, H. (1998). Changes in binge drinking and related problems among American college students between 1993 and 1997: Results of the Harvard School of Public Health college alcohol study. *Journal of American College Health, 47*(2), 57–68.

Windle, M., & Windle, R. C. (2001). Depressive symptoms and cigarette smoking among middle adolescents: Prospective associations and intrapersonal and interpersonal influences. *Journal of Consulting Clinical Psychology, 69,* 215–226.

Wright, E. M., Fagan, A. A., & Pinchevsky, G. M. (2013). The effects of exposure to violence and victimization across life domains on adolescent substance use. *Child Abuse and Neglect, 37,* 899–909.

Wu, P., Goodwin, R. D., Fuller, C., Liu, X., Comer, J. S., Cohen, P., & Hoven, C. W. (2010). The relationship between anxiety disorders and substance use among adolescents in the community. *Journal of Youth and Adolescence, 39,* 177–188.

Empowerment in Coalitions Targeting Underage Drinking: Differential Effects of Organizational Characteristics for Volunteers and Staff

KRISTEN GILMORE POWELL, PhD

SARAH L. GOLD, MAT

N. ANDREW PETERSON, PhD

SUZANNE BORYS, EdD

DONALD HALLCOM, PhD

Social work has adopted the Grand Challenge to reduce and prevent alcohol misuse and related consequences. This study extends previous research through a macro examination of distinct roles within coalitions implementing prevention strategies targeting underage alcohol use. The purpose was to determine whether hypothesized relationships among organizational characteristics, empowerment variables, and perceived effectiveness differed for 2 subgroups (i.e., volunteers and paid staff). The sample was comprised of 357 survey participants affiliated with a statewide substance abuse initiative. Structural equation modeling was used to examine hypothesized relationships between study variables and found differences among subgroups. Results can inform organizational processes within coalitions that focus on engaging different groups to have a stronger impact on community issues, such as substance use consequences.

Underage drinking is a significant public health concern in the United States and is associated with multiple harmful consequences. Alcohol remains the substance mostly widely used by youth. A recent national study found that two out of every three students (64%) have consumed alcohol by the end of high school and 26% have used alcohol by the eighth grade (Johnston, O'Malley, Miech, Bachman, & Schulenberg, 2016). Further, close to half (47%) of 12th-grade students reported having been drunk at least once in their lifetime (Johnston et al., 2016). In addition to troublesome consumption patterns, underage drinking contributes to a wide range of costly consequences affecting not only individuals but also families and communities. Social problems resulting from underage drinking that are concerning to social work practitioners and scholars include motor vehicle crashes, unintentional injuries, alcohol poisonings (Substance Abuse and Mental Health Services Administration [SAMHSA], 2015), drinking and driving (O'Malley & Johnston, 2013), peer violence (Stoddard et al., 2015), and risky sexual behaviors leading to consequences such as unwanted pregnancies and sexually transmitted infections (Khan, Berger, Wells, & Cleland, 2012; Oshri, Tubman, Morgan-Lopez, Saavedra, & Csizmadia, 2013; Salas-Wright, Vaughn, Ugalde, & Todic, 2015).

The American Academy of Social Work and Social Welfare adopted the Grand Challenge to reduce alcohol misuse and its related consequences. This Grand Challenge calls for demonstrable progress within a decade, through sustainable and innovative strategies (Begun, Clapp, & The Alcohol Misuse Grand Challenge Collective, 2016). A recent trend in substance abuse prevention is the adoption of models that are similar to public health models, which target change across populations or communities. Environmental strategies have been endorsed widely by policymakers, scholars, and prevention practitioners to address public health issues. Environmental interventions focus on population-based efforts that change the environment in which individuals make choices (Frieden, 2010; Friend, Carmona, Wilbur, & Levy, 2001; Pettibone, Friend, Nargiso, & Florin, 2013). Typically, a combination of policy efforts, media campaigns, and enforcement strategies work synergistically to impact the environment (Friend, Pettibone, Florin, Vela, & Nargiso, 2015). Environmental strategies that target underage drinking concentrate on reducing access and opportunities to drink, reducing tolerance and attitudes that encourage underage drinking, and increasing penalties for violating alcohol laws

(National Institute on Alcohol Abuse and Alcoholism [NIAAA], 2006). More specifically, environmental strategies that have demonstrated promise for decreasing alcohol use among youth include dram shop liability laws, which hold retail owners or servers liable for harm caused by their patron after their last drink (Scherer, Fell, Thomas, & Voas, 2015); underage alcohol compliance checks, which involve underage individuals under law enforcement supervision attempting to purchase alcohol (Erickson, Smolenski, Toomey, Carlin, & Wagenaar, 2013); mandatory alcohol server training policies and laws (Rammohan et al., 2011; Saltz, 2011; Toomey, Lenk, & Wagenaar, 2007); and public policies affecting price and tax of alcoholic beverages (Wagenaar, Tobler, & Komro, 2010; Xuan et al., 2013).Community-based coalitions play a critical role in the implementation of environmental strategies to combat persistent public health issues. Previous research has studied coalition initiatives using environmental prevention strategies to target substance abuse (Anderson-Carpenter, Watson-Thompson, Chaney, & Jones, 2016; Flewelling & Hanley, 2016; Powell & Peterson, 2014), interpersonal violence (Schober & Fawcett, 2015), youth violence (Morrel-Samuels, Bacallao, Brown, Bower, & Zimmerman, 2016), cardiovascular disease and stroke (Kegler et al., 2015), childhood obesity (Foltz, Belay, Dooyema, Williams, & Blanck, 2015), childhood HIV (Miller et al., 2016), and tobacco use (Bunnell et al., 2012; Rhoades, Beebe, Boeckman, & Williams, 2015). Leading national institutes, including the Institute of Medicine, the Centers for Disease Control and Prevention (CDC), and the SAMHSA, support evidence-based, community-level environmental approaches to addressing today's health and social problems and resulting consequences (CDC, 2011; Florin et al., 2012; Pronk, Hernandez, & Lawrence, 2013). Public health models, such as the Strategic Prevention Framework (SPF; Edwards, Stein-Seroussi, Flewelling, Orwin, & Zhang, 2015; SAMHSA, 2016), are guided by prevention science through concerted efforts to target risk and protective factors that affect the probability of poor health outcomes later in life. Risk and protective factors exist across ages and can be targeted through multiple domains from the individual to community level (Harrop & Catalano, 2016). As Begun, Clapp, and The Alcohol Misuse Grand Challenge Collective (2016) suggested, there is a critical need for multisector collaboration to implement multilevel approaches to target the grand challenge of reducing alcohol misuse and its consequences. Coalitions are well-positioned to build capacity among multiple sectors and work to improve community-level health problems, including underage drinking. This study investigates the organizational characteristics that might affect critical members of multisector coalitions working at the macro level to combat underage drinking and improve the resulting community consequences.

CONCEPTUAL FRAMEWORK

Figure 1 shows the conceptual framework for this study. It shows that empowering organizational characteristics of prevention coalitions are hypothesized to have direct effects on coalition members' perceived effectiveness, as well as indirect effects through their influence on members' empowerment.

Further, this model presents the hypothesis that these organizational characteristics of coalitions and individuals' empowerment will differentially influence perceived effectiveness of two district groups—specifically coalition staff and volunteers. Empowerment is a fundamental concept within the Social Work Code of Ethics, calling social workers to foster empowerment among vulnerable populations by addressing environmental barriers that negatively affect people's health and well-being on a macro level (National Association of Social Workers, 2008).

Two central theoretical frameworks from the empowerment literature guided the study. The first framework is a model of psychological empowerment (PE) proposed by Zimmerman (1995), which refers to empowerment at the individual level of analysis and includes one's beliefs about their own competence, ability to exercise control, and understanding of the sociopolitical environment. This framework contains three components: (a) *intrapersonal empowerment*, or how one thinks about oneself in terms of perceived control, self-efficacy, competence, and mastery; (b) *interactional empowerment*, or the possession of a critical awareness of one's environment and a set of skills and understandings about social and political processes; and (c) *behavioral empowerment*, or one's actions such as community involvement, organizational participation, and coping skills (Zimmerman, 1995). This PE framework guided previous studies of individual and community-based health promotion (Christens, Peterson, Reid, & Garcia-Reid, 2015; Holden, Evans, Hinnant, & Messeri, 2005; Peterson, Lowe, Aquilino, & Schneider, 2005; Speer & Hughey, 1995). Much of the previous research has focused on the

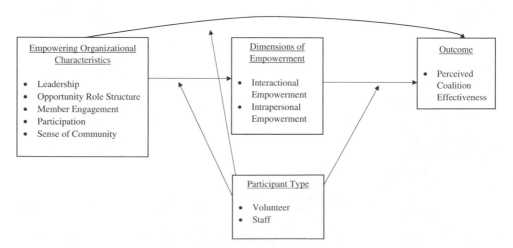

FIGURE 1 Conceptual framework for the study.

intrapersonal component of PE. To align our work with previous research, we focused on intrapersonal empowerment and also extend research with the inclusion of interactional empowerment (see Figure 1, presented as the two dimensions of empowerment).

The second theoretical framework is a model of organizational empowerment (OE) proposed by Peterson and Zimmerman (2004). Zimmerman (2000) originally defined OE as the organizational efforts that generate opportunities for members' PE and the organizational effectiveness necessary for goal achievement. Peterson and Zimmerman (2004) extended this definition to propose an OE framework containing three components. First, the *intraorganizational component* of OE refers to the internal structure and functioning of groups or organizations that might foster an infrastructure for members to engage in proactive behaviors that are needed to obtain goals. Second, the *interorganizational component* includes the linkages between organizations, such as networking, collaboration, and resource procurement. Third, the *extraorganizational component* includes efforts by community-based groups and organizations to influence the larger environment of which they are a part. Consistent with much of the previous empirical work in this area, our study focuses on the *intraorganizational* component of OE by examining organizational characteristics within the infrastructure of the coalitions that might foster members' empowerment and lead to perceived goal attainment. Previous research has examined various organizational characteristics of coalitions, including coalition capacity, member engagement, leadership (i.e., Powell & Peterson, 2014), skills improvement (Kegler, Norton, & Aronson, 2007), and sustainability of coalitions' efforts (Gloppen et al., 2016). As Figure 1 shows, the conceptual framework includes five empowering organizational characteristics (i.e., leadership, opportunity role structure [ORS], member engagement, participation, and sense of community).

Figure 1 also depicts participant type (i.e., volunteer, staff) as the final dimension of the conceptual framework. Previous literature has suggested that different factors are important for empowerment and participation in community-level initiatives for different subgroups. Studies have examined the importance of volunteer participation for successful and sustainable urban neighborhood health initiatives (Foster-Fishman et al., 2006; Peterson, Speer, & Peterson, 2011) and engagement of youth leaders in community development initiatives (Christens & Dolan, 2011). Foster-Fishman and colleagues (2009) developed an explicit process model to examine who participates at the community or neighborhood level, specifically leaders versus followers. This study extends this literature through the specific examination of relationships between organizational characteristics, empowerment, and perceived effectiveness and how these might vary among different coalition member groups. The sequence of events has been suggested in previous studies (i.e., Powell & Peterson, 2014), but this research is in the early stages of exploration. Further, no paths for these variables have been suggested for different groups. Using individual and OE theory (Peterson & Zimmerman, 2004; Zimmerman, 1995) to test our conceptual framework (Figure 1), this article answers this overall research question: By testing the hypothesized path model, do the relationships among organizational characteristics, empowerment, and perceived effectiveness differ among two groups within substance abuse prevention coalitions?

Results of this study could be useful to researchers and prevention practitioners as they develop interventions that enhance the capacity of coalitions targeting the harmful consequences of underage drinking. Further, this study is a good first step in assessing coalitions' effectiveness through members' perceptions. As seen in previous studies on environmental strategies, it often takes multiple years before movement within long-term outcomes is detected (Oesterle et al., 2015; Rhoades et al., 2015; Scherer et al., 2015). In the meantime, it is important to assess structures, functioning, and members' empowerment and perceived effectiveness in reaching coalition goals to prevent underage drinking.

METHOD

Procedures, Setting, and Participants

This study used a cross-sectional design to analyze secondary survey data collected in 2013, for the evaluation of a statewide substance abuse prevention initiative within a Northeastern U.S. state. The sampling frame for this study was the membership rosters for 17 community coalitions. A census of each coalition was attempted by recruiting participants who were coalition staff or members to complete a Web-based, self-administered survey. The coordinators of each coalition were sent a letter with a description of the study and a request to send a Web-based survey link to their coalition member list, including all paid staff and members. All 17 coordinators agreed to send the survey out to their membership. Data were collected through this survey, which contained 48 items. Participants' consent was obtained on the first screen of the Web-based survey.

A total of 406 participants completed surveys. The individual response rates of each coalition ranged from 11% to 88%. It is important to note that several coalitions sent the survey to their entire agency electronic mailing list and expected only a small number of responders, primarily those people considered active members in their coalition. For example, one coalition sent the survey to 250 people (their agency's listserv) and the resulting response rate was low (22%). This was most likely due to the fact that the actual number of active coalition members was much smaller than 250 people. The difference between the agency list and the number of active coalition members affected the ability to calculate a true response rate, which is reflected in the lower end of the response rate range. With this in mind, a total of 1,456 were included in the sampling frame for all coalitions and resulted in an overall response rate of 28%. The final sample for analysis ($n = 357$) included only those participants who answered whether they were involved as paid staff or as a volunteer. The participants were staff and members of regionally based, substance abuse prevention coalitions. These coalitions were trained in prevention science and funded by multiple sources (i.e., state funding, federal subawards from SAMHSA, etc.) to lead individual and community-level efforts to target the risk and protective factors of underage drinking (the coalitions must also target prescription drug misuse in the efforts). Coalition training within the prevention science framework included the development of logic models, which link their data-driven efforts to risk and protective factors with selected short- and long-term outcomes (Harrop & Catalano, 2016). The regional coalitions collaborate and link local community key players (i.e., law enforcement, schools, volunteer alliance groups, local government, etc.) as part of their capacity-building efforts to ensure multisector and multilevel approaches in the prevention of underage alcohol misuse and related consequences.

Demographic information self-reported by survey respondents included age, gender, race, ethnicity, highest level of education, and total household income. Participants ($n = 357$) were paid staff (46%) and volunteer members (54%) associated with the coalitions. Most of the participants were female (72%), identified as White (70%), and not of Latino or Hispanic origin (96%). Eleven percent of the sample reported being age 23 to 29; 13% were 30 to 39 years old; 27% were 40 to 49; 30% were 50 to 59; 19% were 60 to 69; and less than 2% were 70 to 74. The majority of the sample completed a bachelor's degree (39%) or master's degree (42%).

Measures

The survey instrument was developed using existing, validated scales designed to assess organizational characteristics, including leadership, ORS, sense of community, participation, and engagement; intrapersonal and interactional empowerment; and perceived effectiveness.

LEADERSHIP AND OPPORTUNITY ROLE STRUCTURE

This study used Maton's Organizational Characteristics Scale (Maton, 1988) to measure perceptions of two organizational characteristics in community-based organizations: (a) leadership, and (b) ORS. First, the leadership subscale measured the extent to which survey respondents rated the formal or informal leaders within a group as interpersonally and organizationally talented, committed, and dedicated to the coalition as well as supportive and responsive to members. Five items were used to measure participants' perceptions of leadership (e.g., "The leaders are very committed and dedicated to the regional coalition"). Second, the ORS subscale measured the extent to which members were encouraged to undertake a variety of formal positions or roles within their coalition and to take charge of different aspects of group functioning (Maton, 1988). The ORP subscale included five items (e.g., "Positions of responsibility are spread among members of the regional coalition"). For both measures, a 6-point, Likert-type rating scale was used and ranged from *strongly disagree* to *strongly agree*. The mean of the five leadership items comprised the overall score. Higher scores represented greater leadership (Cronbach's α = .78, M = 5.37, SD = .74). The five items for ORS were coded and calculated the same way (Cronbach's α = .88, M = 4.94, SD = .85).

SENSE OF COMMUNITY

The study used the revised version of the Community Organization Sense of Community (COSOC) scale (Hughey, Speer, & Peterson, 1999; Peterson et al., 2008) to measure participants' self-reported levels of connectedness. The COSOC items are positioned toward community-level organizations, which fit the study sample used here. This study included eight items from the COSOC using a phrase completion response option format (Hodge & Gillespie, 2007). This technique involves the presentation of an incomplete sentence fragment (i.e., I feel _____ to others in the regional coalition), which is then followed by two opposing phrases (i.e., very unconnected, very connected) that can be used to complete the sentence fragment. The phrases were configured to anchor each end of a 10-point scale. The mean of these items comprised the overall score (Cronbach's α = .94, M = 8.10, SD = 1.73).

MEMBER PARTICIPATION AND ENGAGEMENT

The extent to which members participate in their coalitions on a regular basis was measured by one item asking them to rate how often they participate on a 5-point scale ranging from *not at all* to *5 or more times a month* (M = 2.32, SD = .83) The assessment of coalition member engagement was based on a study by Kegler and Swan (2011). Survey participants were asked in which roles from a list of 10 they had participated (e.g., served as an officer, helped to implement activities, helped to plan for sustainability, recruited at least one new person to the coalition). Responses were summed and represented level of engagement by total number of roles.

INTRAPERSONAL EMPOWERMENT

The study included the Sociopolitical Control Scale–Revised (SPCS–R), developed and tested by Peterson and colleagues (2006) to measure intrapersonal PE. The SPCS–R was based on Zimmerman's (1995) model of PE and the original Sociopolitical Control Scale (SPCS; Zimmerman & Zahniser, 1991). This scale was designed to assess the dimensions of leadership competence (i.e., people's self-perceptions of their skill at organizing a group of people) and policy control (i.e., people's self-perceptions of their ability to influence policy decisions in a local community) as defined by Zimmerman and Zahniser (1991). Whereas the original SPCS included negatively and positively worded items, the revised scale included all positively worded items and it was found to have good internal consistency (Cronbach's α ranged from .78–.81). The study used all 17 items of the SPCS–R using a phrase completion response option format (Hodge & Gillespie, 2007). This technique involves the presentation of an incomplete sentence fragment (i.e., When trying to solve a problem in my community, I like to _____), which is then followed by two opposing phrases (i.e., wait and see if others will deal with it, work on the problem right away) that can be used to complete the sentence fragment. The phrases were configured to anchor each end of a 10-point scale. A total of eight of these items were used to measure the leadership competence component of PE and the other nine items were used to measure the policy control component of PE. The mean of these items comprised the overall score (Cronbach's α = .93, M = 7.96, SD = 1.09).

INTERACTIONAL EMPOWERMENT

Respondents' interactional empowerment was measured through the assessment of skills development as a result of participating within the coalitions (Christens, 2012; Zimmerman, 1995). Based on a study by Kegler and Swan (2011), survey participants were asked the extent to which 13 skills had been improved as a result of their participation within their coalition (e.g.,, assessing needs and assets, writing grants, facilitating groups, resolving conflict). Participants were asked to rate their improved skills as a result of coalition participation on a 4-point Likert type scale ranging from *not at all* to *a great deal* [of improvement]. The mean of these items comprised the overall score (Cronbach's α = .96, M = 2.95, SD = .67).

PERCEIVED EFFECTIVENESS

This study used a perceived effectiveness scale, developed with guidance from the framework of Sowa and colleagues (2004) called the Multidimensional and Integrated Model of Nonprofit Organizational Effectiveness (MIMNOE). The MIMNOE encompasses two different dimensions of effectiveness: management (i.e., managerial structure and process of managing) and program effectiveness (i.e., program services, capacity, and outcomes; Sowa et al., 2004). The scale of perceived effectiveness contained 13 items (e.g., "The regional coalition has a good mission statement that describes its reason for being," and "I am satisfied with how the regional coalition performs"), using a 6-point, Likert-type scale rating system ranging from *strongly disagree* to *strongly agree*. The mean of these items comprised the overall score (Cronbach's α = .91, M = 4.79, SD = .69).

Data Analysis

Structural equation modeling (SEM) was performed to examine whether the proposed links between organizational characteristics, two dimensions of individual empowerment, and perceived effectiveness differed between paid coalition staff and volunteer coalition members. This analysis is similar to traditional path analysis; however, SEM allows for simultaneous estimation of equations rather than a series of regression equations. Multiple-group analysis procedures of IBM AMOS 22 (Arbuckle, 2011) were used to test a nonrestricted model in which the parameter estimates were allowed to differ across the two subgroups, and a restricted model in which all estimated parameters were required to be equal across the two subgroups of participants. The multigroup analysis was employed to test whether different models were operating for volunteers and paid staff. In each model, the organizational characteristic of leadership was considered an exogenous variable (Powell & Peterson, 2014). Paths were also hypothesized for several other variables using a path model generating approach: ORS, sense of community, participation, coalition engagement, interactional empowerment, and intrapersonal empowerment. The sample size did not provide an adequate participants-to-parameters ratio to test the measurement model simultaneously in this study.

RESULTS

The purpose of this study was to determine whether the hypothesized linkages among organizational characteristics, empowerment variables, and perceived effectiveness differed for coalition volunteers compared to paid coalition staff. Model comparison tests indicated that the nonrestricted model fit the data better than the restricted model, $\Delta\chi^2 = 56.28$, $\Delta df = 25$, $p < .01$. The nonrestricted model provided a good model-to-data fit, $\chi^2(4) = .801$, $p = .938$, comparative fit index (CFI) = 1.0, normed fit index (NFI) = 0.999, root mean square error of approximation (RMSEA) = 0.000. Based on these results, we concluded that coalition volunteers and paid staff were different from one another in terms of the hypothesized relationships among organizational characteristics, empowerment variables, and perceived effectiveness. The models presented in Figures 2 and Figures 3 show significant paths ($p < .01$) for both subgroups as well as distinctly significant paths unique to each of the two groups (dashed lines indicated significant paths unique to the corresponding subgroup). The path coefficients presented are statistically significant standardized beta weights.

Before reporting on distinct linkages between the two groups, results indicate several significant paths for both groups of paid staff and coalition volunteers. Findings indicated that for both groups, ORS had a direct, positive effect on perceived effectiveness but also an indirect effect through mediation of sense of community. Individuals who reported higher scores representing more opportunities for roles also tended to report higher perceptions of coalition effectiveness.

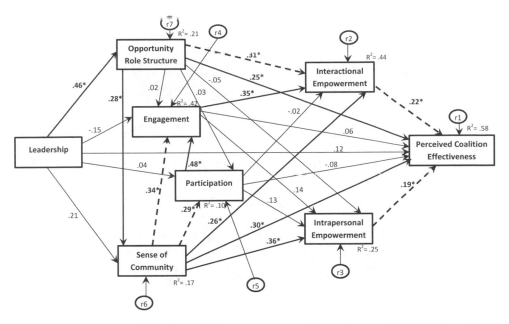

FIGURE 2 Path diagram for the multiple-group structural equation model: Staff. *Note*: These paths are statistically significant standardized regression weights, $p < .01$. Dashed lines represent significant relationships that were unique for staff. Bolded lines represent significant relationships that were common for both staff and volunteers.

Additionally, those with higher ORS tended to have a higher sense of community, which led to higher perceived coalition effectiveness. For both groups, leadership had a positive, indirect effect on perceived effectiveness through the mediated effect of opportunities for roles. Those respondents who gave higher ratings of coalition leadership tended to have higher ratings for ORS, which led to higher perceived effectiveness. Finally, results indicated that engagement was found to have a positive, direct effect on interactional empowerment among paid staff and volunteers. These findings indicate that among both groups, respondents who reported higher levels of engagement also tended to report greater interactional empowerment as compared to those who reported lower levels of engagement.

Analysis of the parameter values and their significance for each of the two subgroups showed several direct and indirect significant effects among the study variables that were unique for paid staff only. First, results show that among staff members (Figure 2), both dimensions of empowerment had positive, direct effects on perceived effectiveness. These findings suggest that for paid staff only, those respondents who reported higher perceived interactional empowerment tended to report greater perceived effectiveness ($\beta = .22$, $p < .01$, $SE = .077$). Similarly, those staff respondents who reported higher perceived intrapersonal empowerment tended to report greater perceived effectiveness ($\beta = .19$, $p < .01$, $SE = .038$).

Second, ORS was found to predict perceived effectiveness indirectly through its relationship with interactional empowerment for paid staff (Figure 2). These

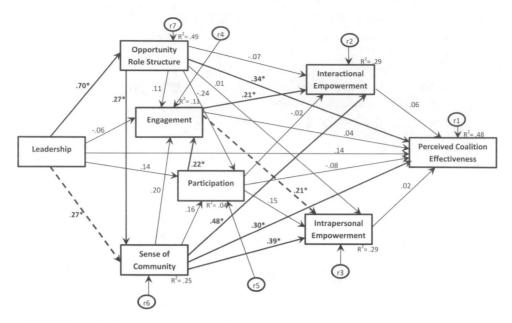

FIGURE 3 Path diagram for the multiple-group structural equation model: Volunteers. *Note*: These paths are statistically significant standardized regression weights, *p* < .01. Dashed lines represent significant relationships that were unique for volunteers. Bolded lines represent significant relationships that were common for both staff and volunteers.

findings suggest that for paid staff, those respondents who reported more opportunities for roles within the coalition tended to report greater interactional empowerment as compared to those who perceived fewer opportunities for roles (β = .31, *p* < .01, *SE* = .059), which led to higher levels of perceived effectiveness. Finally, participation within the coalition was found to mediate the effect of sense of community on engagement among paid staff (Figure 2). These findings suggest for paid staff only, those respondents who reported a higher sense of community tended to report greater participation in their coalition (β = .29, *p* < .01, *SE* = .062), which led to higher levels of engagement (β = .48, *p* < .01, *SE* = .233).

Results showed several direct and indirect significant effects among study variables that were significant for volunteers only (Figure 3). Uniquely important for volunteers, results showed that sense of community is a mediator for leadership and its impact on empowerment and perceived effectiveness. These findings suggest that for volunteers (Figure 3), those respondents who rated leadership of the coalitions higher tended to have higher sense of community (β = .27, *p* < .01, *SE* = .224), which led to higher levels of perceived effectiveness (β = .30, *p* < .01, *SE* = .031). Similarly, those volunteer respondents who had higher ratings of leadership tended to have a higher sense of community, which led to higher levels of empowerment, both intrapersonal (β = .39, *p* < .01, *SE* = .045) and interactional empowerment (β = .48, *p* < .01, *SE* = .029). The direct, positive effect of engagement on respondents' level of intrapersonal empowerment was also uniquely significant for volunteers (Figure 3). This finding suggests that volunteers who reported higher levels of engagement within their coalition tended to have higher ratings of intrapersonal empowerment ($\beta = .21$, $p < .01$, $SE = .034$).

DISCUSSION

With growing reliance on coalition efforts in public health initiatives including the prevention of alcohol misuse, it is important to understand capacity and other organizational characteristics that affect empowerment of coalition members. By identifying ways to foster individual empowerment and perceived effectiveness, coalitions could make a stronger impact on the community issues, such as substance misuse and related societal consequences. Although past research has assessed coalition capacity, no study to date has examined how empowerment-related mechanisms might function differently for volunteers and staff. This study provides important findings that might help engage and nurture participation from both coalition members and staff. Results show that when staff members have a higher sense of their own abilities, competencies, and feelings of mastery within their coalitions, they perceive greater coalition effectiveness. This finding was unique to staff only, giving us a more detailed representation of distinct groups' functioning within coalitions as well as extending empowerment research with the link to an outcome (i.e., perceived effectiveness). Further, the study showed that staff members' opportunities to take on specific roles within the coalition was important in fostering empowerment and higher perceived effectiveness. This study also highlighted the importance of sense of community among staff members on their levels of engagement. These findings help prevention leaders as they design interventions that foster empowering organizational characteristics that might led to more empowered staff members. For example, we might strategically structure coalitions so that many staff persons gain opportunities to hold task-related roles (Maton, 1988). Similarly, we might focus on organizational processes that incorporate diversity of interests and backgrounds to foster a sense of connectedness (Hughey et al., 1999).

The results showed the importance of fostering leadership and a sense of community among volunteers to increase empowerment and perceived effectiveness among this district group. This finding somewhat supports the study by Powell and Peterson (2014), in which leadership was found to have only an indirect effect on perceived effectiveness through several mediators. This result also contributes to the evidence suggesting that sense of community is a significant contributor to empowerment (Hughey, Peterson, Lowe, & Oprescu, 2008; Speer, Peterson, Armstead, & Allen, 2013) and furthers empirical knowledge applying the conceptual models of Zimmerman (1995) through the inclusion of two components of PE (i.e., interaction and intrapersonal empowerment). Prevention leaders might develop capacity interventions that are distinct for community volunteers, using these findings. For example, we might structure coalition-building efforts in a way that fosters a strong leadership through skill development and capacity building.

Finally, engagement was an important organizational process that fostered interactional empowerment for both groups. This suggests that it is important for all coalition members to have the opportunity to engage in multiple and important aspects of the organization such as needs assessment and planning, evaluating progress, and sustainability planning (Kegler & Swan, 2011), which in turn fosters higher levels of interactional empowerment. This study also supports previous evidence that talented and dedicated leadership predicts individuals' perceptions of organizational effectiveness indirectly through ORS as the mediator (Powell & Peterson, 2014) for both groups. These findings present organizational character-istics that could foster empowerment and effectiveness for all types of coalition members.

Limitations of the Study

Although this research adds to the body of current literature, there are several noteworthy limitations to this study related to the sample and methods. First, causal interpretation of the study might be limited by the cross-sectional design of the study. Further research to explore characteristics of coalition members and staff over time and control for rival explanations might help us better understand the relationships suggested in the current model. Second, it is important to note that effectiveness was measured by self-rated items. Although this scale included items about reaching project goals and intended outcomes, it only measures perceptions of coalitions' effectiveness toward prevention of underage drinking. It often takes many years to detect measurable change resulting from environmental, commu-nity-level interventions (Oesterle et al., 2015; Rhoades et al., 2015; Scherer et al., 2015). Additionally, it has been suggested that although community-level change is the ultimate indicator of effectiveness, measures of coalition functioning might act as a plausible proxy, supporting the belief that higher functioning groups will have a great chance in goal attainment (Zakocs & Edwards, 2006). Therefore, this study is a step toward measuring long-term goal attainment. Future research should include measures of goal achievement and other outcome measures relevant to effectiveness.

Third, the sample in this study was not diverse in several demographic categories. The survey sample consisted mostly of participants who self-identified as female (72%), White (62%), and not of Latino or Hispanic origin (96%). The number of participants who self-identified within different minority groups was very small. Although some coalitions are likely less diverse than others, caution should be applied regarding the generalizability of the findings due to the diversity issue. Future research might include sampling techniques that can ensure the collection of a more diverse sample representative of the population from which it is drawn.

Implications

This study takes an important step in our understanding of organizational characteristics that foster empowerment and increase perceived effectiveness among two groups of coalition members. Practically, these results offer lessons for prevention leaders and funders as they tailor interventions to strengthen capacity for more effective prevention strategies. Previous research has found that specialized training in prevention science increases the impact and sustainability of coalition-based initiatives. For example, a study of the Communities that Care model (Gloppen et al., 2016) found that sustainability was greater for coalitions that received training dedicated to the prevention science model. This study might guide the development of training in prevention science models that would address the specific needs of different subgroups such as staff and sector volunteers that might facilitate more empowered membership. Practitioners might consider these important differences between subgroups and adapt their strategies to the unique strengths and needs of their coalition members (e.g.,, skills development training geared to those in the prevention field vs. community volunteers, providing opportunities for different types of roles within the coalition, etc.).

In a review of the literature on coalition effectiveness, Zakocs and Edwards (2006) found multiple indicators including strong leadership, member engagement, and group cohesion. This study extends their work by describing factors that are important to different groups within coalition structures. Coalition functioning is an indicator of the ability to attain organizational goals. This study can guide prevention leaders in ways to foster empowered members working with a high-functioning group. More specifically, findings suggest the need to support volunteers and staff in distinct ways to sustain efforts and reach intended long-term community outcomes. Future research might include sustainability measures and goal attainment to extend the examination of organizational characteristics that might foster empowerment among the different sectors involved in creating lasting and effective coalitions to combat underage drinking.

FUNDING

This research was supported in part by a grant from the New Jersey Division of Mental Health and Addiction Services to Rutgers University. The views expressed are those of the authors and do not necessarily represent the views of the funding agency.

REFERENCES

Anderson-Carpenter, K. D., Watson-Thompson, J., Chaney, L., & Jones, M. (2016). Reducing binge drinking in adolescents through implementation of the strategic prevention framework. *American Journal of Community Psychology, 57*, 36–46. doi:10.1002/ajcp.12029

Arbuckle, J. L. (2011). *Amos 20 user's guide*. Retrieved from http://public.dhe.ibm.com/software/analytics/spss/documentation/amos/20.0/en/Manuals/IBM_SPSS_Amos_User_Guide.pdf

Begun, A. L., Clapp, J. D., & The Alcohol Misuse Grand Challenge Collective. (2016). Reducing and preventing alcohol misuse and its consequences: A Grand Challenge for social work. *The International Journal of Alcohol and Drug Research, 5*(2), 73–83. doi:10.7895/ijadr.v5i2.223

Bunnell, R., O'Neil, D., Soler, R., Payne, R., Giles, W. H., Collins, J., & Bauer, U. (2012). Fifty communities putting prevention to work: Accelerating chronic disease prevention through policy, systems and environmental change. *Journal of Community Health, 37*, 1081–1090. doi:10.1007/s10900-012-9542-3

Centers for Disease Control and Prevention. (2011). *A national strategy to revitalize environmental public health services*. Retrieved from https://www.cdc.gov/nceh/ehs/docs/nationalstrategy2003.pdf

Christens, B. D. (2012). Toward relational empowerment. *American Journal of Community Psychology, 50*, 114–128. doi:10.1007/s10464-011-9483-5

Christens, B. D., & Dolan, T. (2011). Interweaving youth development, community development, and social change through youth organizing. *Youth & Society, 43*, 528–548. doi:10.1177/0044118X10383647

Christens, B. D., Peterson, N. A., Reid, R. J., & Garcia-Reid, P. (2015). Adolescents' perceived control in the sociopolitical domain a latent class analysis. *Youth & Society, 47*, 443–461. doi:10.1177/0044118X12467656

Edwards, J. M., Stein-Seroussi, A., Flewelling, R. L., Orwin, R. G., & Zhang, L. (2015). Sustainability of state-level substance abuse prevention infrastructure after the completion of the SPF SIG. *The Journal of Primary Prevention, 36*, 177–186. doi:10.1007/s10935-015-0382-7

Erickson, D. J., Smolenski, D. J., Toomey, T. L., Carlin, B. P., & Wagenaar, A. C. (2013). Do alcohol compliance checks decrease underage sales at neighboring establishments? *Journal of Studies on Alcohol and Drugs, 74*, 852. doi:10.15288/jsad.2013.74.852

Flewelling, R. L., & Hanley, S. M. (2016). Assessing community coalition capacity and its association with underage drinking prevention effectiveness in the context of the SPF SIG. *Prevention Science, 17*, 830–840. doi:10.1007/s11121-016-0675-y

Florin, P., Friend, K. B., Buka, S., Egan, C., Barovier, L., & Amodei, B. (2012). The interactive systems framework applied to the strategic prevention framework: The Rhode Island experience. *American Journal of Community Psychology, 50*, 402–414. doi:10.1007/s10464-012-9527-5

Foltz, J. L., Belay, B., Dooyema, C. A., Williams, N., & Blanck, H. M. (2015). Childhood obesity research demonstration (CORD): The cross-site overview and opportunities for interventions addressing obesity community-wide. *Childhood Obesity, 11*(1), 4–10. doi:10.1089/chi.2014.0159

Foster-Fishman, P. G., Fitzgerald, K., Brandell, C., Nowell, B., Chavis, D., & Van Egeren, L. A. (2006). Mobilizing residents for action: The role of small wins and strategic supports. *American Journal of Community Psychology, 38*, 213–220. doi:10.1007/s10464-006-9081-0

Foster-Fishman, P. G., Pierce, S. J., & Van Egeren, L. A. (2009). Who participates and why: Building a process model of citizen participation. *Health Education & Behavior, 36,* 550–569. doi:10.1177/1090198108317408

Freisthler, B., Kepple, N. J., Sims, R., & Martin, S. E. (2013). Evaluating medical marijuana dispensary policies: Spatial methods for the study of environmentally-based interventions. *American Journal of Community Psychology, 51,* 278–288. doi:10.1007/s10464-012-9542-6

Frieden, T. R. (2010). A framework for public health action: The health impact pyramid. *American Journal of Public Health, 100,* 590–595. doi:10.2105/AJPH.2009.185652

Friend, K., Carmona, M., Wilbur, P., & Levy, D. (2001). Youths' social sources of cigarettes: The limits of youth-access policies. *Contemporary Drug Problems, 28,* 507–526. doi:10.1177/009145090102800309

Friend, K., Pettibone, K., Florin, P., Vela, J., & Nargiso, J. (2015). Environmental change strategies targeting drug abuse prevention. *Drugs: Education, Prevention and Policy, 22,* 311–315. doi:10.3109/09687637.2014.977229

Gloppen, K. M., Brown, E. C., Wagenaar, B. H., Hawkins, J. D., Rhew, I. C., & Oesterle, S. (2016). Sustaining adoption of science-based prevention through Communities that Care. *Journal of Community Psychology, 44,* 78–89. doi:10.1002/jcop.21743

Harrop, E., & Catalano, R. F. (2016). Evidence-based prevention for adolescent substance use. *Child and Adolescent Psychiatric Clinics of North America, 25,* 387–410. doi:10.1016/j.chc.2016.03.001

Hodge, D. R., & Gillespie, D. F. (2007). Phrase completion scales: A better measurement approach than Likert scales? *Journal of Social Service Research, 33*(4), 1–12. doi:10.1300/J079v33n04_01

Holden, D. J., Evans, W. D., Hinnant, L. W., & Messeri, P. (2005). Modeling psychological empowerment among youth involved in local tobacco control efforts. *Health Education & Behavior, 32,* 264–278. doi:10.1177/1090198104272336

Hughey, J., Peterson, N. A., Lowe, J. B., & Oprescu, F. (2008). Empowerment and sense of community: Clarifying their relationship in community organizations. *Health Education & Behavior, 35,* 651–663. doi:10.1177/1090198106294896

Hughey, J., Speer, P. W., & Peterson, N. A. (1999). Sense of community in community organizations: Structure and evidence of validity. *Journal of Community Psychology, 27,* 97–113. doi:10.1002/(ISSN)1520-6629

Johnston, L. D., O'Malley, P. M., Miech, R. A., Bachman, J. G., & Schulenberg, J. E. (2016). *Monitoring the future: National survey results on drug use, 1975–2015. 2015 Overview: Key findings on adolescent drug use.* Retrieved from http://www.monitoringthefuture.org/pubs/monographs/mtf-overview2015.pdf

Kegler, M. C., Honeycutt, S., Davis, M., Dauria, E., Berg, C., Dove, C., … Hawkins, J. (2015). Policy, systems, and environmental change in the Mississippi delta: Considerations for evaluation design. *Health Education & Behavior, 42*(Suppl. 1), 57S–66S. doi:10.1177/1090198114568428

Kegler, M. C., Norton, B. L., & Aronson, R. (2007). Skill improvement among coalition members in the California Healthy Cities and Communities Program. *Health Education Research, 22,* 450–457. doi:10.1093/her/cyl109

Kegler, M. C., & Swan, D. W. (2011). Advancing coalition theory: The effect of coalition factors on community capacity mediated by member engagement. *Health Education Research, 27*, 572–584. doi:10.1093/her/cyr083

Khan, M. R., Berger, A. T., Wells, B. E., & Cleland, C. M. (2012). Longitudinal associations between adolescent alcohol use and adulthood sexual risk behavior and sexually transmitted infection in the United States: Assessment of differences by race. *American Journal of Public Health, 102*, 867–876. doi:10.2105/AJPH.2011.300373

Maton, K. (1988). Social support, organizational characteristics of empowering community settings: A multiple case study approach. *American Journal of Community Psychology, 23*, 631–656. doi:10.1007/BF02506985

Miller, R. L., Janulis, P. F., Reed, S. J., Harper, G. W., Ellen, J., & Boyer, C. B. & Adolescent Medicine Trials Network for HIV/AIDS Interventions. (2016). Creating youth-supportive communities: Outcomes from the Connect-to-Protect® (C2P) structural change approach to youth HIV prevention. *Journal of Youth and Adolescence, 45*, 301–315.

Morrel-Samuels, S., Bacallao, M., Brown, S., Bower, M., & Zimmerman, M. (2016). Community engagement in youth violence prevention: Crafting methods to context. *The Journal of Primary Prevention, 37*, 189–207. doi:10.1007/s10935-016-0428-5

National Association of Social Workers. (2008). *Code of ethics of the National Association of Social Workers*. Washington, DC: NASW Press. Retrieved from http://www.naswdc.org/pubs/code/code.asp

National Institute on Alcohol Abuse and Alcoholism. (2006). *Underage drinking: Why do adolescents drink, what are the risks, and how can underage drinking be prevented?* (Alcohol Alert No. 67). Rockville, MD: Author.

O'Malley, P. M., & Johnston, L. D. (2013). Driving after drug or alcohol use by U.S. high school seniors, 2001–2011. *American Journal of Public Health, 103*, 2027–2034. doi:10.2105/AJPH.2013.301246

Oesterle, S., Hawkins, J. D., Kuklinski, M. R., Fagan, A. A., Fleming, C., Rhew, I. C., … Catalano, R. F. (2015). Effects of Communities that Care on males' and females' drug use and delinquency 9 years after baseline in a community-randomized trial. *American Journal of Community Psychology, 56*, 217–228. doi:10.1007/s10464-015-9749-4

Oshri, A., Tubman, J. G., Morgan-Lopez, A. A., Saavedra, L. M., & Csizmadia, A. (2013). Sexual sensation seeking, co-occurring sex and alcohol use, and sexual risk behavior among adolescents in treatment for substance use problems. *The American Journal on Addictions, 22*, 197–205. doi:10.1111/j.1521-0391.2012.12027.x

Peterson, N. A., Lowe, J. B., Aquilino, M. L., & Schneider, J. E. (2005). Linking social cohesion and gender to intrapersonal and interactional empowerment: Support and new implications for theory. *Journal of Community Psychology, 33*, 233–244. doi:10.1002/jcop.20047

Peterson, N. A., Lowe, J. B., Hughey, J., Reid, R. J., Zimmerman, M. A., & Speer, P. W. (2006). Measuring the intrapersonal component of psychological empowerment: Confirmatory factor analysis of the sociopolitical control scale. *American Journal of Community Psychology, 38*(3–4), 287–297.

Peterson, N. A., Speer, P. W., Hughey, J., Armstead, T. L., Schneider, J. E., & Sheffer, M. A. (2008). Community organizations and sense of community: Further development in theory and measurement. *Journal of Community Psychology, 36*, 798–813. doi:10.1002/jcop.20260

Peterson, N. A., Speer, P. W., & Peterson, C. H. (2011). Pathways to empowerment in substance abuse prevention: Citizen participation, sense of community, and police responsiveness in an urban U.S. setting. *Global Journal of Community Psychology Practice, 1*(3), 23–31.

Peterson, N. A., & Zimmerman, M. A. (2004). Beyond the individual: Toward a nomological network of organizational empowerment. *American Journal of Community Psychology, 34*, 129–145. doi:10.1023/B:AJCP.0000040151.77047.58

Pettibone, K. G., Friend, K. B., Nargiso, J. E., & Florin, P. (2013). Evaluating environmental change strategies: Challenges and solutions. *American Journal of Community Psychology, 51*, 217–221. doi:10.1007/s10464-012-9556-0

Powell, K. G., & Peterson, N. A. (2014). Pathways to effectiveness in substance abuse prevention: Empowering organizational characteristics of community-based coalitions. *Human Service Organizations: Management, Leadership & Governance, 38*, 471–486. doi:10.1080/23303131.2014.935839

Pronk, N. P., Hernandez, L. M., & Lawrence, R. S. (2013). An integrated framework for assessing the value of community-based prevention: A report of the Institute of Medicine. *Preventing Chronic Disease, 10*. doi:10.5888/pcd10.120323

Rammohan, V., Hahn, R. A., Elder, R., Brewer, R., Fielding, J., & Naimi, T. S., & Task Force on Community Preventive Services. (2011). Effects of dram shop liability and enhanced overservice law enforcement initiatives on excessive alcohol consumption and related harms: Two community guide systematic reviews. *American Journal of Preventive Medicine, 41*, 334–343.

Rhoades, R. R., Beebe, L. A., Boeckman, L. M., & Williams, M. B. (2015). Communities of excellence in tobacco control: Changes in local policy and key outcomes. *American Journal of Preventive Medicine, 48*, S21–S28. doi:10.1016/j.amepre.2014.10.002

Salas-Wright, C. P., Vaughn, M. G., Ugalde, J., & Todic, J. (2015). Substance use and teen pregnancy in the United States: Evidence from the NSDUH 2002–2012. *Addictive Behaviors, 45*, 218–225. doi:10.1016/j.addbeh.2015.01.039

Saltz, R. F. (2011). Enlisting bars and restaurants in the prevention of intoxication and subsequent harms: Why it matters. *American Journal of Preventive Medicine, 41*, 353–354. doi:10.1016/j.amepre.2011.06.028

Scherer, M., Fell, J. C., Thomas, S., & Voas, R. B. (2015). Effects of dram shop, responsible beverage service training, and state alcohol control laws on underage drinking driver fatal crash ratios. *Traffic Injury Prevention, 16*(Suppl. 2), S59–S65. doi:10.1080/15389588.2015.1064909

Schober, D. J., & Fawcett, S. B. (2015). Using action planning to build organizational capacity for the prevention of intimate partner violence. *Health Education & Behavior, 42*, 449–457. doi:10.1177/1090198114564501

Sowa, J. E., Selden, S. C., & Sandfort, J. R. (2004). No longer unmeasurable? A multidimensional integrated model of nonprofit organizational effectiveness. *Nonprofit and Voluntary Sector Quarterly, 33*, 711–728. doi:10.1177/0899764004269146

Speer, P. W., & Hughey, J. (1995). Community organizing: An ecological route to empowerment and power. *American Journal of Community Psychology, 23,* 729–748. doi:10.1007/BF02506989

Speer, P. W., Peterson, N. A., Armstead, T. L., & Allen, C. T. (2013). The influence of participation, gender, and organizational sense of community on psychological empowerment: The moderating effects of income. *American Journal of Community Psychology, 51,* 103–113. doi:10.1007/s10464-012-9547-1

Stoddard, S. A., Epstein-Ngo, Q., Walton, M. A., Zimmerman, M. A., Chermack, S. T., Blow, F. C., … Cunningham, R. M. (2015). Substance use and violence among youth: A daily calendar analysis. *Substance Use & Misuse, 50,* 328–339. doi:10.3109/10826084.2014.980953

Substance Abuse and Mental Health Services Administration. (2015). *2015 report to Congress on the prevention and reduction of underage drinking.* Retrieved from https://www.stopalcoholabuse.gov/media/ReportToCongress/2015/report_-main/2015_RTC_Volume_I.pdf

Substance Abuse and Mental Health Services Administration. (2016). *Applying the strategic prevention framework.* Retrieved from http://www.samhsa.gov/capt/applying-strategic-prevention-framework

Toomey, T. L., Lenk, K. M., & Wagenaar, A. C. (2007). Environmental policies to reduce college drinking: An update of research findings. *Journal of Studies on Alcohol and Drugs, 68,* 208–219. doi:10.15288/jsad.2007.68.208

Wagenaar, A. C., Tobler, A. L., & Komro, K. A. (2010). Effects of alcohol tax and price policies on morbidity and mortality: A systematic review. *American Journal of Public Health, 100,* 2270–2278. doi:10.2105/AJPH.2009.186007

Xuan, Z., Nelson, T. F., Heeren, T., Blanchette, J., Nelson, D. E., Gruenewald, P., & Naimi, T. S. (2013). Tax policy, adult binge drinking, and youth alcohol consumption in the United States. *Alcoholism: Clinical and Experimental Research, 37,* 1713–1719. doi:10.1111/acer.12152

Zakocs, R. C., & Edwards, E. M. (2006). What explains community coalition effectiveness? A review of the literature. *American Journal of Preventive Medicine, 30,* 351–361. doi:10.1016/j.amepre.2005.12.004

Zimmerman, M. A. (1995). Psychological empowerment: Issues and illustrations. *American Journal of Community Psychology, 23,* 581–599. doi:10.1007/BF02506983

Zimmerman, M. A. (2000). Empowerment theory: Psychological, organizational and community levels of analysis. In J. Rappaport, & E. Seidman (Eds.), *Handbook of community psychology* (pp. 43–63). New York, NY: Kluwer Academic/Plenum Publishers.

Zimmerman, M. A., & Zahniser, J. H. (1991). Refinements of sphere-specific measures of perceived control: Development of a sociopolitical control scale. *Journal of Community Psychology, 19,* 189–204. doi:10.1002/(ISSN)1520-6629

What Lies Beneath: Trauma Events, PTSD, and Alcohol Misuse in Driving Under the Influence Program Clients

MELINDA HOHMAN, PhD

MELANIE BARKER, LCSW, MPH

SUSAN WOODRUFF, PhD

The prevention and reduction of alcohol misuse is one of the Grand Challenges of Social Work. Addressing client needs beyond alcohol misuse can improve client outcomes. Driving under the influence program clients (N = 1,248) were screened for trauma events and posttraumatic stress disorder (PTSD). Results found that males more often reported having been assaulted with a weapon or that they caused injury to someone else. Females more often reported sexual assault and other unwanted sexual experience. About 26% overall screened positive for PTSD. Social workers need to be alert to various types of trauma and help clients identify the connection between trauma and alcohol misuse.

The prevention and reduction of alcohol misuse as well as the social problems caused by this misuse is one of the Grand Challenges of Social Work (Begun, Clapp, & The Alcohol Misuse Grand Challenge Collective, 2016). One area of misuse that can affect anyone in the population is that of driving under the influence (DUI) of alcohol or other drugs (AOD), either as the driver, passenger, pedestrian, or occupants of other cars. In 2014, about one third of all fatal car crashes in the United States involved a driver who was impaired by alcohol, accounting for 9,967 deaths. DUI-based crashes caused about 326,000 injuries and more than 1 million people were arrested for driving under the influence of alcohol or drugs that same year (Jewett, Shults, Banerjee, & Bergen, 2015; National Highway Traffic and Safety Administration, 2015). Most DUI participants (97%) have been arrested for impairment due to alcohol use, but it is difficult to discern how many have mixed alcohol with drug use prior to the arrest unless they are actually tested for drugs in addition to alcohol (S. Woodruff, personal communication, January 29, 2017).

DUI rates in California peaked in 2008 and have slowly declined to about 8% of the state's population. In 2013, 160,388 individuals over age 18 were arrested for DUI with 133,525 convictions (Daoud, Tashima, & Grippe, 2015). Despite a declining rate, recidivism remains a problem. A longitudinal study of California DUI drivers over a 19-year period found that 33% of male and 24% of female first-time offenders had a subsequent DUI offense (Daoud et al., 2015). Treatment following a DUI conviction, one of several sanctions that can be imposed by the court, was enacted into law in 1978 with the goal of reducing repeat offenses for clients with first-time or multiple DUI convictions. A recent report of a quasi-experimental study of the effectiveness of California's DUI program indicated that those assigned to a DUI program were significantly less likely to have a DUI in the subsequent year than those who were not assigned (Daoud et al., 2015). In 2013, 126,331 clients presented to 264 DUI treatment programs across the state of California (Zhang, 2015).

Treatment programs provide assessment and referral as well as education, group, and individual counseling, with various programs lasting 3, 6, 9, 12, 18, or 30 months, depending on the type of conviction and previous convictions (California Department of Health Care Services, 2016). Clients might also be mandated to attend 12-step meetings, such as Alcoholics Anonymous. The goals of these programs are to not only reduce DUI recidivism, but also AOD-related high-risk behaviors, to encourage clients to reduce AOD misuse in general, and to increase clients' well-being across life areas (California Association of DUI Treatment Providers, n.d.). Certified AOD counselors who might also be social workers provide treatment (Daoud et al., 2015) and DUI programs are self-funded through client payment. These types of programs have shown modest success in reducing reoffense of DUI (Nochajski & Stasiewicz, 2006).

The clients who attend DUI programs are typically not social drinkers who made a poor decision to get behind the wheel while intoxicated, but rather tend to resemble a clinical population (McCutcheon et al., 2009; Palmer, Ball, Rounsaville, & O'Malley, 2007). Research has found high rates of lifetime AOD use disorders in those who participate in DUI programs (91% males, 85% females), with rates and severity of AOD symptoms being higher among those with a repeat offense (Lapham et al., 2001; LaPlante, Nelson, Odegaard, LaBrie, & Shaffer, 2008). DUI program clients also have high rates of psychiatric comorbidities, with posttraumatic stress disorder (PTSD) being one of the most common (Dreissen et al., 2008; Peller, Najavits, Nelson, LaBrie, & Shaffer, 2010). Using diagnostic measures, studies have found lifetime rates of PTSD among DUI program clients to be high, especially in females (27–35%) as compared to males (9–12%; Lapham, C'de Baca, McMillan, & Lapidus, 2006; Lapham et al., 2001; LaPlante et al., 2008; McCutcheon et al., 2009). PTSD is concerning, as it has been found to be linked to poor treatment response and outcomes, including recidivism (McCutcheon et al., 2009; Peller et al., 2010; Shaffer et al., 2007).

To receive a diagnosis of PTSD, one must have experienced a trauma event and be experiencing PTSD-related symptoms, such as intrusive thoughts about the event, intense anxiety, or reckless behavior (American Psychiatric Association, 2013). Trauma is defined as, "an event, series of events, or set of circumstances that is experienced … as physically or emotionally harmful or threatening and has lasting adverse effects on the individual's functioning and physical, social, emotional, or spiritual well-being" (Substance Abuse and Mental Health Services Administration [SAMHSA], 2014a, p. 7). SAMHSA (2014b) divides trauma events into three categories: those caused naturally such as an earthquake, wildfire, or hurricane; those caused by people that are accidental such as a car accident or accidental gun shooting; and those caused intentionally, such as combat, sexual assault, stabbing, home invasion, or food tampering. Trauma can be caused by experiencing one of these events, witnessing the event itself, or even learning about it through hearing others' descriptions (American Psychiatric Association, 2013).

Trauma event screens are given to identify the specific traumas that clients have experienced, observed, or both. About 70% of the general population has experienced one event (Volpicelli, Balaraman, Hahn, Wallace, & Bux, 2009) and the rate is higher among DUI program clients. Peller and colleagues (2010) found that 82% of the DUI sample reported at least one past trauma event, with males being more likely to report assaulting others, being assaulted, or participating in combat. Females were more likely to report intimate partner violence and sexual assault. These gender-related findings were similar to those from a study by Bailey, Webster, Baker, and Kavanagh (2012) of clients in treatment for alcohol use disorders and major depression. Using a trauma event screen, 71.6% reported at least one trauma over their lifetime. About half of the sample reported an "other traumatic event," the definition of which was not included in the screen nor specified by the researchers.

High rates of trauma events have been found to be linked to alcohol misuse and to alcohol treatment dropout (Odenwald & Semrau, 2012). Although it is unclear as to whether trauma occurs first and then alcohol is used to medicate the resulting PTSD or if trauma occurs due to being vulnerable while under the influence, researchers tend to support the former with trauma events preceding AOD use (Van Dam, Vedel, Ehrin, Vedel, & Emmelkamp, 2012). Not everyone develops PTSD in relation to experiencing or observing a trauma event and PTSD symptoms and intensity can differ based on the type of trauma event experienced (Wanklyn et al., 2016). For instance, in a study comparing three types of trauma (sexual assault, sudden unexpected death of a loved one, and motor vehicle accident) in college students with PTSD, sexual assault produced the highest scores on a PTSD screen, followed by sudden death of a loved one, and then motor vehicle accident. The students who had been sexually assaulted scored highest on the avoidance and numbing symptoms on the PTSD screen, followed by reexperiencing and arousal symptoms (Kelley, Weathers, McDevitt-Murphy, Eakin, & Flood, 2009).

In treatment settings for substance use, behavioral health and AOD providers are encouraged to develop trauma-informed care (TIC) for their clients to increase positive treatment outcomes (SAMHSA, 2014b). TIC includes educating social workers and counselors about trauma and its potential impacts, creating policies and procedures that do not retraumatize clients, and screening for trauma history and possible PTSD to further assess and refer clients as needed for trauma treatment. Social workers are also called on to educate clients about the relationship between their personal trauma(s) and alcohol misuse as a means to prevent further alcohol misuse, and in this case, drinking and driving (SAMHSA, 2014b). Understanding the types of trauma experienced and the resultant PTSD has implications for the types of referral and possible treatment provided (Dworkin, Mota, Schumacher, Vinci, & Coffey, 2016; Kelley et al., 2009).

PURPOSE OF THE STUDY

Studies have examined the rates of PTSD in clients in DUI programs but few studies have reported the types of trauma events of these same clients and their relation to PTSD. The purpose of this study is to gain an understanding of the explicit types of trauma experienced and witnessed by DUI program clients, how this might vary by gender, and the relationship of trauma events to PTSD. Determining predictors of PTSD will alert social workers to the importance of these events, allow them to more thoroughly assess trauma in clients, and make timely referrals, if needed, for trauma treatment. Understanding variance in trauma events and effects by gender could also aid in program design and planning, or as stated in the Grand Challenge, allow for innovation for a sustainable solution (Begun et al., 2016).

Research questions for this study are as follows:

1. What types of traumatic events do DUI program clients experience or witness and do these vary by gender?
2. What is the relationship of these events and multiple events on PTSD severity and do these vary by gender?
3. What are the predictors of scoring positively on a PTSD screen among DUI program clients?

METHOD

This study is based on secondary data collected during the client intake process at a DUI program based in an urban area in the U.S. Southwest. This program has been in existence for about 25 years and serves about 2,500 clients per month. Clients are mandated to attend the program as part of their sentencing or as part of requirements to reobtain their driver's license, which are typically removed. Depending on the number of previous DUIs and type of conviction, the program ranges from 3 to 18 months (DeYoung, 1997). Clients might also be court-ordered to attend support meetings such as Alcoholics Anonymous. About 225 new clients receive an intake process each month. University institutional review board permission was obtained for this study.

Sample

During the study period of March through October 2015, 1,735 men and women participated in the intake process. Of those, 59 were non-English speakers, and thus were ineligible to be given the trauma screens. Out of a final sample size of 1,676, 1,248 completed the trauma screens, for a response rate of 74%, which is acceptable or even very good, for sample representation (Rubin & Babbie, 2014). Subsequent analysis of responders versus nonresponders detected no differences between groups on age, education, race, marital status, gender, military service; and blood alcohol content (BAC) on arrest. Number of previous DUIs was statistically significant, with first-time DUI program clients more likely to fill out the trauma screens, $\chi^2 = 6.65$, $p < .05$.

The client sample was comprised of 896 males (71.8%) and 352 females (28.2%). Over half of the clients were White (60.0%), followed by Latino (19.0%), Asian (8.0%), biracial and "other" self-identified (7.5%), and African American (5.0%). As Table 1 shows, female clients were significantly more likely to be White and less likely to be African American than were male clients, $\chi^2 = 17.32$, $p < .001$. Females were also significantly more likely to be divorced, whereas males were more likely to be single or never married, $\chi^2 = 11.64$, $p < .05$. Female clients were also significantly more likely to be unemployed or work less than 30 hr a week as compared to their male counterparts, $\chi^2 = 8.63$, $p < .05$. Males as compared to females were significantly more likely to have military experience, either as current active duty or reserves military or as a veteran, $\chi^2 = 21.38$, $p < .001$.

Males and females in the sample were similar in age (about 35 years). Both had about 15 years of education. For most of the clients (75%), this was their first DUI conviction or program. There were no differences between males and females in the number of prior DUI offenses. Females had a statistically significantly higher BAC at arrest (.17) as compared to males (.15), $t(1,035) = -4.65$, $p < .001$.

TABLE 1 Bivariate Analyses of Demographic and Driving Under the Influence (DUI) Characteristics, by Gender

	Male		Female	
	n	%	*n*	%
Race**				
White	493	55.0	230	65.3
Latino/a	180	20.1	63	17.9
African American	73	8.1	11	3.1
Asian/Pacific Islander	71	7.9	27	7.7
Other/biracial	79	8.8	21	6.0
Marital status*				
Single/never married	586	65.4	202	57.4
Married	138	15.4	54	15.3
Divorced	116	12.9	69	19.6
Separated	25	2.8	14	4.0
Widowed/other	31	3.5	13	3.7
Employed*				
≥ 30 hours a week	387	43.2	142	29.5
≤ 29 hours a week	307	34.3	104	29.5
Unemployed, looking for work	127	14.2	71	20.2
Not in the labor force	75	8.4	35	9.9
Military status***				
None	765	85.4	333	94.6
Active/reserves	41	4.6	9	2.6
Veteran	90	10.0	10	2.8
Prior DUI offense				
0	661	73.8	267	75.9
1	161	18.0	64	18.2
2 or more	74	8.3	21	6.0
	M	*SD*	*M*	*SD*
Age	34.98	11.23	35.09	11.93
Years of education	14.73	3.72	15.18	4.04
BAC at arrest**	.15	.05	.17	.07

Note: $N = 1,248$. BAC = blood alcohol content.
*$p < .05$. **$p < .01$. ***$p < .001$.

Data Collection

In the intake session, clients filled out paperwork with demographic and DUI informational questions. The DUI program provided TIC and thus screened for PTSD and trauma events as one step in the process. Clients were also provided with the trauma assessment screens, which are administered by self-report, following the suggested protocol of SAMHSA (2014a, 2014b). The screens, their purpose, and the voluntary nature of completing these screens were explained by a counselor prior to their distribution to clients. Data from the screening were entered by staff into a data file for program evaluation purposes. To maintain anonymity, all identifying data including names and birth dates were removed from the data before being provided to the researchers. Client case numbers did remain in the data.

MEASURESDEMOGRAPHIC AND ALCOHOL SEVERITY MEASURES

Clients were asked to report their birth date, race, gender, education, marital status, and whether they had military experience (veteran, active duty, reserves, or none of the above). They also reported the number of prior DUI convictions and their BAC at the current conviction, which were used as proxy measures for severity of alcohol misuse. Prior research has found that rates of alcohol use disorder increase with number of DUIs and BAC (Siegal et al., 2000). The number of DUI convictions is indicative of patterned alcohol use in situations that are physically dangerous and BAC is indicative of tolerance, both of which are alcohol use disorder criteria (American Psychiatric Association, 2013). For anonymity purposes, birth dates were removed from the data file and only a numerical age was provided.

LIFE EVENTS CHECKLIST–5

The Life Events Checklist–5 (LEC–5; Weathers et al., 2013) is a 17-item checklist of various events considered to be traumatic and related to PTSD. Respondents are asked to check whether a particular item, over the course of their lifetime, (a) has happened to them, (b) been witnessed, (c) heard about it, or (d) been a part of their work. For this study, we selected the first two categories. Sample items include, "Assaulted with a weapon," "Natural disaster," and "Life-threatening illness or injury." Because the screen is self-reported, clients are free to interpret items however they want, although some of the items have an explanation. For example, "Assaulted with a weapon" also states "for example, being shot, stabbed, threatened with a knife, gun, bomb." Also, clients can report accidental death "happened to me" on the scale, which most likely means that they "witnessed" it. At the DUI program, a clinical interviewer follows up with clients and asks about the reported items for further discussion, if necessary. The original LEC scale has been shown to have good test–retest reliability and strong convergence with other measures of trauma (Gray, Litz, Hsu, & Lombardo, 2004). No psychometric tests have been conducted on the LEC–5, which is a minimally modified version of the LEC (Weathers et al., 2013). One limitation of the LEC–5 is that it does not include items specific to child abuse or intimate partner violence (Gray et al., 2004) however some of the items might capture this. It should also be noted that the screen does not ask for the number of times experienced for each event, just whether or not the event has ever been experienced.

PTSD CHECKLIST–CIVILIAN VERSION

The PTSD Checklist–Civilian Version (PCL–C; Weathers, Litz, Huska, & Keane, 1994) is a 17-item self-report scale that is a screening tool for civilians regarding PTSD. It is based on *Diagnostic and Statistical Manual of Mental Disorders* (4th ed. [*DSM–IV*]; American Psychiatric Association, 1994) PTSD criteria and was designed to be administered along with a trauma event screen (Weathers et al., 2013). Clients are asked how much they have been bothered by the various items, which are "responses to stressful life experiences," during the last month. Clients respond on a Likert scale ranging from 1 (*not at all*) to 5 (*extremely*). Sample items include, "Feeling distant or cut off from other people," "Feeling very upset when something reminded you of a stressful experience from the past," and "Trouble falling or staying asleep." Items are summed, giving a range of 17 to 85. Cut scores, indicating a need for further diagnostic assessment, can range from 30 to 60, depending on the need and context of the scale administration setting (McDonald & Calhoun, 2010). A cut point score of 30 to 35 is for people in a general population, for screening purposes, or in situations where people might underreport symptoms (Weathers et al., 2013), such as might be found in a DUI setting (Nochajski & Stasiewicz, 2005). For clinical purposes, the DUI program in this study chose a cut score of 30. The screen has been shown to have acceptable reliability, good internal consistency, and suitable convergent validity (Ruggiero, Del Ben, Scotti, & Rabalais, 2003; Wilkens, Lang, & Norman, 2011).

Analyses

Chi-square and independent sample *t*-test analyses were used to test for statistically significant differences between males and females on demographic, BAC, and items from the LEC–5. A 2 × 2 analysis of variance (ANOVA) was performed to determine significant differences between males and females and their PCL scores on the LEC–5, based on experiencing or witnessing an event. Finally, a logistic multivariate regression (Agresti, 2002) was performed to assess the independent associations between demographic, alcohol use severity, and LEC–5 items with the PTSD screen score, after PTSD was recoded into a dichotomous variable (either positive for PTSD or negative, based on the PCL–C cutoff score). Variables that had a significant relationship with the PCL–C in the bivariate analyses were entered into the multivariate analysis. All analyses were conducted with the Statistical Package for the Social Sciences (SPSS), version 24.

RESULTS

Experienced Events ("Happened to Me"): Overall and by Gender

Eighty percent of the sample reported events that "happened to me" on at least one of the 17 events on the LEC–5. The number of unique events experienced ranged from 0 to 15, with a mean of 2.67 events (SD = 2.52). Males and females did not differ with regard to the number of events they had experienced, and again, it should be noted that the LEC–5 does not ask for the frequency of each event.

The total number of reported events and scores on the PCL–C were significantly and positively correlated, both for males (r = .49, p < .001) and females (r = .57, p < .001). The number of events was not correlated with the alcohol misuse measures for either males or females. The number of DUIs was significantly correlated with BAC for males (r = .13, p < .01). For females, the number of DUIs was also significantly correlated with BAC (r = .16, p < .01) and BAC was significantly correlated with scores on the PCL–C (r = .14, p < .05).

Table 2 presents the percentages of clients who indicated "Yes" to experiencing various events by gender. Males and females did not differ significantly in their experience of 10 of the 17 events. Overall, males and females reported relatively high rates of experiencing transportation accidents not necessarily related to the DUI (57.0%), physical assault (36.0%), and other stressful events (25.0%). On the other hand, overall rates were relatively low for captivity (1.3%), sudden violent death (4.3%), and severe human suffering (4.3%).

Males were significantly more likely than females to report having been in a serious accident (of any kind), and were more likely to report having been assaulted with a weapon. Males were also more likely to report that they caused injury, harm, or death to someone else as compared to females. Female clients were over six times more likely than males to report having been sexually assaulted, and over three times more likely than males to have had other unwanted sexual experiences. Males were over three times more likely to have experienced combat or a war zone as compared to females. A third of the female clients reported experiencing "other stressful events" at a significantly higher rate than the male clients (about 25%).

Witnessed Events: Overall and by Gender

Clients were also asked to endorse whether they had witnessed the various items on the LEC–5. Almost 55% of the sample reported witnessing at least one event. The number of events witnessed ranged from 0 to 17, with a mean of 1.67 events (SD = 2.41). Males had a higher mean number of witnessed events (1.76) compared to women (1.44), t(1,246) = 2.19, p < .05.

As shown in Table 2, males and females did not differ significantly in witnessing 13 of the 17 events. Among the most prevalent witnessed events for both males and females were witnessing a transportation accident (21.0%), witnessing a life-threatening illness or injury (17.0%), and witnessing a natural disaster (14.0%). Rarer witnessed events that did not differ for

TABLE 2 Chi-Square Analysis of Life Events Checklist–5 by Gender

	Experienced				Witnessed			
	Male		Female		Male		Female	
	n	%	n	%	n	%	n	%
Fire or explosion	118	13.2	42	11.9	203	22.7	53	15.1*
Natural disaster	308	34.4	124	35.2	129	14.4	39	11.1
Exposure to toxic substance	72	8.0	19	5.4	31	3.5	5	1.4
Transportation accident	518	57.8	210	59.7	198	22.1	63	17.9
Serious accident	183	20.4	49	13.9**	147	16.4	40	11.4*
Life-threatening illness or injury	100	11.2	35	9.9	151	16.9	68	19.3
Physical assault	326	36.4	115	32.7	172	19.2	45	12.8**
Assaulted with a weapon; serious injury, harm, or death	174	19.4	35	9.9***	94	10.5	24	6.8*
I caused to someone else sudden violent death	55	6.1	12	3.4*	37	4.1	8	2.3
(e.g., homicide, suicide)	38	4.2	18	5.1	82	9.2	42	11.9
Sudden accidental death	44	4.9	22	6.3	95	10.6	35	9.9
Severe human suffering	39	4.4	14	4.0	82	9.2	25	7.1
Sexual assault	28	3.1	68	19.3***	14	1.6	11	3.1
Other unwanted sexual experience	61	6.8	82	23.3***	28	3.1	14	4.0
Combat, war-zone exposure	68	7.6	8	2.3***	23	2.6	5	1.4
Captivity	12	1.3	5	1.4	15	1.7	2	0.6
Other stressful event	221	24.7	116	33.0**	76	8.5	28	8.0

Note: N = 1,248.
*$p < .05$. **$p < .01$. ***$p < .001$.

males and females were witnessing of captivity (1.5%), witnessing a sexual assault (2.0%), and witnessing combat (2.3%). With regard to witnessed events that differed by gender, males were significantly more likely to report that they had witnessed a fire or explosion and more likely to report witnessing a serious accident than females. Reports of having witnessed physical assaults and assaults with a weapon were significantly higher for males than females.

Experienced and Witnessed Events and PCL–C Scores by Gender

The mean PCL–C score for the entire sample was 26.06 ($SD = 12.93$) with a range of 17 to 85. Using a clinical cutoff score of 30, 195 of the males (23.5%) and 91 of the females (27.7%) fell into the category of needing a further assessment for PTSD (i.e., screened positive). There was not a statistically significant difference between males and females on the percent falling at or above the cut point.

As shown in Table 3, a series of 2 × 2 ANOVA tests were performed to assess whether there were differences in PCL–C scores (a) between those who experienced a specific event or not (i.e., experienced main effect), (b) between males and females (i.e., gender main effect), or (c) if there was an Experience× Gender interaction. An interaction would indicate that the effect of experiencing the event on PTSD scores (i.e., PCL–C) would differ for males and females. Captivity was not included as an event in the analysis because of its infrequent occurrence. Other than the transportation accident and natural disaster events, those who reported experiencing any of the other events fell above the clinical cutoff score of 30 as a group. Those who endorsed experiencing an event consistently scored significantly higher on the PCL–C than those not experiencing the event, as evidenced by statistically significant experience main effects for every event. Three events yielded significant Experience × Gender interactions: fire or explosion, $F = 4.83$, $p < .05$; physical assault, $F = 5.60$, $p < .05$; and sudden accidental death, $F = 15.16$, $p < .001$. Males reported greater adverse effects of experiencing a fire or explosion than females, as measured by their PCL–C scores. On the other hand, females were more greatly affected (i.e., higher PCL–C scores) than males by experiencing physical assault and sudden accidental death.

As for those who endorsed witnessing various items, PCL–C scores on all of the events except transportation accident and physical assault were significantly higher for those who witnessed versus did not witness (i.e., witnessed main effect). There were no differences on any item by gender nor were there any interactions between witnessing and gender.

Multivariate Logistic Regression Analysis

The PCL–C total score was recoded into a categorical dichotomous variable using the clinical cutoff of 30. Those who scored 30 and above were considered positive for PTSD whereas those who scored under 30 were considered negative. Bivariate analysis of demographic and alcohol use severity variables found that only BAC, $t(376.49) = -2.51$, $p < .05$; military or veteran status, $\chi^2 = 13.19$, $p < .01$; and having a previous DUI conviction, $\chi^2 = 6.11$, $p < .05$, were significantly related to screening positive for PTSD (gender was not significantly related to the PTSD categorical variable). These variables, along with experiencing and witnessing events that were significantly related to the PCL–C score at the bivariate level, were entered in a logistic regression to determine independent predictors of having a positive PTSD screen.

Results, shown in Table 4, indicate that higher BACs were associated with greater odds of having a positive PTSD screen ($p = .04$). Military service and previous DUIs were not significant in the multivariate model. The majority of experiencing and witnessing events were not significant in the multivariate model: Nine of the experienced events and 12 of the witnessed events were not statistically significant. Experiences including exposure to toxic substances or radiation, life-threatening illness (marginal), physical assault, serious injury caused by

TABLE 3 2 × 2 Analysis of Variance of Life Events Checklist–5 and PTSD Checklist–Civilian Version Scores by Gender

Fire or explosion								
Yes	33.84	17.71	30.46	15.77[a, c]	28.69	13.78	29.31	13.97[a]
No	24.41	11.31	26.53	12.91	24.82	12.33	26.58	13.17
Natural disaster								
Yes	27.57	13.54	29.13	15.13[a]	29.88	14.24	29.32	13.77[a]
No	24.67	12.22	25.83	12.07	24.97	12.37	26.73	13.25
Exposure toxic substance								
Yes	36.19	18.78	42.11	18.45[a,b]	35.79	18.05	34.40	24.57[a]
No	24.76	11.67	26.08	12.38	25.32	12.39	26.89	13.10
Transportation accident								
Yes	27.44	14.24	29.06	13.78[a]	27.17	12.48	28.21	13.07
No	23.24	9.88	23.97	12.00	25.26	12.82	26.73	13.38
Serious accident								
Yes	31.14	15.43	35.60	18.06[a,b]	29.07	15.19	32.43	17.37[a]
No	24.28	11.59	25.54	11.74	25.01	12.13	26.36	12.63
Life-threatening illness or injury								
Yes	35.56	16.11	36.03	18.93[a]	29.17	14.37	30.89	13.54[a]
No	24.44	11.71	26.00	12.16	24.98	12.31	26.05	13.54
Physical assault								
Yes	31.05	18.05	35.25	16.69[a,b,c]	27.32	12.83	28.34	12.43
No	22.65	9.46	22.91	8.78	25.30	12.72	26.80	13.45
Assaulted with a weapon								
Yes	33.31	17.64	38.70	15.22[a]	32.92	16.60	32.52	17.27[a]
No	23.88	10.54	25.70	12.45	24.84	11.97	26.59	12.91
Serious injury, harm, or death I caused to someone else								
Yes	39.93	20.21	42.30	21.65[a]	36.11	17.73	39.75	23.59[a]
No	24.84	11.68	26.52	12.73	25.22	12.31	26.69	12.86
Sudden violent death (e.g., homicide, suicide)								
Yes	38.82	19.44	43.88	20.43[a]	34.59	17.15	36.08	16.70[a]
No	25.12	12.10	26.14	12.28	24.79	11.88	25.75	12.29
Sudden accidental death								
Yes	27.63	12.44	42.31	18.80[a,b,c]	32.75	16.63	33.71	16.79[a]
No	25.58	12.78	26.07	12.34	24.84	11.95	26.23	12.66
Severe human suffering								
Yes	46.57	16.72	48.62	20.25[a]	34.76	17.39	39.22	18.48[a]
No	24.77	11.75	26.12	12.20	24.78	11.85	26.07	12.42
Sexual assault								
Yes	37.85	15.94	37.81	16.49[a]	38.08	17.84	33.80	16.69[a]
No	25.29	12.46	24.44	11.01	25.49	12.58	26.80	13.17
Other unwanted sexual experience								
Yes	36.10	18.20	37.25	16.40[a]	36.64	15.46	33.31	16.23[a]
No	24.90	11.91	23.92	10.45	25.34	12.53	26.75	13.15
Combat or war-zone exposure								
Yes	37.73	20.38	40.17	21.40[a]	35.10	17.81	42.40	23.10[a]
No	24.71	11.42	26.76	13.04	25.44	12.53	26.77	13.02
Other stressful event								
Yes	33.56	15.95	34.30	16.35[a]	33.89	14.08	36.27	15.94[a]
No	23.05	10.25	23.48	9.81	24.88	12.35	26.21	12.78

Note: Scores ≥ 30 are indicative of the need for further assessment of posttraumatic stress disorder. Range = 17–85. [a]Statistically significant differences between experienced events or not, $p < .05$. [b]Statistically significant differences between male and female, $p < .05$. [c]Statistically significant Experiences × Gender interaction, $p < .05$.

TABLE 4 Multivariate Logistic Regression of Predictors of Screening Positive for Posttraumatic Stress Disorder

Variable	p	Adjusted OR	95% CI
Active vs. no military	ns	0.94	[.43, 2.05]
Veteran vs. no military	ns	0.71	[.21, 2.37]
1 DUI vs. none previously	ns	0.68	[.35, 1.35]
2+ DUI vs. none previously	ns	0.50	[.23, 1.07]
BAC	.04	1.03	[1.00, 1.06]
Experienced			
Fire or explosion	ns	1.26	[.74, 2.16]
Natural disaster	ns	0.77	[.51, 1.16]
Exposure to toxic substance	.02	2.26	[1.14, 4.47]
Transportation accident	ns	1.17	[.79, 1.74]
Serious accident	ns	0.93	[.58, 1.49]
Life-threatening illness	.05	1.75	[.99, 3.08]
Physical assault	.002	1.93	[1.28, 2.89]
Assaulted with a weapon	ns	1.10	[.66, 1.84]
Serious injury I caused	.027	2.49	[1.11, 5.61]
Homicide, suicide	ns	1.18	[.46, 2.99]
Sudden accidental death	ns	0.54	[.22, 1.35]
Severe human suffering	.009	4.77	[1.48, 15.40]
Sexual assault	ns	1.75	[.88, 3.49]
Other unwanted sex	.004	2.34	[1.31, 4.19]
Combat or war-zone	ns	2.12	[.85, 5.31]
Other stressful event	.000	3.17	[2.16, 4.67]
Witnessed			
Fire or explosion	ns	0.94	[.59, 1.49]
Natural disaster	ns	1.38	[.83, 2.29]
Exposure to toxic substance	ns	2.26	[1.14, 4.47]
Serious accident	ns	.81	[.25, 2.63]
Life-threatening illness	ns	1.11	[.67, 1.80]
Assaulted with a weapon	ns	0.75	[.40, 1.42]
Serious injury I caused	ns	0.95	[.36, 2.53]
Homicide, suicide	.007	2.36	[1.26, 4.40]
Sudden accidental death	ns	0.90	[.49, 1.67]
Severe human suffering	ns	1.40	[.75, 2.61]
Sexual assault	ns	0.51	[.14, 1.82]
Other unwanted sex	ns	1.39	[.50, 3.89]
Combat or war-zone	ns	0.63	[.18, 2.21]
Other stressful event	.004	2.39	[1.32, 4.33]

Note: $n = 960$. DUI = driving under the influence; BAC = blood alcohol content.

client, severe human suffering, other unwanted sex, and other stressful events each independently were related to a higher risk of a positive PTSD screen. Reports of experiencing severe human suffering in particular was a strong predictor, with clients reporting that event being 4.8 times more likely to screen positive for PTSD. As for those witnessing adverse events, two events were independent predictors in the model. Those who had witnessed a suicide or homicide, and those who witnessed an "other stressful event" were 2.3 times more likely to screen positive than their counterparts who had not witnessed.

DISCUSSION

This study found that 80% of the sample reported experiencing one or more traumatic events, which is similar to the findings of Peller et al. (2010) of 82% of DUI program clients reporting one or more events, and higher than the 70% rate in the general population. The mean number of unique trauma events in this sample was 2.67.

The most frequently reported experienced event was transportation accident, followed by natural disaster and physical assault. Males were significantly more likely to report being in a serious accident and intentionally caused events such as assaulted with a weapon, causing injury to someone else, or being in combat. Females were more likely than males to report sexual assault and other unwanted sexual experience, which is consistent with other studies regarding gender differences in traumatic events (Bailey et al., 2012). Unlike previous research, males and females reported experiencing a physical assault at similar rates.

Although there were no statistically significant differences between males and females on several items, some of the overall findings of the screening had clinical implications. Sixty-six clients during this study period reported having experienced "sudden accidental death" and 130 reported witnessing this event. Fifty-six reported having experienced "sudden violent death [for example, homicide or suicide]" and 124 reported witnessing this event. Social workers who are clinical counselors interviewed clients about these items and indicated that the reporting of "experiencing" these events was related to clients' own suicide attempts or being with someone who died violently in the clients' presence.

Other LEC–5 items were unexpected to the counselors. For instance, "exposure to toxic substance" was reported by 91 clients who worked in the biotech industry or in medical laboratories. Although fewer in number ($n = 17$), captivity was described to counselors as being kidnapped in other countries, being sex trafficked, or in a forced marriage. The item "other stressful event" was significantly more likely to be endorsed by females at almost one third of the sample and by one quarter by males. Clinically, the counselors found this to be a very good item to have on the measure. Counselors reported that clients stated things like, "My PTSD in general" or "My life right now" or that the DUI event itself was traumatizing. In the study by Bailey et al. (2012) half of the clients endorsed this same item. The counselors and social workers liked this item and indicated that overall, the LEC–5 itself was opening doors to conversations that they had never had in the past.

Despite having a high percentage of clients reporting trauma, even with a low PTSD cut point, this study identified fewer clients reporting PTSD symptoms than the Bailey et al. (2012) study (25.5% vs. 38.0%). However, it should be noted that the Bailey study included an AOD treatment sample and not a

DUI sample. Some studies have surmised that due to its involuntary nature, DUI program clients might be likely to underreport alcohol use and other problems (Nochajski & Stasiewicz, 2005). Studies of lifetime PTSD in DUI samples have reported lower rates for males than this study (9–12% vs. 23.5%), but similar rates to this study for females (27–35% vs. 27.7%; (Lapham et al., 2006; Lapham et al., 2001; McCutcheon et al., 2009). Our lower PTSD cut point might be identifying false positives in male clients as compared to a thorough diagnostic assessment as in these other studies.

When PTSD scores were significantly related to individual LEC–5 items, experiencing the event was invariably associated with higher PTSD. Females had higher PTSD scores as compared to males on the exposure to toxic substance, serious accident, and physical assault. Only fire or explosion, physical assault, and sudden accidental death had statistically significant differences by experience and gender. Although it is beyond the scope of this study to determine how the events intercorrelated with each other, one can assume that the highest PTSD scores of being in combat, exposure to toxic substances, experiencing sudden accidental death, and severe human suffering could all be related to one another, thus increasing the PTSD score on the PCL.

As for the predictors of a positive PTSD screen, BAC was marginally related ($p = .04$) such that those who screened positive had higher BACs than those screening negative. PTSD and alcohol misuse commonly cooccur, with one explanatory mechanism suggesting that individuals with PTSD drink to cope with negative affect (Radomski & Read, 2016). More strongly predictive of PTSD than BAC, however, were experiencing severe human suffering, witnessing homicide or suicide, serious injury I caused, exposure to toxic substance, other unwanted sex, and the "other stressful event." Social workers who are screening clients for events might be alerted that these could possibly be related to PTSD. In TIC, social workers who provide in-depth interviews based on screening content are advised to discuss the links between trauma, PTSD, and alcohol use with clients as well as their impacts on program completion (SAMHSA, 2014a, 2014b). Clients are to be referred for concurrent trauma treatment to maximize AOD treatment benefits.

Implications

One practice implication that has come out of this study is the need for the DUI program to establish a female-only treatment group to allow for discussion of the intentional violence of sexual and physical assault in the women's lives. Due to the significant amount of reporting experiencing "severe human suffering" and "life-threatening illness or injury," the program is considering offering a grief and loss support group as an adjunct to regular services.

Discussions around the role of violence, trauma, and alcohol use have informally increased in regular individual and group sessions and it is recommended that it be added into the group curriculum to formally address the trauma–alcohol misuse connection. For some counselors this has been difficult, as these topics are beyond the scope of "traditional" substance use treatment content. The program has added TIC to in-service training as well as the results of this study.

Research findings are suggesting that that the type of PTSD treatment offered should be based on the type of event experienced, such as exposure therapy for combat, or cognitive behavioral methods for sexual assault (Dworkin et al., 2016; Kelley et al., 2009). Referrals to different types of treatment will need to be based on the knowledge of what other community providers are offering.

Limitations and Future Research

One limitation of this study, which is found in research examining trauma and alcohol use (Van Dam et al., 2012), is that we cannot establish a causal link between these two variables. It is unknown if clients have problematic AOD use due to experienced or witnessed trauma events or if AOD use puts clients at risk to be involved in traumatic events such as fighting and assaults.

The LEC–5 has numerous limitations. The trauma events are based on self-report in a mandated setting, which might cause underreporting. These events are also open to client interpretation, which could vary. These data cannot determine the impact of events experienced as a child or as adult, nor are intimate partner violence, incarceration, the actual DUI arrest itself, or family harm and disruption addressed in the scale. It cannot be determined whether events were discrete occurrences, occurred together, or were cumulative. Other studies have expanded on the LEC by asking participants to indicate the number of times a specific event was experienced, to write out a description of the worst one, and to assess how their PTSD symptoms were related to the worst event (Kelley et al., 2009). Because this was a community-based sample, the agency did not want to burden clients with a longer, more extensive screening.

Future studies could examine details of client case notes to determine what gets discussed with counselors and how trauma events relate to PTSD and alcohol use. Research could also screen for childhood trauma (e.g., the Adverse Childhood Experiences questionnaire; Felitti & Anda, 2010) to examine its relationship with alcohol misuse and subsequent relapse and recidivism among DUI program clients. Studies also need to determine how screening data are used by social workers and counselors and the impact of receiving TIC on DUI program clients. Further, it is important to determine if trauma discussion and referral make an impact to reduce alcohol misuse and drinking and driving, thus the need for longitudinal and prospective studies.

CONCLUSION

A Grand Challenge of Social Work is to reduce alcohol misuse and its social consequences. Understanding what lies beneath problematic use and the trauma–alcohol misuse connection could be a step in the direction of increasing successful intervention outcomes. This study found violence (physical and sexual assault) and grief and loss (severe human suffering) events in a subset of a sample of DUI program clients as well as related PTSD. These concerns are currently being addressed through programmatic changes, discussions about the link between trauma and alcohol use, and referral for trauma treatment.

REFERENCES

Agresti, A. (2002). *Categorical data analysis* (2nd ed.). New York, NY: Wiley.

American Psychiatric Association. (1994). *Diagnostic and statistical manual of mental disorders* (4th ed.). Washington, DC: Author.

American Psychiatric Association. (2013). *Diagnostic and statistical manual of mental disorders* (5th ed.). Arlington, VA: Author.

Bailey, K., Webster, R., Baker, A. L., & Kavanagh, D. J. (2012). Exposure to dysfunctional parenting and trauma events and posttraumatic stress profiles among a treatment sample with coexisting depression and alcohol use problems. *Drug and Alcohol Review, 31*, 529–537. doi:10.1111/j.1465-3362.2011.00401.x

Begun, A. L., Clapp, J. D., & The Alcohol Misuse Grand Challenge Collective. (2016). Reducing and preventing alcohol misuse and its consequences: A Grand Challenge for social work. *The International Journal of Alcohol and Drug Research, 5*(2), 73–83. doi:10.7895/ijadr.v5i2.223

California Association of DUI Treatment Providers. (n.d.). *The CADTP organization*. Retrieved from http://www.cadtp.org/about-cadtp

California Department of Health Care Services. (2016). *Driving Under the Influence programs*. Retrieved from http://www.dhcs.ca.gov/individuals/Pages/DUI.aspx

Daoud, S. O., Tashima, H. N., & Grippe, R. (2015b). *Annual report of the California DUI management information system*. Retrieved from http://www.dmv.ca.gov/portal/wcm/connect/77b8b0e3-c20b-42b0-8670-451d9c9262cd/S5-250.pdf?MOD=AJPERES

DeYoung, D. J. (1997). An evaluation of the effectiveness of alcohol treatment, driver license actions and jail terms in reducing drunk driving recidivism in California. *Addiction, 92*, 989–997. doi:10.1111/j.1360-0443.1997.tb02978.x

Dreissen, M., Schulte, S., Luedecke, C., Schaefer, I., Sutmann, F., Ohlmeier, M. … The TRAUMA B-Study Group. (2008). Trauma and PTSD in patients with alcohol, drug, or other dual dependence: A multi-center study. *Alcoholism: Clinical and Experimental Research, 32*, 481–488. doi:10.1111/j.1530-0277.2007.00591.x

Dworkin, E. R., Mota, N. P., Schumacher, J. A., Vinci, C., & Coffey, S. F. (2016). The unique associations of sexual assault and intimate partner violence with PTSD symptom clusters in a traumatized substance-abusing sample. *Psychological*

Trauma: Theory, Research, Practice and Policy. Advance online publication. doi:10.1037/tra0000212

Felitti, V. J., & Anda, R. F. (2010). The relationship of adverse childhood experiences to adult medical disease, psychiatric disorders and sexual behavior: Implications for healthcare. In R. Lanius, E. Vermetten, & C. Pain (Eds.), *The impact of early life trauma on health and disease: The hidden epidemic* (pp. 77–87). Cambridge, UK: University of Cambridge Press.

Gray, M. J., Litz, B. T., Hsu, J. L., & Lombardo, T. W. (2004). Psychometric properties of the Life Events Checklist. *Assessment, 11,* 330–341. doi:10.1177/1073191104269954

Jewett, A., Shults, R. A., Banerjee, T., & Bergen, G. (2015). Alcohol-impaired driving among adults—United States, 2012. *MMWR Morbidity and Mortality Weekly Report, 64*(30), 814–817. doi:10.15585/mmwr.mm6430a2

Kelley, L. P., Weathers, F. W., McDevitt-Murphy, M. E., Eakin, D. E., & Flood, A. M. (2009). A comparison of PTSD symptom patterns in three types of civilian trauma. *Journal of Traumatic Stress, 22,* 227–235. doi:10.1002/(ISSN)1573-6598

Lapham, S. C., C'de Baca, J., McMillan, G., & Lapidus, J. (2006). Psychiatric disorders in a sample of repeat impaired-driving offenders. *Journal of Studies on Alcohol, 67,* 707–713. doi:10.15288/jsa.2006.67.707

Lapham, S. C., Smith, E., C'de Baca, J., Chang, I., Skipper, B. J., Baum, G., & Hunt, W. C. (2001). Prevalence of psychiatric disorders among persons convicted of driving while impaired. *Archives of General Psychiatry, 58,* 943–1041. doi:10.1001/archpsyc.58.10.943

LaPlante, D. A., Nelson, S. E., Odegaard, S. S., LaBrie, R. D., & Shaffer, H. J. (2008). Substance and psychiatric disorders among men and women repeat driving under the influence offenders who accept a treatment-sentencing option. *Journal of Studies on Alcohol and Drugs, 69,* 209–217. doi:10.15288/jsad.2008.69.209

McCutcheon, V. V., Heath, A. C., Edenberg, H. J., Grucza, R. A., Hesselbrock, V. M., Kramer, J. R., & Bucholz, K. K. (2009). Alcohol criteria endorsement and psychiatric and drug disorders among DUI offenders: Greater severity among women and multiple offenders. *Addictive Behaviors, 34,* 432–439. doi:10.1016/j.addbeh.2008.12.003

McDonald, S. D., & Calhoun, P. S. (2010). The diagnostic accuracy of the PTSD Checklist: A critical review. *Clinical Psychology Review, 30,* 976–987. doi:10.1016/j.cpr.2010.06.012

National Highway Traffic and Safety Administration. (2015). *Alcohol impaired driving.* Retrieved from https://crashstats.nhtsa.dot.gov/Api/Public/ViewPublication/812231

Nochajski, T. H. & Stasiewicz, P. R. (2005). Assessing stages of change in DUI offenders: A comparison of two measures. *Journal of Addictions Nursing, 16,* 57–67. doi: 10.1080/10884600590919127.

Nochajski, T. H., & Stasiewicz, P. R. (2006). Relapse to driving under the influence (DUI): A review. *Clinical Psychology Review, 26,* 179–195. doi:10.1016/j.cpr.2005.11.006

Odenwald, M., & Semrau, P. (2012). Reducing dropout among traumatized alcohol patients in detoxification treatment: A pilot intervention study. *European Addiction Research, 18,* 54–63. doi:10.1159/000333336

Palmer, R. S., Ball, S. A., Rounsaville, B. J., & O'Malley, S. S. (2007). Concurrent and predictive validity of drug use and psychiatric diagnosis among first-time DWI offenders. *Alcoholism: Experimental and Clinical Research, 31,* 619–624.

Peller, A. J., Najavits, L. M., Nelson, S. E., LaBrie, R. A., & Shaffer, H. J. (2010). PTSD among a treatment sample of repeat DUI offenders. *Journal of Traumatic Stress, 23*, 468–473. doi:10.1002/jts.v23·4

Radomski, S. A., & Read, J. P. (2016). Mechanistic role of emotion regulation in the PTSD and alcohol association. *Traumatology, 22*, 113–121. doi:10.1037/trm0000068

Rubin, A., & Babbie, E. (2014). *Research methods for social work* (8th ed.). Belmont, CA: Brooks/Cole.

Ruggiero, K. J., Del Ben, K., Scotti, J. R., & Rabalais, A. E. (2003). Psychometric properties of the PTSD Checklist–Civilian version. *Journal of Traumatic Stress, 16*, 495–502. doi:10.1023/A:1025714729117

Shaffer, H. J., Nelson, S. E., LaPlante, D. A., LaBrie, R. A., Albanese, M., & Caro, G. (2007). The epidemiology of psychiatric disorders among repeat DUI offenders accepting a treatment-sentencing option. *Journal of Consulting and Clinical Psychology, 75*, 795–804. doi:10.1037/0022-006X.75.5.795

Siegal, H. A., Falck, R. S., Carlson, R. G., Rapp, R. C., Wang, J., & Cole, P. A. (2000, May). *The hardcore drunk driving offender.* Paper presented at the 15th International Conference on Alcohol, Drugs & Traffic Safety, Stockholm, Sweden.

Substance Abuse and Mental Health Services Administration. (2014a). *SAMHSA's concept of trauma and guidance for a trauma-informed approach* (HHS Publication No. [SMA] 14-4884). Rockville, MD: Author.

Substance Abuse and Mental Health Services Administration. (2014b). *Trauma-informed care in behavioral health services* (Treatment Improvement Protocol [TIP] Series 57, HHS Publication No. [SMA] 14-4816). Rockville, MD: Author.

van Dam, D., Vedel, E., Ehrin, T., Vedel, E., & Emmelkamp, P. M. (2012). Psychological treatments for concurrent posttraumatic stress disorder and substance use disorders: A systematic review. *Clinical Psychology Review, 32*, 202–214. doi:10.1016/j.cpr.2012.01.004

Volpicelli, J., Balaraman, G., Hahn, J., Wallace, H., & Bux, D. (1999). The role of uncontrollable trauma in the development of PTSD and alcohol addiction. *Alcohol Research and Health, 23*, 256–262.

Wanklyn, S. G., Pukay-Martin, N. D., Belus, J. M., St. Cyr, K., Girard, T. A., & Monson, C. M. (2016). Trauma types as differential predictors of posttraumatic stress disorder (PTSD), major depressive disorder (MDD), and the comorbidity. *Canadian Journal of Behavioral Science, 48*, 296–305. doi:10.1037/cbs0000056

Weathers, F. W., Blake, D. D., Schnurr, P. P., Kaloupek, D. G., Marx, B. P., & Keane, T. M. (2013). *The Life Events Checklist for DSM–5 (LEC–5).* Washington, DC: National Center for PTSD. Retrieved from http://www.ptsd.va.gov

Weathers, F. W., Litz, B. T., Huska, J. A., & Keane, T. M. (1994). *PTSD Checklist–Civilian version.* Boston, MA: National Center for PTSD, Behavioral Science Division.

Wilkens, K. C., Lang, A. J., & Norman, S. B. (2011). Synthesis of the psychometric properties of the PTSD Checklist (PCL) military, civilian, and specific versions. *Depression and Anxiety, 28*, 596–606. doi:10.1002/da.20837

Zhang, S. (2015). *Program performance benchmarks and DUI integrated GIS map.* Retrieved from https://www.google.com/webhp?sourceid=chrome-instant&ion=1&espv=2¡UTF-8#q=program+performance+benchmarks+and+DUI

Technology-Based Interventions and Trainings to Reduce the Escalation and Impact of Alcohol Problems

STELLA M. RESKO, PhD

SUZANNE BROWN, PhD and JAMES J. LISTER, PhD

STEVEN J. ONDERSMA, PhD

REBECCA M. CUNNINGHAM, MD

MAUREEN A. WALTON, PhD

There has been a rapid increase in the development of technological innovations to reduce the escalation and impact of alcohol problems among adolescents and adults. Technology-based interventions offer the possibility of reaching individuals who otherwise might not seek treatment, (e.g., those in remote areas, those not perceiving a need for treatment, or others who might resist treatment). This article describes 4 case examples of technology-based interventions for risky drinking: (a) a freely available and interactive Web site that provides individualized feedback and information on risky drinking patterns; (b) a brief intervention for adolescents that provides individualized feedback to teens regarding their alcohol use; (c) a computer-delivered screening and brief intervention for alcohol use among pregnant women; and (d) a simulation program for training social workers in screening and brief intervention. These case examples highlight how technology could have a role in addressing the Alcohol Misuse Grand Challenge.

Social work researchers have identified alcohol misuse as one of the most important and compelling social issues facing society (Begun, Clapp, & The Alcohol Misuse Grand Challenge Collective, 2016), due in part to its tremendous health and social consequences. The World Health Organization (2004) has identified myriad consequences of alcohol misuse across the globe. These include lost workplace productivity, unemployment, workplace accidents, and family consequences, such as fetal alcohol spectrum disorders, family violence, and mental health issues among the family members of individuals who misuse alcohol. The negative outcomes of alcohol misuse are especially concerning for adolescents and young adults, for whom brain development, specifically frontal lobe maturity, is incomplete, leaving youth more likely to engage in substance misuse and impulsive behaviors associated with alcohol misuse such as risky sexual behaviors, violence, mental health issues, and higher risks for early death (Casey, Jones, & Somerville, 2011). Social workers encounter problems related to alcohol misuse across all practice settings and among clients across the developmental spectrum (Begun et al., 2016). Simply ignoring problems related to alcohol misuse could result in barriers to meaningful change in other domains as well (Perron & Vaughn, 2013). For this reason, the American Academy of Social Work and Social Welfare has identified reducing and preventing alcohol misuse and its consequences as one of its Grand Challenges for social work policy and practice.

DEVELOPING INTERVENTIONS TO ADDRESS ALCOHOL MISUSE

In recent years, considerable progress has been made in understanding the etiology of alcohol use disorders and developing evidence-based treatments (Begun et al., 2016; Warren & Hewitt, 2010). Therapies for alcohol use disorders include a growing number of pharmacological treatments such as naltrexone (Revia or Vivitrol), acomprosate (Campral), and disulfiram (Antabuse; Douaihy, Kelly, & Sullivan, 2013). Treatment providers often use these pharmacological therapies in conjunction with behavioral interventions. The evidence base for these behavioral therapies addressing alcohol misuse has been growing. Researchers have identified numerous psychosocial therapies that are widely considered effective in dealing with substance use disorders. These include motivational interviewing, motivational enhancement therapy, cognitive-behavioral therapy, and community reinforcement approaches (Marsch, Carroll, & Kiluk, 2014).

Despite these advances, many individuals with alcohol use disorders do not receive treatment. Estimates suggest that 86% of the 21.7 million people aged 12 or older who needed substance use treatment in 2015 did not receive any services (Center for Behavioral Health Statistics and Quality [CBHSQ], 2016). Small portions of young people with substance use disorders, 11.2% of adolescents aged 12 to 17 and 10.4% of young adults aged 18 to 25, receive any type of services for substance misuse (CBHSQ, 2016). The dissemination of evidence-based interventions has been a particular challenge for the social work profession and the substance use treatment field more generally (Begun et al., 2016). Lack of clinician knowledge and skills have been cited as reasons for the difficulty in implementing evidence-based practices (Corrigan, Steiner, McCracken, Blaser, & Barr, 2001). Lack of agency resources and infrastructure to support the dissemination of evidence-based interventions has been another barrier to their use in substance abuse treatment settings (Gotham, 2004). Because of these shortcomings, interventions that are easy to use and cost-effective, such as technologically based techniques, might offer one possibility for increasing access to evidence-based interventions.

TECHNOLOGY-BASED INTERVENTIONS FOR ALCOHOL MISUSE

There has been a rapid increase in the development of technological innovations to help reduce the escalation and impact of alcohol problems among adolescents and adults (see Table 1 for examples). Interventions using information and communication technologies include computer-based interventions, educational Web sites, interactive Web-based tools (e.g., dynamic, modular programs often modeled after face-to-face interventions), interventions on mobile devices (e.g., tablets, phones), online counseling and support groups, gaming, and text messaging support. Researchers have also used technology to support more traditional face-to-face social work (Berzin, Singer, & Chan, 2015). Information and communication technologies, for example, can augment a face-to-face intervention by providing clients with computerized feedback on alcohol use during a therapist-delivered intervention (Resko, Walton, Chermack, Blow, & Cunningham, 2012; Walton et al., 2010) or providing supportive text messages following up a traditional intervention session (Berzin et al., 2015). Studies have demonstrated that technology-based interventions for substance misuse can achieve high levels of acceptability from clients and can make them more comfortable when addressing sensitive topics (Choo, Ranney, Wong, & Mello, 2012).

Interventions that use information- and communication-based technologies are appealing, particularly as the use of technological innovations has grown. According to Pew Research, 89% of the U.S. population currently use the Internet or own a smartphone (Poushter, 2016). Facebook, which is the most popular social media platform, is used by 79% of online adults (68% of the U.S. population; Greenwood, Perrin, & Duggan, 2016). Many populations, including adolescents and young adults, have widely adopted technology. Approximately 99% of adults ages 18 to 34 in the United States use the Internet and the majority (92%) also own a smartphone (Poushter, 2016).

The appeal of technology-based interventions has increased as racial and socioeconomic disparities in technology use have narrowed. In the United States in 2016, 88% of Whites, 88% of Hispanics, and 85% of African Americans used the Internet (Pew, 2017). This contrasts with 2000, when 53% of Whites and 38% of African Americans in the United States used the Internet (Pew, 2017). Although disparities related to socioeconomic status remain, the disparities in Internet use based on income have gotten smaller since 2000 (see Figure 1). In 2000, the lowest income group (< $30,000) had rates of Internet use that were 47% lower than the rate for Americans with incomes over $75,000. In 2016, 79% of individuals with incomes below $30,000 were Internet users, a rate that is 19% lower than rates for Americans with incomes over $75,000 (Pew, 2017). Technology-based interventions could offer the possibility of broader access to evidence-based behavioral

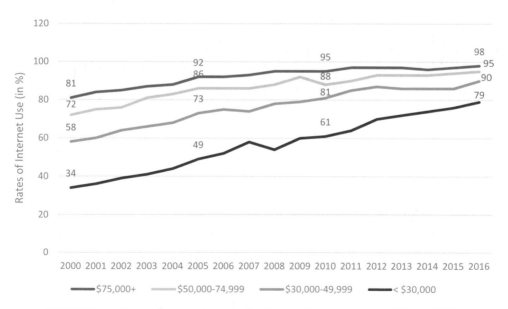

FIGURE 1   Rates of Internet use in the United States by income (Pew, 2017).

TABLE 1 Examples of Technology-Based Interventions for Alcohol Use Disorders

Intervention	Description	Target Population	Outcomes
Brief Orientation Week Ecological Momentary Intervention (Riordan, Conner, Flett, & Scarf, 2015)	Text-message intervention implemented during Orientation Week	University students	Reduced alcohol consumption among female students
Electronic Check-Up to Go (E-CHUG; Walters, Vader, & Harris, 2007)	Online assessment, information, and personalized feedback	Young adults (age 18–21)	Reduced consumption and frequency of intoxication among high-risk drinkers
Electronic Screening and Brief Intervention (E-SBI; Bendtsen, Johansson, & Åkerlind, 2006)	Web-based screening and personalized feedback	College students (age 18–24)	Greater motivation to change drinking among students with risky drinking patterns
Web-based feedback (Bewick et al., 2010)	8-week electronic personalized feedback and social norms information on drinking behavior	College-age young adults (age 18–24)	Reduction in drinking over a 24-week period
Texting to Reduce Alcohol Consumption (Suffoletto, Callaway, Kristan, Monti, & Clark, 2013)	12-week short weekly text message feedback following emergency room in-person screening	High-risk young adults (age 18–25)	Decreased number of binge drinking days over 3 months

| Increasing Readiness to Change (Mason, Benotsch, Way, Kim, & Snipes, 2014) | 4–6 personalized booster messages daily for 4 consecutive days | College students with problem alcohol use | Significantly increased participants' readiness to change |
| Supportive Text Messaging (Agyapong, Ahern, McLoughlin, & Farren, 2012) | Twice-daily supportive text messages for 3 months | Adults with depression and alcohol use disorder | Improvements in depression and global functioning |

treatments (Marsch et al., 2014; Ondersma, Chase, Svikis, & Schuster, 2005). There is a potential to reach broader segments of the U.S. population, including more adolescents and young adults. It provides opportunities to reach groups like sexual minority youth (Berzin et al., 2015), individuals in rural communities, or individuals without health insurance, who traditionally have not had broad access to substance use treatment (Campbell, Muench, & Nunes, 2014). It also provides an opportunity to reach individuals who do not recognize a need for alcohol treatment (Muench, 2014). These types of communication are portable, flexible, and easy to disseminate, creating the potential to reach far greater numbers of individuals who need treatment and ultimately to have a greater overall impact than traditional face-to-face interventions (Berzin et al., 2015; Litvin, Abrabtes, & Brown, 2013).

Technology-based interventions bring the possibility of reaching individuals who might otherwise not seek treatment or prefer to do so using technology. This could be particularly helpful for individuals in remote areas without access to treatment (Berzin et al., 2015; Copeland, 2011). Social workers often provide services for clients who do not perceive a need for treatment or others who might resist treatment due to the stigma associated with alcohol use or seeking help (Resko, Brown, Mendoza, Crosby, & González-Prendes, 2016). This delivery method might help in such situations (Copeland, 2011; Ondersma, Grekin, & Svikis, 2011). Privacy concerns can be a barrier to substance use treatment (CBHSQ, 2016) and the possibility of accessing interventions autonomously can help increase the comfort level of clients and allow for anonymity (Marsch & Dallery, 2012; Ondersma et al., 2011). This has been some of the appeal of text-based interventions for adolescents and young adults. These approaches might be particularly helpful with sensitive or stigmatized behaviors such as alcohol consumption (Marsch & Dallery, 2012). Technology could similarly aid social workers in reaching individuals who engage in substance use but do not self-report use (Ondersma et al., 2011). For example, many substance-use interventions with adolescents or with pregnant women or new mothers are reliant on self-reports of substance use. Adolescents frequently underreport (Delaney-Black et al., 2010) and interventions reliant on these reports might miss a substantial portion of adolescents who could benefit from these services. Concerns regarding child custody or the criminal justice system can prevent pregnant women or women with children from disclosing alcohol or other substance use or seeking treatment (Ondersma et al., 2011). Technological innovations might help promote wider use of indirect interventions that engage clients in discussions of change (e.g., focused on "parenting strengths" or "health and wellness") without assuming alcohol or drug use or offending clients (Ondersma et al., 2011).

The temporal flexibility of technology-based interventions might help overcome the rigid structures and time frames of traditional services, allowing for "on-demand," ubiquitous access to therapeutic support (Berzin et al., 2015; Litvin et al., 2013). Waiting lists are a contemporary reality of many substance use treatment programs, particularly for those that serve individuals with limited resources (Carr et al., 2008). Long waiting times can be a barrier to accessing treatment. Individuals seeking assistance for substance use problems are less likely to enter treatment when they have to wait for services, and often continue to use alcohol and drugs while waiting, which places them at heightened risk for health complications (e.g., overdoses, injuries, exposure to infectious diseases; Carr et al., 2008). Those who seek treatment at night or on weekends might also relapse because they are unable to endure waiting for treatment providers to open during regular business hours (Boyer, Smelson, Fletcher, Ziedonis, & Picard, 2010). Technology-enhanced services could eliminate waits by providing services 24/7.

Using technology to deliver evidence-based interventions for alcohol misuse could also enable wider dissemination of treatment to audiences in diverse settings (Marsch & Dallery, 2012). Web-based interventions, for example, can be offered in the home or integrated into community organizations, schools, workplaces, emergency rooms, and primary or specialty care clinics, as well as via mobile devices. Technology has the potential to address some of the challenges associated with the delivery of science-based interventions, as it allows complex interventions to be delivered at a low cost, without substantially increasing demands on staff time or training needs (Marsch & Dallery, 2012). This is particularly helpful when providing treatment for alcohol misuse in busy settings (e.g., primary care clinics, emergency departments) where substance use problems have not traditionally been the focus. Technology-based interventions have the potential to be more cost-effective than face-to-face interventions (Berzin et al., 2015; Ondersma et al., 2005). Although these interventions might have greater initial costs, the marginal cost per additional user is low, unlike conventional face-to-face interventions (Khadjesari, Murray, Hewitt, Hartley, & Godfrey; 2011; Tebb et al., 2016).

Technology-based interventions also are more likely to be implemented with fidelity, because they rely less on clinician skills, motivation, and performance (Resko et al., 2012; Tebb et al., 2016). Technological advances allow interventions to be delivered with a standardized approach, while also providing individually tailored messages (Litvin et al., 2013; Tebb et al., 2016). These benefits could be seen in interventions delivered through computers or the Web, as well as face-to-face interventions that are augmented by technology (e.g., face-to-face interventions that use computer-based prompts or personalized feedback).

Social work has an important role to play in the development and use of technology to prevent and intervene with alcohol misuse. Social workers encounter substance misuse in a broad range of practice settings (Begun et al., 2016), and substance misuse affects individuals and families throughout the life span. Social work has identified the importance of harnessing technology for social good as one of its Grand Challenge agendas for the coming decade (Berzin et al., 2015).

Social workers provide more than 50% of prevention and treatment services in the substance abuse and mental health fields (National Association of Social Workers, 2009). Therefore, it is vital that social workers be knowledgeable about innovations in intervention implementation, especially interventions that target hard-to-reach populations, such as technology-based intervention techniques.

In the following sections, we describe three examples of technology-based interventions addressing problematic alcohol use: Rethinking Drinking, SafER-teens and electronic screening, and a brief intervention for alcohol use in pregnancy (e-SBI). We also describe a Web-based client simulation program for training social workers in screening and brief intervention for adolescent alcohol misuse. These health care settings are increasingly important for social workers, as treatment for alcohol and drug use disorders extends beyond specialty treatment providers to settings where substance use problems are seen but have not traditionally been the focus of services (Office of National Drug Control Policy, 2015; Perron & Vaughn, 2013).

Rethinking Drinking

The National Institute on Alcohol Abuse and Alcoholism (NIAAA), a part of the National Institutes of Health, developed the Rethinking Drinking initiative (see https://www.rethinkingdrinking.niaaa.nih.gov/). It is a freely available and interactive Web site that has evidence-based information on alcohol for the general public and health professionals such as social workers. NIAAA designed many of the resources for individuals who drink more than their low-risk limits.[1] Rethinking Drinking suggests strategies for individuals who are ready to cut down on their drinking (e.g., keeping track of how much they drink, measuring drinks, setting goals) and recommends other approaches for those who are not ready (e.g., weighing reasons for or against making a change). The Web site includes interactive tools providing information on several alcohol-related topics (e.g., what is a standard drink, how many standard drinks are in various-sized containers, the caloric content of alcohol, blood alcohol concentration levels and symptoms of alcohol use disorders). Several of the interactive tools provide individualized feedback and can help people better understand their drinking patterns, whether they exhibit signs of a possible drinking problem, and whether and how to change their behaviors. A few resources can be downloaded and printed, including a 16-page educational booklet available in English or Spanish (see http://pubs.niaaa. nih.gov/publications/RethinkingDrinking/Rethinking_Drinking.pdf).

---

[1]   NIAAA's low-risk drinking guidelines recommend no more than four drinks in a single day for males and no more than 14 drinks in a week. For females and individuals over age 65 (male or female), the low-risk drinking guideline recommends no more than three drinks in a single day and seven drinks in a week. These guidelines are not recommended for individuals who are underage, pregnant or trying to become pregnant, planning to drive or operate machinery, or taking medications that interact with alcohol, and have health conditions made worse by alcohol.

Researchers conducting several medication trials (e.g., Litten et al., 2013) have used the Rethinking Drinking resources (e.g., online modules) as part of the behavioral therapy in their studies. Other researchers have incorporated the Rethinking Drinking materials into standard practice by providing a printed copy of the brochure or information about the Web site to all patients who received either an in-person or a computer intervention (e.g., Book et al., 2013).

The Rethinking Drinking tools have also been used to educate health professionals on screening and treatment for alcohol use disorders. In a study of Screening, Brief Intervention, and Referral to Treatment (SBIRT) training in primary care settings, Ornstein and colleagues (2013) provided primary care treatment providers with information about the Rethinking Drinking Web site. A training program on SBIRT for registered nurses (RN-SBIRT) included similar content, and involved a live demonstration of the Rethinking Drinking Web site (Broyles, Kraemer, Kengor, & Gordon, 2013). The interactive tools on the Rethinking Drinking site might be particularly helpful in educating social workers and social work students on alcohol misuse. In a general course on substance misuse designed for master's-level social work students, we have used an assignment that incorporates Rethinking Drinking (see the Appendix for our sample Web-based assessment and drinking feedback assignment). This experiential and writing assignment has students complete the online assessment, receive personalized feedback, and then write a brief paper (two to three pages).

SafERteens

SafERteens is a brief intervention for adolescents that uses motivational interviewing and normative resetting[2] to decrease alcohol use and aggression among adolescents receiving care in emergency departments (EDs; Walton et al., 2010). The urban ED represents an underutilized venue for delivering substance use and violence interventions to adolescents (Cunningham et al., 2009). The interactive, one-session intervention is tailored to the adolescent's gender and level of involvement in alcohol use, binge drinking, fighting, and weapon carrying. The one-session intervention is administered on site in the ED by a therapist (i.e., research social worker) or a computer. The therapist and computer interventions were designed to have similar content, but with different modes of presentation (Walton et al., 2010). As part of efforts to enhance the cultural relevance of the intervention, it was developed with input from urban youth and uses culturally relevant visuals (e.g., racially diverse virtual peers), content

---

[2] Normative resetting addresses perceptions that substance use is very common among one's peers. Addressing these descriptive social norms is particularly important for adolescent substance use prevention (Eisenberg, Toumbourou, Catalano, & Hemphill, 2014).

(e.g., goals and values), and language tailored to the communities where it is delivered. In both the therapist- and computer-based delivery of the SafERteens intervention, adolescent patients complete a computer-based screening and receive feedback on their drinking and involvement with violence in an open, nonjudgmental manner. The intervention is grounded in harm reduction principles, which are well suited for adolescents (Monti, Barnett, O'Leary, & Colby, 2001). Consistent with motivational interviewing (Miller & Rollnick, 2012), SafERteens emphasizes uncovering a discrepancy between current behavior and future goals and increasing problem recognition, motivation, and self-efficacy (Walton et al., 2010). The intervention includes sections that address the adolescent's goals; provide personalized feedback regarding alcohol use, participation in violence, and weapon use; provide a decisional balance exercise for the potential benefits of deciding to reduce or stop drinking and fighting; provide five role-play situations; and provide a referral (Walton et al., 2010). In both delivery mechanisms of the SafERteens intervention, the role-plays are individualized to each participant based on responses from the screening survey, addressing topics such as anger management, conflict resolution, alcohol refusal skills, and avoiding drinking and driving (Walton et al., 2010).

In the therapist-delivered intervention, tablet computers guide the process and display content and tailored feedback to prompt discussions (Cunningham et al., 2012; Walton et al., 2010). The research social workers who delivered the intervention were initially trained on motivational interviewing techniques and the specific SafERteens intervention and received additional supervision and training throughout the study (Walton et al., 2010). The use of tablet computers standardized the delivery of the intervention by the therapist. This helps to ensure greater levels of fidelity to the intervention (Resko et al., 2012) and can be helpful in EDs and other busy clinical settings (Cunningham et al., 2012).

The computer SafERteens intervention is a stand-alone interactive program with touch screens and audio via headphones (Cunningham et al., 2012; Cunningham et al., 2009). A virtual buddy guides patients through the computer program and provides feedback on choices made. The buddy is a virtual peer selected by the participant and helps the adolescent identify reasons to avoid drinking and aggression.

The three-armed SafERteens study (n = 235 for control group, n = 237 for computer intervention, and n = 254 for therapist intervention) has demonstrated positive results as an ED-based brief intervention for youth involved with violence or alcohol use. At 6 months after the intervention, participants in the therapist intervention showed self-reported reductions in alcohol consequences (therapist, −32.2%; control, −17.7%; odds ratio = 0.56, 95% CI [0.34, 0.91]) compared with controls; participants in the computer intervention also reported reductions in alcohol consequences (computer, −29.1%; control, −17.7%; odds ratio = 0.57; 95% CI [0.34, 0.95]; Walton et al., 2010). These differences, however, were not maintained at 1 year (Cunningham et al., 2012); further, this program did not reduce alcohol consumption, likely reflecting low drinking levels among adolescents in the study. The SafERteens therapist intervention has demonstrated more lasting changes related to violence; changes in attitudes, self-efficacy, and reductions in violent behaviors, peer victimization, and violence-related consequences were maintained at 1 year following the intervention (Cunningham et al., 2012). In terms of costs, the SafERteens therapist intervention cost about $17 per violent event or consequences averted (Sharp et al., 2014). Further, both the therapist and computer interventions showed promise for reducing dating violence victimization (Cunningham et al., 2013).

To reduce alcohol misuse and violence on a broader scale, future studies are needed to discover methods for improving these outcomes, particularly those related to alcohol misuse, and to further understand the effectiveness of the SafERteens behavioral intervention when delivered by social workers and other clinical staff (i.e., nonresearch staff). In this regard, a study is underway to integrate and translate this brief intervention, focusing primarily on violence, into a practical program incorporated into routine clinical practice in the ED. This study will use ED staff to conduct screenings for violent behaviors and delivery of a brief intervention; the original program is also being augmented by automatic delivery of tailored text messages (containing reminders of content discussed during the intervention session) over a 2-month period. To address the practical barrier of lack of 24/7 availability of on-site ED staff to deliver interventions, the study will also test remote delivery by off-site therapists using Health Insurance Portability and Accountability Act compliant technology. These efforts will determine the reach, effectiveness, adoption, implementation, and maintenance of the SafERteens BI (Glasgow, Lichtenstein, & Marcus, 2003). Additional information about the SafERteens intervention, including training materials (e.g., role-play videos of interventions), is available at www.SafERteens.org.

Electronic Screening and Brief Intervention to Reduce Alcohol Use in Pregnancy

The third technology-based intervention we describe is an electronic screening and brief intervention designed to reduce alcohol use during pregnancy (e-SBI; Ondersma et al., 2015). Because the e-SBI for pregnant women has been developed more recently, less research has been published on it. The e-SBI intervention is based on the principles of self-determination theory (Ryan & Deci, 2000) and motivational interviewing (Miller & Rollnick, 2012). The intervention emphasizes the use of the nonspecific or common therapy factors such as empathy, optimism, and being nonjudgmental (see Wampold & Imel, 2015). The intervention is tailored to women's race and ethnic identities (e.g., uses culturally diverse actors in the intervention videos, uses culturally relevant language and content) and alcohol risk perceptions. In addition, the computer-delivered technology uses techniques to create a life-like feel (referred to as *ethopoeia*) that has been shown to elicit social responses from participants (Nass & Moon, 2000) and that might enhance motivation (Mumm & Mutlu, 2011) as well as working alliance and engagement (Bickmore, Gruber, & Picard, 2005) with computer-delivered interventions. For example, this software uses an animated narrator that displays emotion, speaks aloud, refrains from placing judgment on participants, and seeks out the perspectives of participants throughout the brief intervention.

This intervention aims to cultivate self-directed change and improve attitudes and behaviors with regard to seeking treatment for alcohol use. The 20-min session features a brief set of videos, which include an African American physician describing the effects of alcohol use during pregnancy and a testimonial from a mother who details the benefits of choosing to stop drinking during pregnancy. In addition to the videos, the intervention has other components that focus on (a) information regarding the risks of drinking alcohol during pregnancy, (b) assisting the participant in weighing the costs and benefits that changing alcohol use behavior might have, and how it relates to strongly held personal goals or values, (c) providing normed feedback about the prevalence of alcohol use during pregnancy and consequences or gains should the participant stop drinking during pregnancy, and (d) offering participants the option of setting a specific change goal for their alcohol use throughout their pregnancy.

The e-SBI for pregnant women has demonstrated acceptability among two samples of primarily African American pregnant women. The women in each study rated the e-SBI intervention favorably with regard to ease of use, helpfulness, and general appeal (scores of 4.7–5.0 on a 1–5 Likert scale; Ondersma et al., 2015; Tzilos, Sokol, & Ondersma, 2011). It also has shown preliminary efficacy in a small Stage I clinical trial during which women were randomized to either e-SBI ($n = 24$) or a control condition ($n = 24$; Ondersma et al., 2015). Although the study had limited statistical power, women who received the intervention reported less frequent alcohol use during pregnancy and improved pregnancy outcomes (e.g., birth weight). The e-SBI intervention demonstrated medium-sized intervention effects that did not reach statistical significance ($p < .10$ and $p < .20$), which is likely related to being underpowered (Ondersma et al., 2015).

Patient Simulation for Training in Adolescent Screening and Brief Intervention

The independent research organization NORC at the University of Chicago, partnered with the Council on Social Work Education, Center for Clinical Social Work, American Association of Colleges of Nursing, and New York–based technology company Kognito to develop a curriculum and training materials for integrating adolescent SBIRT education into undergraduate and graduate courses in social work and nursing (McPherson, Goplerud, & Adam, 2015). As part of these efforts, they developed an online simulation that enables learners to practice conducting brief interventions for alcohol misuse with virtual adolescent patients.

The Web-based training program includes information about SBIRT and three interactive role-playing situations that feature emotionally responsive virtual patients with problems at different levels of severity (e.g., weekly alcohol use or high-risk use, monthly alcohol use or moderate-risk use) and contexts (e.g., primary care, ED, school social worker or nurse, office setting). These simulated role-play conversations can be delivered on computers, tablets, and mobile devices and use gaming technology to prepare social workers and other professionals to effectively lead real-life conversations related to substance misuse (McPherson et al., 2015). Initial feedback from social work students has shown that the use of virtual clients can help students feel less self-conscious when learning new practice skills (Walters et al., 2016). The simulation helps health professionals screen young patients for substance use, and to conduct brief interventions, using the principles of motivational interviewing (McPherson et al., 2015). Participants who complete the online training receive scores and considerable feedback on their performances. The simulation can be completed by students on their own (e.g., as a homework assignment) or in class (e.g., in multiple small groups or by the class as a whole; Walters et al., 2016). Through financial support from the Conrad N. Hilton Foundation, the simulation has been made available to educators for free or at reduced cost through the Adolescent SBIRT Learning Collaborative (http://sbirt.webs.com/learning-collaborative). Several universities (e.g., the University of Pittsburgh, the University of Southern California, and Wayne State University) are currently evaluating the effectiveness of this SBIRT training for social workers and nurses.

DISCUSSION AND FUTURE DIRECTIONS

Alcohol is a complex biopsychosocial problem that affects individuals, families, and communities across the life span (Begun et al., 2016). Social workers, along with other substance-use prevention and treatment professionals have a growing collection of evidence-based psychosocial interventions available for the treatment of alcohol use disorders. Social workers frequently work with individuals experiencing substance misuse problems and have important roles in the treatment of alcohol and drug disorders that include providing substance abuse treatment and prevention services.

Considerable opportunities exist for leveraging technology in the delivery of evidence-based social work interventions to promote widespread reach and impact (Berzin et al., 2015; Marsch & Dallery, 2012). As the examples reviewed here demonstrate, this line of intervention is promising and underscores the potential public health impact of technology-based therapeutic tools.

With the growing emphasis on cost-effective care and the integration of treatment for alcohol and drug use into other areas of health care in which providers might have limited expertise in treating individuals with substance use disorders (Office of National Drug Control Policy, 2015; Perron & Vaughn, 2013), technology-based therapeutic tools could become increasingly important and clinically useful. These tools as well as other technologies (e.g., short message service or text messages) are well positioned to meet these unmet needs in this new model of care (Marsch & Dallery, 2012). Interventions like the computer SafERteens or the e-SBI that are delivered via computers, mobile devices, or other emerging technologies might be cost-effective approaches that help social workers reach underserved populations in diverse settings. Technology-enhanced interventions, like the therapist-delivered SafERteens brief intervention, could be helpful in ensuring that therapeutic services provided in busy clinical settings are consistently high in quality (Cunningham et al., 2012). Such interventions provide an opportunity for social workers to develop and study multidisciplinary solutions to alleviate alcohol misuse and its related consequences. Social workers have important roles in this effort, and should consider utilizing or adapting technology to enhance intervention and prevention for alcohol misuse.

To fully realize the potential of technology-delivered interventions for alcohol misuse, several areas of inquiry remain important. Efforts are needed to reduce economic barriers that prevent social service agencies from using technology-based interventions (Campbell et al., 2014). Although such interventions can have relatively low costs per client, they can present considerable barriers for social service agencies with limited financial resources. Research is needed to ensure technology-based interventions are optimally designed to produce maximal behavior changes. Efficient and effective methods should be identified to integrate technology-based interventions into systems of care in a manner that is most responsive to the needs of clients (Marsch & Dallery, 2012). Social workers can play an important role in this process. Finding ways to increase the reach of technology-based interventions is important. Several of the case examples described here have had success in getting individuals to complete technology-based interventions in health care settings. For mobile interventions or Web sites like Rethinking Drinking, efforts are needed to enhance the use of stand-alone interventions. We need to learn more about the mechanisms underlying behavior change from technology-delivered interventions (Ondersma et al., 2011; Resko et al., 2012; Walton et al., 2010). Further research along these lines will be important in isolating mechanisms that are useful in predicting treatment responses, and in ensuring that key ingredients are present, as these interventions become widely available (Begun et al., 2016; Marsch & Dallery, 2012).

FUNDING

This article was supported by grants from the National Institute on Alcohol Abuse and Alcoholism.

REFERENCES

Agyapong, V. I. O., Ahern, S., McLoughlin, D. M., & Farren, C. K. (2012). Supportive text messaging for depression and comorbid alcohol use disorder: Single-blind randomised trial. *Journal of Affective Disorders, 141*, 168–176. doi:10.1016/j.jad.2012.02.040

Begun, A. L., Clapp, J. D., & The Alcohol Misuse Grand Challenge Collective. (2016). Reducing and preventing alcohol misuse and its consequences: A Grand Challenge for social work. *The International Journal of Alcohol and Drug Research, 5*(2), 73–83. doi:10.7895/ijadr.v5i2.223

Bendtsen, P., Johansson, K., & Åkerlind, I. (2006). Feasibility of an email-based electronic screening and brief intervention (e-SBI) to college students in Sweden. *Addictive Behaviors, 31*, 777–787. doi:10.1016/j.addbeh.2005.06.002

Berzin, S. C., Singer, J., & Chan, C. (2015). *Practice innovation through technology in the digital age: A Grand Challenge for social work*. Retrieved from http://aaswsw.org/wp-content/uploads/2013/10/Practice-Innovation-through-Technology-in-the-Digital-Age-A-Grand-Challenge-for-Social-Work-GC-Working-Paper-No-12.pdf

Bewick, B. M., West, R., Gill, J., O'May, F., Mulhern, B., Barkham, M., & Hill, A. J. (2010). Providing web-based feedback and social norms information to reduce student alcohol intake: A multisite investigation. *Journal of Medical Internet Research, 12*(5), e59. doi:10.2196/jmir.1461

Bickmore, T., Gruber, A., & Picard, R. (2005). Establishing the computer–patient working alliance in automated health behavior change interventions. *Patient Education and Counseling, 59*(1), 21–30.

Book, S. W., Thomas, S. E., Smith, J. P., Randall, P. K., Kushner, M. G., Bernstein, G. A., … Randall, C. L. (2013). Treating individuals with social anxiety disorder and at-risk drinking: Phasing in a brief alcohol intervention following paroxetine. *Journal of Anxiety Disorders, 27*, 252–258. doi:10.1016/j.janxdis.2013.02.008

Boyer, E. W., Smelson, D., Fletcher, R., Ziedonis, D., & Picard, R. W. (2010). Wireless technologies, ubiquitous computing and mobile health: Application to drug abuse treatment and compliance with HIV therapies. *Journal of Medical Toxicology, 6*, 212–216. doi:10.1007/s13181-010-0080-z

Broyles, L. M., Kraemer, K. L., Kengor, C., & Gordon, A. J. (2013). A tailored curriculum of alcohol Screening, Brief Intervention, and Referral to Treatment (SBIRT) for nurses in inpatient settings. *Journal of Addictions Nursing, 24*, 130–141. doi:10.1097/JAN.0b013e3182a4cb0b

Campbell, A. N., Muench, F., & Nunes, E. V. (2014). Technology-based behavioral interventions for alcohol and drug use problems. In L. A. Marsch, S. E. Lord, & J. Dallery (Eds.), *Behavioral healthcare and technology: Using science-based innovations to transform practice* (pp. 40–55). Oxford, UK: Oxford University Press.

Carr, C. J., Xu, J., Redko, C., Lane, D. T., Rapp, R. C., Goris, J., & Carlson, R. G. (2008). Individual and system influences on waiting time for substance abuse treatment. *Journal of Substance Abuse Treatment, 34,* 192–201. doi:10.1016/j.jsat.2007.03.005

Casey, B. J., Jones, R. M., & Somerville, L. H. (2011). Breaking and accelerating of the adolescent brain. *Journal of Research on Adolescence, 21*(1), 21–33. doi:10.1111/j.1532-7795.2010.00712.x

Center for Behavioral Health Statistics and Quality. (2016). *Key substance use and mental health indicators in the United States: Results from the 2015 National Survey on Drug Use and Health* (HHS Publication No. SMA 16-4984, NSDUH Series H-51). Retrieved from http://www.samhsa.gov/data/sites/default/files/NSDUH-FFR1-2015/NSDUH-FFR1-2015/NSDUH-FFR1-2015.pdf

Choo, E. K., Ranney, M. L., Wong, Z., & Mello, M. J. (2012). Attitudes toward technology-based health information among adult emergency department patients with drug or alcohol misuse. *Journal of Substance Abuse Treatment, 43,* 397–401. doi:10.1016/j.jsat.2012.09.005

Copeland, J. (2011). Application of technology in the prevention and treatment of substance use disorders and related problems: Opportunities and challenges. *Substance Use & Misuse, 46*(1), 112–113. doi:10.3109/10826084.2011.521423

Corrigan, P. W., Steiner, L., McCracken, S. G., Blaser, B., & Barr, M. (2001). Strategies for disseminating evidence-based practices to staff who treat people with serious mental illness. *Psychiatric Services, 52,* 1598–1606. doi:10.1176/appi.ps.52.12.1598

Cunningham, R. M., Chermack, S. T., Zimmerman, M. A., Shope, J. T., Bingham, C. R., Blow, F, C., & Walton, M. A. (2012). Brief motivational interviewing intervention for peer violence and alcohol use in teens: One-year follow-up. *Pediatrics, 129,* 1083–1090. doi:10.1542/peds.2011-3419

Cunningham, R. M., Walton, M. A., Goldstein, A., Chermack, S. T., Shope, J. T., Raymond Bingham, C., … Blow, F. C. (2009). Three month follow up of brief computerized and therapist interventions for alcohol and violence among teens. *Academic Emergency Medicine, 16,* 1193–1207. doi:10.1111/j.1553-2712.2009.00513.x

Cunningham, R. M., Whiteside, L. K., Chermack, S. T., Zimmerman, M. A., Shope, J. T., Bingham, C. R., … Walton, M. A. (2013). Dating violence: Outcomes following a brief motivational interviewing intervention among at-risk adolescents in an urban ED. *Academic Emergency Medicine, 20,* 562–569. doi:10.1111/acem.12151

Delaney-Black, V., Chiodo, L. M., Hannigan, J. H., Greenwald, M. K., Janisse, J., Patterson, G. … Sokol, R. J. (2010). Just say "I don't": Lack of concordance between teen report and biological measures of drug use. *Pediatrics, 126,* 887–893. doi:10.1542/peds.2009-3059

Douaihy, A. B., Kelly, T. M., & Sullivan, C. (2013). Medications for substance use disorders. *Social Work in Public Health, 28,* 264–278. doi:10.1080/19371918.2013.759031

Eisenberg, M. E., Toumbourou, J. W., Catalano, R. F., & Hemphill, S. A. (2014). Social norms in the development of adolescent substance use: A longitudinal analysis of the International Youth Development Study. *Journal of Youth and Adolescence, 43,* 1486–1497. doi:10.1007/s10964-014-0111-1

Glasgow, R. E., Lichtenstein, E., & Marcus, A. C. (2003). Why don't we see more translation of health promotion research to practice? Rethinking the efficacy-to-effectiveness transition. *American Journal of Public Health*, *93*, 1261–1267. doi:10.2105/AJPH.93.8.1261

Gotham, H. J. (2004). Diffusion of mental health and substance abuse treatments: Development, dissemination, and implementation. *Clinical Psychology: Science and Practice*, *11*, 60–176.

Greenwood, S., Perrin, A., & Duggan, M. (2016). *Social media update 2016*. Retrieved from http://www.pewinternet.org/2016/11/11/social-media-update-2016/

Khadjesari, Z., Murray, E., Hewitt, C., Hartley, S., & Godfrey, C. (2011). Can stand alone computer based interventions reduce alcohol consumption? A systematic review. *Addiction*, *106*, 267–282. doi:10.1111/add.2011.106.issue-2

Litten, R. Z., Ryan, M. L., Fertig, J. B., Falk, D. E., Johnson, B., Dunn, K. E., ... Kampman, K. (2013). A double-blind, placebo-controlled trial assessing the efficacy of varenicline tartrate for alcohol dependence. *Journal of Addiction Medicine*, *7*(4), 277–286.

Litvin, E. B., Abrantes, A. M., & Brown, R. A. (2013). Computer and mobile technology-based interventions for substance use disorders: An organizing framework. *Addictive Behaviors*, *38*, 1747–1756. doi:10.1016/j.addbeh.2012.09.003

Marsch, L. A., Carroll, K. M., & Kiluk, B. D. (2014). Technology-based interventions for the treatment and recovery management of substance use disorders: A JSAT special issue. *Journal of Substance Abuse Treatment*, *46*(1), 1–4. doi:10.1016/j.jsat.2013.08.010

Marsch, L. A., & Dallery, J. (2012). Advances in the psychosocial treatment of addiction: The role of technology in the delivery of evidence-based psychosocial treatment. *The Psychiatric Clinics of North America*, *35*, 481–493. doi:10.1016/j.psc.2012.03.009

Mason, M., Benotsch, E. G., Way, T., Kim, H., & Snipes, D. (2014). Text messaging to increase readiness to change alcohol use in college students. *The Journal of Primary Prevention*, *35*(1), 47–52. doi:10.1007/s10935 013-0329-9

McPherson, T., Goplerud, E., & Adam, C. (2015). Integrating adolescent substance abuse screening, brief intervention and treatment in health professions education. *Addiction Science & Clinical Practice*, *10*(2), 1. doi:10.1186/1940-0640-10-S2-O36

Miller, W. R., & Rollnick, S. (2012). *Motivational interviewing: Helping people change*. New York, NY: Guilford.

Monti, P. M., Barnett, N. P., O'Leary, T. A., & Colby, S. M. (2001). Motivational enhancement for alcohol-involved adolescents. In P. M. Monti, S. M. Colby, & T. A. O'Leary (Eds.), *Adolescents, alcohol, and substance abuse: Reaching teens through brief interventions* (pp. 145–182). New York, NY: Guilford.

Muench, F. (2014). The promises and pitfalls of digital technology in its application to alcohol treatment. *Alcohol Research*, *36*(1), 131–142.

Mumm, J., & Mutlu, B. (2011). Designing motivational agents: The role of praise, social comparison, and embodiment in computer feedback. *Computers in Human Behavior*, *27*(5), 1643–1650.

Nass, C., & Moon, Y. (2000). Machines and mindlessness: Social responses to computers. *Journal of Social Issues*, *56*(1), 81–103.

National Association of Social Workers. (2009). *Social work speaks: NASW policy statements, 2009–2012* (8th ed.). Washington, DC: NASW Press.

Office of National Drug Control Policy. (2015). *National drug control strategy.* Retrieved from https://www.whitehouse.gov/sites/default/files/ondcp/policy-and-research/2015_national_drug_control_strategy.pdf

Ondersma, S. J., Beatty, J. R., Svikis, D. S., Strickler, R. C., Tzilos, G. K., Chang, G., ... Sokol, R. J. (2015). Computer delivered screening and brief intervention for alcohol use in pregnancy: A pilot randomized trial. *Alcoholism: Clinical and Experimental Research, 39*, 1219–1226. doi:10.1111/acer.12747

Ondersma, S. J., Chase, S. K., Svikis, D. S., & Schuster, C. R. (2005). Computer-based brief motivational intervention for perinatal drug use. *Journal of Substance Abuse Treatment, 28*, 305–312. doi:10.1016/j.jsat.2005.02.004

Ondersma, S. J., Grekin, E. R., & Svikis, D. (2011). The potential for technology in brief interventions for substance use, and during-session prediction of computer-delivered brief intervention response. *Substance Use & Misuse, 46*, 77–86. doi:10.3109/10826084.2011.521372

Ornstein, S. M., Miller, P. M., Wessell, A. M., Jenkins, R. G., Nemeth, L. S., & Nietert, P. J. (2013). Integration and sustainability of alcohol screening, brief intervention, and pharmacotherapy in primary care settings. *Journal of Studies on Alcohol and Drugs, 74*, 598–604. doi:10.15288/jsad.2013.74.598

Perron, B. E., & Vaughn, M. G. (2013). Conclusions and future directions. In M. G. Vaughn & B. E. Perron (Eds.), *Social work practice in the addictions* (pp. 261–264). New York, NY: Springer.

Pew Research Center. (2017). *Internet/broadband fact sheet.* Retrieved from http://www.pewinternet.org/fact-sheet/internet-broadband/

Poushter, J. (2016). *Smartphone ownership and Internet usage continues to climb in emerging economies.* Retrieved from http://www pewglobal.org/2016/02/22/smartphone-ownership-and-internet-usage-continues-to-climb-in-emerging-economies/

Resko, S. M., Brown, S., Mendoza, N. S., Crosby, S., & González-Prendes, A. (2016). Perceived treatment needs among women with co-occurring substance use disorders and PTSD. *Journal of Dual Diagnosis, 12*, 271–281. doi:10.1080/15504263.2016.1248309

Resko, S. M., Walton, M. A., Chermack, S. T., Blow, F. C., & Cunningham, R. M. (2012). Therapist competence and treatment adherence for a brief intervention addressing alcohol and violence among adolescents. *Journal of Substance Abuse Treatment, 42*, 429–437. doi:10.1016/j.jsat.2011.09.006

Riordan, B. C., Conner, T. S., Flett, J. A., & Scarf, D. (2015). A brief orientation week ecological momentary intervention to reduce university student alcohol consumption. *Journal of Studies on Alcohol and Drugs, 76*, 525–529. doi:10.15288/jsad.2015.76.525

Ryan, R. M., & Deci, E. L. (2000). Self-determination theory and the facilitation of intrinsic motivation, social development, and well-being. *American Psychologist, 55*(1), 68–78. doi:10.1037/0003-066X.55.1.68

Sharp, A. L., Prosser, L. A., Walton, M., Blow, F. C., Chermack, S. T., Zimmerman, M. A., & Cunningham, R. (2014). Cost analysis of youth violence prevention. *Pediatrics, 133*, 448–453. doi:10.1542/peds.2013-1615

Suffoletto, B., Callaway, C. W., Kristan, J., Monti, P., & Clark, D. B. (2013). Mobile phone text message intervention to reduce binge drinking among young adults: Study protocol for a randomized controlled trial. *Trials*, *14*(1), 93. doi:10.1186/1745-6215-14-93

Tebb, K. P., Erenrich, R. K., Jasik, C. B., Berna, M. S., Lester, J. C., & Ozer, E. M. (2016). Use of theory in computer-based interventions to reduce alcohol use among adolescents and young adults: A systematic review. *BMC Public Health*, *16*(1), 517. doi:10.1186/s12889-016-3183-x

Tzilos, G. K., Sokol, R. J., & Ondersma, S. J. (2011). A randomized Phase I trial of a brief computer-delivered intervention for alcohol use during pregnancy. *Journal of Women's Health*, *20*, 1517–1524. doi:10.1089/jwh.2011.2732

Walters, A., McPherson, T., Adam, C., Copeland, V., Mayeda, S., & Resko, S. M., (2016, October). *Integrating adolescent SBIRT throughout social work and nursing education*. Panel presentation at the annual meeting of the Council on Social Work Education, Atlanta, GA.

Walters, S. T., Vader, A. M., & Harris, T. R. (2007). A controlled trial of web-based feedback for heavy drinking college students. *Prevention Science*, *8*(1), 83–88. doi:10.1007/s11121-006-0059-9

Walton, M. A., Chermack, S. T., Shope, J. T., Bingham, C. R., Zimmerman, M. A., Blow, F. C., & Cunningham, R. M. (2010). Effects of a brief intervention for reducing violence and alcohol misuse among adolescents: A randomized controlled trial. *Journal of the American Medical Association*, *304*, 527–535. doi:10.1001/jama.2010.1066

Wampold, B. E., & Imel, Z. E. (2015). *The great psychotherapy debate: The evidence for what makes psychotherapy work*. New York, NY: Routledge.

Warren, K. R., & Hewitt, B. G. (2010). NIAAA: Advancing alcohol research for 40 years. *Alcohol Health & Research World*, *33*(1), 5.

World Health Organization. (2004). *Global status report on alcohol*. Geneva, Switzerland: WHO Department of Mental Health and Substance Abuse.

APPENDIX

Web-Based Assessment and Feedback on Alcohol Use

Experiential component: Complete the Rethinking Drinking Web-based tools

Rethinking Drinking, http://rethinkingdrinking.niaaa.nih.gov/, is an evidence-based, online alcohol intervention and personalized feedback tool. It was developed by researchers at the National Institute on Alcohol Abuse and Alcoholism. You will complete the following interactive tools that provide information, assessment, and personalized feedback on alcohol use: What counts as a drink? Check your drinking pattern, Calculators for cocktail content, drink size, alcohol calorie content, alcohol spending, and blood alcohol concentration.

Written component: Write a two- to three-page summary of your reactions to the program, personalized assessment and feedback you completed and received. Is your feedback consistent with or different from what you thought? Will it affect your future behavior? Is it useful? How might Web-based programs be useful in addressing problematic substance use? Was the Web-based program you completed relevant to the needs of different groups (e.g., men, women, young adults, older adults, racial or ethnic minorities)? What recommendations would you have for improving such programs?

Options for instructors: Instructors can have students complete the tool to check drinking patterns more than one time to see how the feedback differs for men and women with various levels of alcohol use. Instructors may allow students to select modules themselves or instruct students to complete specific modules/interactive tools. Other Web or app-based interventions, such as the electronic check up to go (e-CHUG), may be available at some universities and can be used for this assignment.

Effects and Durability of an SBIRT Training Curriculum for First-Year MSW Students

JOAN M. CARLSON, PhD

JON AGLEY, PhD

RUTH A. GASSMAN, PhD

ANGELA M. McNELIS, PhD

RHONDA SCHWINDT, DNP

JULIE VANNERSON, MD

DAVID CRABB, MD

KHADIJA KHAJA, PhD

Screening, Brief Intervention, and Referral to Treatment (SBIRT) is an evidence-based process for identification, prevention, and treatment of alcohol misuse. The purpose of this study was to examine the effects of an alcohol-focused training on first-year MSW students' (n = 71) knowledge, attitudes, and beliefs about SBIRT. Changes in item means were assessed using repeated-measures analysis of variance (critical α = .002). Data indicated a significant and strong main effect for training; perceived competence improved immediately and remained significantly higher 30 days posttraining. Other improvements included knowing what questions to ask patients, ease making alcohol-related statements, and believing that it is rewarding to work with at-risk patients.

Widespread alcohol misuse is a serious risk factor for health, social, and economic problems (World Health Organization [WHO], 2014). In the United States, alcohol use is especially prevalent; nearly 65% of adults age 18 and over are classified as current, regular drinkers (Schoenborn, Adams, & Peregoy, 2013), and the National Survey on Drug Use and Health reports that 52% of Americans age 12 and over currently drink (Center for Behavioral Health Statistics and Quality, 2015). Additionally, a significant number of adults also engage in binge drinking, defined as "a pattern of drinking that brings blood alcohol concentration (BAC) levels to 0.08," typically occurring after five or more drinks for men and four or more drinks for women within 2 hr (National Institute of Alcohol Abuse and Alcoholism, 2016). Estimates of adult (age 18+) prevalence of binge drinking within the past 30 days in the United States range from 17.1% (Centers for Disease Control and Prevention, 2012) to nearly 25% (Substance Abuse and Mental Health Services Administration [SAMHSA], 2014). At the same time, the majority of adults who engage in excessive drinking do not meet the criteria for an alcohol use disorder (Esser et al., 2014), while still consuming alcohol at levels indicative of alcohol misuse. Especially given the Social Work Grand Challenge of Reducing and Preventing Alcohol Misuse and Its Consequences (Begun, Clapp, & The Alcohol Misuse Grand Challenge Collective, 2016), it is important to address alcohol use that occurs across a spectrum of levels, use patterns, and contexts.

The consequences of heavy drinking include a multitude of short- and long-term adverse effects that increase the likelihood of injury and early death, with nearly 88,000 persons dying annually in the United States from alcohol-related causes (Stahre, Roeber, Kanny, Brewer, & Zhang, 2014). Recently, WHO reported a causal link between harmful alcohol use and infectious diseases, including tuberculosis and HIV/AIDS (WHO, 2014). Alcohol misuse has become the fourth leading preventable cause of death in the United States (Stahre et al., 2014).

Excessive alcohol use also places an enormous economic burden on the United States, costing an estimated $249.0 billion in 2010, with the U.S.

government covering $100.7 billion, or 40.4%, of those costs. The median cost of alcohol use per state is $3.5 billion, with binge drinking accounting for more than 70% of the economic burden in all states. These costs have remained steady since 2006, even through the economic recession from 2007 to 2009 (Sacks, Gonzales, Bouchery, Tomedi, & Brewer, 2015).

Given the magnitude and scope of this problem in the United States, more approaches are needed to reduce alcohol misuse and alcohol use disorders across the spectrum to address at-risk, harmful, excessive or binge, and dependent alcohol use, as well as other synonymous classifications of use identified by multiple groups and organizations (Reid, Fiellin, & O'Connor, 1999). To this end, a variety of synergistic approaches, including primary, secondary, and tertiary prevention, are indicated (DiMartini, Rogal, & Potts, 2015).

According to the National Association of Social Workers (NASW, 2013), "Social workers are in a unique position to influence the delivery of services by addressing the acute and chronic needs of clients with Substance Use Disorders (SUDs)" (p. 6) NASW went on to say, "By developing and applying evidence-informed approaches that incorporate established interventions and evolving techniques based on emerging research findings, social workers can markedly improve treatment services for clients and their families" (p. 6). Social workers are well suited because they work across a variety of health and human service settings. The Institute of Medicine (1990) original endorsement and vision of Screening, Brief Intervention, and Referral to Treatment (SBIRT) in its report *Broadening the Base of Treatment for Alcohol Problems*, was for SBIRT to occur outside the specialty treatment sector within a range of community organizations providing general services that persons with drinking problems frequent. It is advantageous for social workers to deal with the individual and societal effects of alcohol given they are already well versed in evidence-based practices that address support for individuals and families dealing with "divorce, child and adult abuse, unemployment, accidents, crimes, hospitalization, loss of workforce productivity and high economic costs," which are often related to alcohol addiction (Dziegieleski, 2005, p. 125). Further, 10% of violent crimes in the United States are linked to alcohol or other substances, with social workers serving on the front lines to address this in their various roles in domestic violence shelters, child welfare and human service agencies, prisons, hospitals, mental health clinics, community-based agencies, treatment centers, victim advocacy agencies, homeless shelters, schools, hospice, sexual assault services, and so on (Dziegieleski, 2005). Although a large number of social workers are trained to provide mental health and substance abuse services, many other social workers provide services to individuals and families where alcohol can be a primary component of the presenting problem.

SCREENING, BRIEF INTERVENTION, AND REFERRAL TO TREATMENT

SBIRT is an evidence-based process to facilitate prevention and treatment of alcohol and other substance use, and typically utilizes motivational interviewing (MI) as a supportive skill set (Babor et al., 2007). Recent analyses of SBIRT for alcohol have demonstrated cost savings and health improvement in both emergency and outpatient health care settings (Barbosa, Cowell, Bray, & Aldridge, 2015). To facilitate implementation and dissemination of SBIRT, SAMHSA funded 17 5-year training programs for physicians in 2008 and 2009 that continue to produce substantive information on training outcomes for medical residents. Social workers have only been a specified target of SAMHSA SBIRT training programs since 2013, so comparatively fewer studies have been performed regarding training methods and outcomes for this group of health professionals. Recent work has included assessments of knowledge acquisition via training (e.g., Gotham, Knopf-Amelung, Krom, Stilen, & Kohnle, 2015) and qualitative assessments of SBIRT integration into curricular activities such as field work practice (e.g., Ogden, Vinjamuri, & Kahn, 2016).

Social work curricula can include evidence-based education to address the needs of clients who drink in harmful ways or have substance use disorders. Several of the recent competency standards the Council on Social Work Education (CSWE, 2015) established specifically state that social work curricula must teach students to engage in practice-informed research and research-informed practice; engage with individual families, groups, organizations, and communities; assess individuals, families, groups, organizations, and communities; and evaluate practice with individuals, families, groups, organizations, and communities. SBIRT training incorporated into curricula affords the opportunity to meet these standards while preparing students to meet the needs of clients and patients.

SBIRT has been shown to be effective at reducing alcohol consumption (Bertholet, Daeppen, Wietlisbach, Fleming, & Burand, 2005; Cherpitel, Moskalewicz, Swiatkiewicz, Ye, & Bond, 2009 and shows marked improvement in general and mental health (Madras et al., 2009). It is also valuable for benefitting a large number of clients at significant cost savings (Quanbeck, Lang, Enami, & Brown, 2010; Solberg, Maciosek, & Edwards, 2008). A variety of attitudes and beliefs are related, or have been hypothesized to relate to utilization of SBIRT skills in clinical practice (e.g., Gassman, 2003, 2007). Curricular evaluation assesses the extent to which specific training structures achieve positive change in desired attitudes and beliefs.

Although causality cannot be established in a nonexperimental design, this type of work is important in iteratively building the knowledge base to support social work training in SBIRT. Thus, the purpose of this study was to examine the effects of an alcohol-focused SBIRT training structure on first-year MSW students' attitudes and beliefs about SBIRT.

SBIRT Training

The three-step, multipronged, and sequential curriculum for this project included the following components. First, MSW students received a set of distinctive, informational, state-of-the-art Microsoft PowerPoint presentations defining SBIRT and providing examples of screening and brief interventions in clinical settings. The presentations addressed SBIRT's value for patients and clients, payers, policymakers, physicians, nurses, and social workers, along with allied health and human service professionals. Students reviewed this content as part of self-directed learning that prepared them for subsequent components of the training. Second, students completed three separate 1-hr interactive Flash-based, self-paced, online educational modules on alcohol, marijuana, and MI that included an interactive quiz requiring a score of 85% or higher for passing on each of the modules. Third, students attended a 4-hr face-to-face MI training that included simulated role-play for integrating each of the stages of change (Prochaska & DiClemente, 1983): precontemplation, contemplation, preparation, action, and maintenance; this component offered students multiple opportunities to practice SBIRT and MI skills in a simulated setting.

METHODS

Sample Selection

The SBIRT training program enrolled first-year MSW students at a large, urban, public university during the 2014–2015 academic year ($N = 95$). Most participants identified as female (80%), non-Hispanic (99%), and White (83%). Due to response attrition at 30-day follow-up (82% response rate) and failure to complete the pretest (93% response rate), the sample used for this study was smaller ($n = 71$) than the population that received the training (number verified by 100% baseline instrument completion). Only participants who completed all three survey instruments were included in the sample. To determine whether failure to complete one of the three surveys was associated with a different mean value for any of the specified constructs (described subsequently), we used a series of Mann–Whitney U tests for each of the 19 individual items on the baseline survey ($\alpha = .05$, critical $\alpha = .002$), finding no significant differences. We therefore suggest that, in terms of the metrics assessed in this study, distribution of instrument noncompletion in this survey appears to have been random.

Survey Administration

Data were collected using a longitudinal survey design with three administration points: prior to enrolling in the SBIRT/MI training (paper administration), immediately following the training (paper administration), and 30 days following the training (electronic administration). Surveys contained a number of items designed to assess educational and programmatic goals and included questions required for the federal Government Performance and Results Act (GPRA). University institutional review board approval was obtained to use these data in this research study.

Item Selection

Among other metrics, each of the survey instruments in this study contained 21 performance and satisfaction items designed to support training program improvement and curricular modification. Those items were taken from prior survey research on knowledge, attitudes, and beliefs about SBIRT that were predictive of likely behavioral performance by physicians and nurses (Gassman, 2003, 2007). Recent pilot work also suggests that a subscale derived from these items could predict documented substance use screening in nurses' clinical practice (Agley et al., 2016). However, because not all MSW students had prior clinical experience, two items from Gassman's research were eliminated prior to analyses, as they presupposed clinical experience. Possible responses to each item ranged from 1 (*strongly disagree*) to 5 (*strongly agree*), with the exception of four normative perception items, which used a 4-point scale and allowed for a response of *unsure* (cases with responses of *unsure* were deleted only for analyses involving those specific items).

Data Analyses

INDIVIDUAL ITEM ASSESSMENT

We used repeated-measures analysis of variance (ANOVA, baseline $\alpha = .05$) to determine changes in mean scores for each item across all three measurement points. Although Likert scale data with conceptually continuous interpretation reasonably can be assessed using parametric statistics (Carifio & Perla, 2008), these individual items were assessed using the nonparametric Friedman test to verify the appropriateness of the parametric conclusion (all conclusions were verified, and supplemental test statistics are shared in Table 1). Because this set of analyses involved multiple comparisons, we adjusted the critical alpha level for the overall tests from .05 to .002 per Bonferroni's correction (highlighting tests in Table 1 that surpassed that threshold), although we still report findings with alpha levels between .05 and .002. In instances where the assumption of homogeneity of variance was violated, a Greenhouse–Geisser correction was used. Effect sizes were calculated as partial eta squared (η^2_p). When significant main effects were observed, we calculated tests of mean

TABLE 1 Significant Changes in First-Year MSW Students Across a Screening, Brief Intervention, and Referral to Treatment (SBIRT) Training

Question	Pretest M	Pretest SD	Posttest M	Posttest SD	Follow-Up M	Follow-Up SD	MS	f	p	η^2_p	$\chi^2 (p)^a$
I know what questions to ask patients to obtain information on their alcohol consumption.	3.04	1.03	4.07	0.68	3.85	0.79	25.18	38.96	**<.001**	0.358	46.14 (<.001)
I am comfortable asking about a patient's drinking patterns.	3.73	0.93	4.08	0.69	3.86	0.78	2.52	5.44	.007	0.072	8.91 (.012)
I don't know how to identify at-risk drinkers who have no obvious symptoms of excess consumption.	3.00	1.04	3.39	0.96	3.23	1.02	2.78	3.34	.038	0.046	11.47 (.003)
I know how I would effectively go about helping patients to reduce their drinking.	2.51	0.94	3.66	0.79	3.69	0.73	35.53	70.83	**<.001**	0.503	75.14 (<.001)
I am at ease making these statements.	3.11	1.01	3.72	0.76	3.61	0.78	8.46	16.30	**<.001**	0.189	23.70 (<.001)
Given adequate information and training, care providers (e.g., physicians, nurses, or social workers) can help patients reduce their alcohol consumption.	4.01	0.84	4.35	0.61	4.15	0.75	2.05	5.13	.007	0.068	7.14 (.028)
In general, it is rewarding to work with at-risk drinkers.	3.30	0.76	3.59	0.71	3.59	0.82	2.07	7.40	**.001**	0.096	13.10 (.001)

Note. Analysis of variance significance values shown in bold meet the more stringent criterion ($p < .002$) for multiple comparisons. For a fuller presentation of results, however, significant results between $p = .05$ and $p = .002$ also are included in normal text.
[a]Value generated by the nonparametric Friedman test as verification.

differences to determine whether the pretest mean differed from the posttest, 30-day follow-up test, or both (α = .05, critical α = .017).

GROUPED ITEM ASSESSMENT

Gassman's (2003) paper grouped sets of items by underlying factor to establish six scales; prior to analyzing those scales, we assessed their internal reliability using the present sample of social work students. Only one scale (perceived competence, using four of the original five items) exceeded an internal reliability alpha of .600 at all three points of measurement (pretest α = .849, baseline α = .776, 30-day follow-up α = .885). This might suggest that social workers perceive aspects of these items differently than do physicians or nurses (e.g., interpretation of the question content might be affected by field of study), as lower alpha levels can stem from heterogeneous interpretation of items within a scale (Cronbach & Shavelson, 2004). To assess aggregate change in mean perceived competence as an underlying concept, we calculated a scale variable (i1 + i2 + i4 + i5)/4 and used the same ANOVA process as described in the previous paragraph.

RESULTS

Analyses revealed significant posttraining improvement in item means for the following metrics (see Table 1): knowing what questions to ask patients to obtain information on their alcohol consumption, $F(1.647, 115.293) = 38.96$, $\boldsymbol{p < .001}$, $\eta^2_p = 0.358$; comfort asking about a patient's drinking patterns, $F(1.790, 123.305) = 5.44$, $p = .007$, $\eta^2_p = 0.072$; knowing how to identify at-risk drinkers who have no obvious symptoms of excess consumption, $F(2, 140) = 3.34$, $p = .038$, $\eta^2_p = 0.046$; knowing how to effectively help patients reduce their drinking, $F(1.821, 127.501) = 70.83$, $\boldsymbol{p < .001}$, $\eta^2_p = 0.503$; ease making these sorts of statements, $F(1.742, 121.968) = 16.30$, $\boldsymbol{p < .001}$, $\eta^2_p = 0.189$; endorsement of the belief that it is rewarding to work with at-risk drinkers, $F(2, 140) = 7.40$, $\boldsymbol{p = .001}$, $\eta^2_p = 0.096$; and endorsement of the belief that care providers can help patients reduce alcohol consumption, $F(2, 140) = 5.13$, $p = .007$, $\eta^2_p = 0.068$. Significance levels that exceeded the standard established by Bonferroni's correction to the alpha level are shown in bold.

For significant main effects, we computed pairwise comparisons (see Table 2). Significance levels reported in this paragraph and in Table 2 were adjusted for Bonferroni's correction at the time of calculation and so should be compared to α = .05 instead of a more conservative value. Students endorsed knowing what questions to ask patients to obtain information on their alcohol consumption more strongly both at posttest (Δ = 1.03, $p < .001$)

TABLE 2 Significant Changes From Pretest to Other Administration Times

Question	Pretest M	Posttest Difference	p	Follow-Up Difference	p
I know what questions to ask patients to obtain information on their alcohol consumption.	3.04	1.03	< .001	0.80	< .001
I am comfortable asking about a patient's drinking patterns.	3.73	0.35	.012	—	—
I don't know how to identify at-risk drinkers who have no obvious symptoms of excess consumption.	3.00	−0.39	.043	—	—
I know how I would effectively go about helping patients to reduce their drinking.	2.51	1.16	< .001	1.18	< .001
I am at ease making these statements.	3.11	0.61	< .001	0.49	.001
Given adequate information and training, care providers (e.g., physicians, nurses, or social workers) can help patients reduce their alcohol consumption.	4.01	0.34	.008	—	—
In general, it is rewarding to work with at-risk drinkers.	3.30	0.30	.003	0.30	.005

Note: Analyses included adjustment for Bonferroni correction for multiple pairwise comparisons. Only significant differences are included.

and at 30-day follow-up (Δ = 0.80, p < .001) than at pretest. They also expressed comfort asking about a patient's drinking patterns more strongly at posttest (Δ = 0.35, p = .012), but not at 30-day follow-up. Students reported knowing how to identify at-risk drinkers who have no obvious symptoms of excess consumption more at posttest than at pretest (Δ = 0.39, p = .043; this item was reverse-coded) but not at 30-day follow-up. However, they reported knowing how to effectively help patients reduce their drinking more strongly at posttest (Δ = 1.16, p < .001) and at 30-day follow-up (Δ = 1.18, p < .001) than at pretest, and they also reported ease making these sorts of statements more strongly at posttest (Δ = 0.61, p < .001) and at 30-day follow-up (Δ = 0.49, p = .001) than at pretest. Finally, students endorsed the belief that care providers can help patients reduce alcohol consumption more strongly at posttest than at pretest (Δ = 0.34, p = .008), but not at 30-day follow-up, and they also endorsed the belief that it is rewarding to work with at-risk drinkers more strongly at posttest (Δ = 0.30, p = .003) and at 30-day follow-up (Δ = 0.30, p = .005) than at pretest.

For the perceived competence scale, the data indicated a significant and strong main effect for the training; perceived competence improved immediately and remained significantly higher 30-days posttraining, $F(1.644, 115.099) = 47.44$, $p < .001$, $\eta^2_p = 0.400$.

DISCUSSION

This study identified multiple positive associations between receiving the SBIRT training described herein and constructs related to MSW students' self-efficacy—further, an aggregate scale composed of these and other items measuring perceived competence also increased following the SBIRT training. The association between self-efficacy and performance of tasks is well established (Stajkovic & Luthans, 1998). Researchers have made the case that self-efficacy is an important construct to measure in social work education (Holden, Meenaghan, Anastas, & Metrey, 2002). Given the significant and varied burden placed on many individuals by alcohol consumption, it is logical to conclude that it is important for MSW students to develop a sense of self-efficacy specifically for addressing sensitive issues with clients regarding alcohol use. Findings from this study indicate that the SBIRT and MI training produced short and moderate-term sustained improvements in a number of important areas for first-year MSW students' knowledge, attitudes, and beliefs about SBIRT. We observed the strongest effects for findings that were significant even given the conservative criterion ($\alpha = .002$), including knowing what questions to ask patients to obtain information on their alcohol consumption, knowing how to effectively help patients reduce their drinking, and ease making these sorts of statements. Given that task complexity moderates the relationship between self-efficacy and performance (Stajkovic & Luthans, 1998), it is important to note that we observed improvement in endorsement of multiple nuanced behaviors, such as familiarity with screening questions. Further, although the effect size was comparatively smaller, students reported increased endorsement of the idea that it is rewarding to work with at-risk drinkers, suggesting that the training might have served to attenuate their concerns or negative perceptions of alcohol-using clients (e.g., reduction in stigma). Researchers have found that alcohol-using patients and clients perceive stigma related to their substance use both on the part of the general public and on the part of their health care providers (Fortney et al., 2004), and so increased endorsement of this survey construct among MSW students is notable.

The social work profession frontline role in providing support to family systems affected by alcohol addiction is well documented and makes it well poised to "improve the quality of care for addiction in the U.S." (Daley & Feit, 2013, p. 162). Social workers are equipped to engage and coordinate services for clients facing multiple difficulties, often working closely with those facing addiction and helping them cope with numerous emotional, environmental, and relational challenges (Celeste & Clapp, 1997). Their long-established community resource networks are critical in dealing with and alleviating a wide variety of social problems. It is essential for social work practitioners to be "skilled in recognizing the signs and symptoms of alcohol use and to become aware of the problems and concerns that result when alcohol is abused" (Dziegieleski, 2005, p. 125). Health professionals and social workers have the most recurrent contact with people needing addiction treatment (Wilkey, Lundgren, & Amodeo, 2013).

MSW programs prepare advanced practitioners to provide care to those with the greatest need and all too often the least access to mental health and addiction treatment. Including SBIRT training in social work curricula has strong potential to affect and successfully increase behavior interventions in line with social work practice principles of client-centered care. Graduates fill gaps in health and allied health care by providing assistance to those in urban, suburban, and rural areas. Preliminary indication of advanced preparation and education of SBIRT and MI indicates it is beneficial for screening, preventive, and primary mental health care to meet the growing needs of patients and clients.

Limitations

This investigation had several limitations that need to be acknowledged. Interpretation of our findings must be tempered because data were collected at a single, large, Midwestern, public university. Further studies are necessary to evaluate SBIRT education training from more diverse educational settings. This study was not a randomized trial and lacked a control component, limiting the extent to which causality can be imputed. As such, we can note that the training appears to have been associated with the reported changes in scores, but cannot assert that it was the direct cause of those changes. Finally, this study was limited to self-reporting measures without corroborating objective measures. The self-reporting measures have, however, been used in previous research.

Implications for the Future

Increasing attention has been paid to the role of social workers to address harmful drinking. Given the effectiveness of brief targeted behavioral interventions in a variety of clinical settings, a number of researchers have proposed that screening and brief intervention be integrated into clinical practice (Mitchell et al., 2015). Expanding training to include social workers has strong potential to increase the number of providers while significantly increasing access to behavioral interventions for clients and patients across health care and allied health care settings. Such behavioral interventions, if supported by additional research, have significant implications for preparing students to address the critical needs of clients or patients surrounding harmful alcohol use.

ACKNOWLEDGMENTS

We wish to thank the faculty and students who made this project possible through their kind support and participation.

FUNDING

This investigation and article would not have been possible without financial support from the Substance Abuse and Mental Health Services Administration, U.S. Department of Health and Human Services (Grant No. 1U79TI025375-01).

REFERENCES

Agley, J., McNelis, A. M., Carlson, J. M., Schwindt, R., Clark, C. A., Kent, K. A., ... Crabb, D. W. (2016). If you teach it, they will screen: Advanced practice nursing students' use of screening and brief intervention in the clinical setting. *Journal of Nursing Education, 55*, 231–235. doi:10.3928/01484834-20160316-10

Babor, T. F., McRee, B. G., Kassebaum, P. A., Grimaldi, P. L., Ahmed, K., & Bray, J. (2007). Screening, Brief Intervention, and Referral to Treatment (SBIRT): Toward a public health approach to the management of substance abuse. *Substance Abuse, 28*(3), 7–30. doi:10.1300/J465v28n03_03

Barbosa, C., Cowell, A., Bray, J., & Aldridge, A. (2015). The cost-effectiveness of alcohol Screening, Brief Intervention, and Referral to Treatment (SBIRT) in emergency and outpatient medical settings. *Journal of Substance Abuse Treatment, 53*, 1–8. doi:10.1016/j.jsat.2015.01.003

Begun, A. L., Clapp, J. D., & The Alcohol Misuse Grand Challenge Collective. (2016). Reducing and preventing alcohol misuse and its consequences: A Grand challenge for social work *International Journal of Alcohol and Drug Research, 5*(2), 73–83. doi:10.7895/ijadr.v5i2.223

Bertholet, N., Daeppen, J.-B., Wietlisbach, V., Fleming, M., & Burand, B. (2005). Reduction of alcohol consumption by brief alcohol intervention in primary care: Systematic review and meta-analysis. *Archives of Internal Medicine, 165*, 986–995. doi:10.1001/archinte.165.9.986

Carifio, J., & Perla, R. (2008). Resolving the 50-year debate around using and misusing Likert scales. *Medical Education, 42*, 1150–1152. doi:10.1111/med.2008.42.issue-12

Celeste, B. A., & Clapp, J. D. (1997). Ideology and social work practice in substance abuse settings. *Social Work, 42*, 552–562. doi:10.1093/sw/42.6.552

Center for Behavioral Health Statistics and Quality. (2015). *Behavioral health trends in the United States: Results from the 2014 National Survey on Drug Use and Health* (HHS Publication No. SMA 15-4927, NSDUH Series H-50). Retrieved from https://www.samhsa.gov/data/sites/default/files/NSDUH-FRR1-2014/NSDUH-FRR1-2014.pdf

Centers for Disease Control and Prevention. (2012). Vital signs: Binge drinking prevalence, frequency, and intensity among adults—United States, 2010. *Morbidity and Mortality Weekly Report, 61*(1), 14–19.

Cherpitel, C. J., Moskalewicz, J., Swiatkiewicz, G., Ye, Y., & Bond, J. (2009). Screening, Brief Intervention, and Referral to Treatment (SBIRT) in a Polish emergency department: Three-month outcomes of a randomized, controlled clinical trial. *Journal of Studies on Alcohol and Drugs, 70,* 982–990. doi:10.15288/jsad.2009.70.982

Council on Social Work Education. (2015). *Educational policy and accreditation standards.* Alexandria, VA: Author. Retrieved from http://www.cswe.org/File.aspx?id=81660

Cronbach, L. J., & Shavelson, R. J. (2004). My current thoughts on coefficient alpha and successor procedures. *Educational and Psychological Measurement, 64,* 391–418. doi:10.1177/0013164404266386

Daley, D. C., & Feit, M. D. (2013). The many roles of social workers in the prevention and treatment of alcohol and drug addiction: A major health and social problem affecting individuals, families, and society. *Social Work in Public Health, 28,* 159–164. doi:10.1080/19371918.2013.758960

DiMartini, A., Rogal, S., & Potts, S. (2015). Future directions: The need for early identification and intervention for patients with excessive alcohol use. In J. Neuberger & A. DiMartini (Eds.), *Alcohol abuse and liver disease* (pp. 223–234). West Sussex, UK: Wiley.

Dziegieleski, S. E. (2005). *Understanding substance abuse addiction: Assessment and intervention.* Chicago, IL: Lyceum.

Esser, M. B., Hedden, S. L., Kanny, D., Brewer, R. D., Cfroerer, J. C., & Naimi, T. S. (2014). Prevalence of alcohol dependence among US adult drinkers, 2009–2011. *Preventing Chronic Disease, 11*(E206), 1–11. doi:10.5888/pcd11.140329

Fortney, J., Mukherjee, S., Curran, G., Fortney, S., Han, X., & Booth, B. M. (2004). Factors associated with perceived stigma for alcohol use and treatment among at-risk drinkers. *The Journal of Behavioral Health Services & Research, 31,* 418–429. doi:10.1007/BF02287693

Gassman, R. A. (2003). Medical specialization, profession, and mediating beliefs that predict stated likelihood of alcohol screening and brief intervention: Targeting educational interventions. *Substance Abuse, 24,* 141–156. doi:10.1080/08897070309511544

Gassman, R. A. (2007). Practitioner-level predictors of alcohol problem detection and management activities. *Journal of Substance Use, 12,* 191–202. doi:10.1080/14659890701237215

Gotham, H. J., Knopf-Amelung, S., Krom, L., Stilen, P., & Kohnle, K. (2015). Competency-based SBIRT training for health-care professionals: Nursing and social work students. *Addiction Science and Clinical Practice, 10*(Suppl. 1), A14. doi:10.1186/1940-0640-10-S1-A14

Holden, G., Meenaghan, T., Anastas, J., & Metrey, G. (2002). Outcomes of social work education: The case for social work self-efficacy. *Journal of Social Work Education, 38,* 115–133.

Institute of Medicine. (1990). *Broadening the base of treatment for alcohol problems: Report of a study by a committee of the Institute of Medicine, Division of Mental Health and Behavioral Medicine.* Washington, DC: National Academies Press.

Madras, B. K., Compton, W. M., Avula, D., Stegbauer, T., Stein, J. B., & Clark, H. W. (2009). Screening, brief interventions, referral to treatment (SBIRT) for illicit drug and alcohol use at multiple healthcare sites: Comparison at intake and 6 months later. *Drug and Alcohol Dependence, 99*(1–3), 280–295. doi:10.1016/j.drugalcdep.2008.08.003

Mitchell, A. M., Fioravanti, M., Kane, I., Piskar, K., Hagle, H., & Boucek, L. (2015). A call for universal alcohol, drug screening. *American Journal of Nursing, 115*(6), 11. doi:10.1097/01.NAJ.0000466294.87304.ce

National Association of Social Workers. (2013). *NASW standards for social work practice with clients with substance use disorders.* Washington, DC: Author.

National Institute of Alcohol Abuse and Alcoholism. (2016). *Drinking levels defined.* Retrieved from https://www.niaaa.nih.gov/alcohol-health/overview-alcohol-consumption/moderate-binge-drinking

Ogden, L. P., Vinjamuri, M., & Kahn, J. M. (2016). A model for implementing an evidence-based practice in student fieldwork placements: Barriers and facilitators to the use of "SBIRT." *Journal of Social Service Research, 42*, 425–441. doi:10.1080/01488376.2016.1182097

Prochaska, J. O., & DiClemente, C. C. (1983). Stages and processes of self-change of smoking: Toward an integrative model of change. *Journal of Consulting and Clinical Psychology, 51*, 390–395. doi:10.1037/0022-006X.51.3.390

Quanbeck, A., Lang, K., Enami, K., & Brown, R. L. (2010). A cost–benefit analysis of Wisconsin's Screening, Brief Intervention, and Referral to Treatment program: Adding the employer's perspective. *Wisconsin Medical Journal, 109*(1), 9–14.

Reid, M. C., Fiellin, D. A., & O'Connor, P. G. (1999). Hazardous and harmful alcohol consumption in primary care. *Archives of Internal Medicine, 159*, 1681–1689. doi:10.1001/archinte.159.15.1681

Sacks, J., Gonzales, K., Bouchery, E., Tomedi, L., & Brewer, R. (2015). 2010 national and state costs of excessive alcohol consumption. *American Journal of Preventive Medicine, 49*(5), e73–e79. doi:10.1016/j.amepre.2015.05.031

Schoenborn, C. A., Adams, P. F., & Peregoy, J. A. (2013). *Health behaviors of adults: United States, 2008–2010.* Retrieved from https://www.cdc.gov/nchs/data/series/sr_10/sr10_257.pdf

Solberg, L. I., Maciosek, M. V., & Edwards, N. M. (2008). Primary care intervention to reduce alcohol misuse: Ranking its health impact and cost effectiveness. *American Journal of Preventive Medicine, 34*, 143–152.e3. doi:10.1016/j.amepre.2007.09.035

Stahre, M., Roeber, J., Kanny, D., Brewer, R. D., & Zhang, X. (2014). Contribution of excessive alcohol consumption to deaths and years of potential life lost in the United States. *Preventing Chronic Disease, 11*, E109. doi:10.5888/pcd11.130293

Stajkovic, A. D., & Luthans, F. (1998). Self-efficacy and work-related performance: A meta-analysis. *Psychological Bulletin, 124*, 240–261. doi:10.1037/0033-2909.124.2.240

Substance Abuse and Mental Health Services Administration. (2014). *Results from the 2014 National Survey on Drug Use and Health: Detailed tables.* Table 2.41B-

Alcohol use in lifetime, past year, and past month among persons aged 18 or older, by demographic characteristics: Percentages, 2013 and 2014. Retrieved from https://www.samhsa.gov/data/sites/default/files/NSDUH-DetTabs2014/NSDUH-Det-Tabs2014.pdf

Wilkey, C., Lundgren, L., & Amodeo, M. (2013). Addiction training in social work schools: A nationwide analysis. *Journal of Social Work Practice in the Addictions*, *13*(2), 192–210.

World Health Organization. (2014). *Global status report on alcohol and health 2014.* Retrieved from http://www.who.int/substance_abuse/publications/global_alcohol_report/msb_gsr_2014_1.pdf?ua+1

SBIRT Training in Social Work Education: Evaluating Change Using Standardized Patient Simulation

PAUL SACCO, PhD

LAURA TING, PhD

TAYLOR BERENS CROUCH, MA

LINDSAY EMERY, MS

MELISSA MORELAND, BA

CHARLOTTE BRIGHT, PhD and JODI FREY, PhD

CARLO DiCLEMENTE, PhD

A grand challenge for social work is addressing widespread public health problems of alcohol misuse. MSW students (n = 83) received Screening, Brief Intervention, and Referral to Treatment (SBIRT) training through didactic sessions, role plays, and pre–post video-taped standardized patient (SP) interactions. SBIRT knowledge, self-reported practice behaviors, and confidence were assessed at pretest, 30 days, and 6 months posttest. Videos were coded to assess intervention-adherent behaviors. General linear mixed models analyzed changes. Participants demonstrated increased adherence to SBIRT behaviors, and knowledge, skills, and confidence increased posttraining. Findings suggest SBIRT training increases students' capacity to implement evidence-based interventions designed to reduce alcohol misuse.

According to the 2014 National Survey on Drug Use and Health (Substance Abuse and Mental Health Services Administration [SAMHSA], 2015a) alcohol is the most commonly used substance among Americans aged 12 years and older, with 139.7 million reporting using within the past 30 days, 60.9 million reporting binge episodes (four or five drinks at a time), and 16.3 million classified as heavy alcohol users, far surpassing usage of other dangerous substances. The same survey revealed that in the past month, 27 million people (10.2% of Americans) had used illicit drugs and 66.9 million people age 12 or older were currently using tobacco products (SAMHSA, 2015a).

The negative impacts of alcohol misuse and other substance abuse are well documented. Economically, alcohol misuse results in a collective loss of more than $223 billion per year, largely due to lost income. Medical and health problems, including early death, are both serious financial and public health consequences of alcohol misuse (Research Society on Alcoholism, 2011). Health problems related to alcohol misuse include accidents, injuries, and disease, as well as high comorbidity rates with mental disorders such as depression and bipolar disorder, and significant emotional and cognitive impairments (Begun, Clapp, & The Alcohol Misuse Grand Challenge Collective, 2016).

Alcohol misuse and substance abuse are highly relevant to social workers engaged in providing services to all populations, including individuals, families, or communities. Social workers could specialize in substance use settings, but also might encounter acute or chronic substance use as a contributing factor to many clients' presenting issues when working in a variety of other settings, including health and mental health care, child welfare, services for the aged, criminal justice and correctional facilities, employee assistance programs, or private practice (National Association of Social Workers, 2000; Standards for Social Work Practice with Clients with Substance Use Disorders Work Group, 2013). Therefore, it is imperative that all social workers, regardless of practice setting, be trained in recognizing substance use and be given the tools and skills to provide basic but crucial screening and evaluation. Furthermore, given that the social work profession uses a biopsychosocial framing to understand clients and address problems, the combination of factors associated with alcohol misuse (e.g., biological vulnerability, sensation seeking, and peer influences) is particularly well suited to social work intervention (Begun et al., 2016)

Recently, the Grand Challenges for Social Work initiated by the American Academy of Social Work and Social Welfare further highlighted the importance of social workers addressing alcohol misuse (Begun et al., 2016) to advance social justice and well-being. Addressing the training and educational needs of future social workers to promote competence within the practice area of alcohol and substance misuse is a critical step toward improving the well-being of those we serve. With that purpose in mind, the goal of this study was to examine the effectiveness of a 15-hr stand-alone Screening, Brief Intervention, and Referral to Treatment (SBIRT) training for MSW students.

LITERATURE REVIEW

SBIRT is a recognized evidence-based intervention for reducing the risk of alcohol in the general population (Babor et al., 2007) and has been included in SAMHSA's National Registry of Evidence-Based Programs and Practices (U.S. Department of Health and Human Services, 2014). SBIRT is a public health approach designed to universally screen persons in a variety of medical settings, such as primary care (Agerwala & McCance-Katz, 2012; Mertens et al., 2015; Pitts & Shrier, 2014), emergency departments (Bernstein et al., 2009), and trauma centers (Madras et al., 2009). Practitioners using SBIRT then provide a brief intervention for those at risk for alcohol and other drug problems, and offer a referral to formal treatment to those with more severe substance use disorders (SAMHSA, 2015b). SBIRT was originally designed for primary care in medicine; however, its use has expanded beyond the medical and public health fields and is being used in employee assistance (McPherson, Goplerud, Derr, Mickenberg, & Courtemanche, 2010), school-based (Mitchell et al., 2012), and criminal justice (Prendergast & Cartier, 2013) programs, all of which are settings that employ social workers. Social work is clearly a profession that can benefit from this model (Bliss & Pecukonis, 2009).

Traditionally, social work students have believed that they must be working in addiction treatment centers or with substance abuse as the primary issue to learn and apply these screening and intervention techniques. However, SBIRT represents a paradigm shift in social work, integrating universal screening from a public health model. Training aims to make apparent the connection between universal social work skills and SBIRT techniques, using motivational interviewing approaches that allow the social worker to guide the client in behavioral change to prevent the occurrence of more severe and debilitating substance-related conditions and consequences (SAMHSA, 2015b). SBIRT provides social workers with early assessment and intervention tools for clients they might encounter in a wide range of settings beyond those that typically serve clients with substance abuse problems. Given the plurality of social workers in helping positions with persons at all levels of risk, this shift has the potential to lead to greater integration of behavioral health into all areas of social work practice.

Screening and brief intervention practice is an effective and feasible approach for social workers. Bliss and Pecukonis (2009) praised the simplicity of the screening and brief intervention approach and argued that this model provides social workers who do not specialize in substance abuse with a starting point to be able to work comfortably and knowledgeably with clients who present with less severe substance use issues. A more complex and time-intensive approach might, in fact, deter social workers from attempting to address substance use problems at all, which would be a disservice to their clients and a departure from their duty to serve vulnerable people. A brief method also does not preclude the use of additional, more comprehensive tools in the treatment of individuals with more serious substance use patterns. SBIRT, therefore, is a model that can be adopted and integrated in various social work practice settings and used universally with all clients once social workers are trained.

Standardized Patients

The use of standardized patients (SPs) in teaching and training students has been common in medical and nursing education (Baer et al., 2004; Barwick, Bennett, Johnson, McGowan, & Moore, 2012; Madson, Loignon, & Lane, 2009), but few studies have used SPs and simulation for social work education (Logie, Bogo, Regehr, & Regehr, 2013). One major advantage of using SPs is the ability to methodically and systematically present behaviors and scenarios relevant to training goals. Duckham, Huang, and Tunney (2013) argued the merits of using SPs in social work education over student-to-student role plays as part of experiential learning and noted its effectiveness in developing clinical skills. However, the use of SPs has also been criticized. One disadvantage and criticism of using SPs is that behaviors presented by the actors might not be realistic in terms of how actual clients might respond in situations beyond their scripts. If trainees present the SPs with unexpected responses, the actors might be unable to respond readily, let alone spontaneously, but are limited by the scripted responses, which restricts the interaction and learning experience (Miller, Yahne, Moyers, Martinez, & Pirritano, 2004).

Logie and colleagues (2013) reviewed the limited research on the use of SPs in social work education (none specifically on SBIRT) and found students were generally receptive to the learning experience. Others note that evaluating student interactions with SPs might be an evidence-based method to assess direct practice skills in students (Rawlings, 2012) as long as the assessment in itself is reliable and valid. DiClemente, Crouch, Norwood, Delahanty, and Welsh (2015) addressed the need for reliable and valid measures of behavioral interactions through the development of a coding scheme used with medical residents learning SBIRT with SPs. Other studies training medical residents in SBIRT have used SPs (Swiggart, Ghulyan, & Dewey, 2012; Wamsley et al., 2013; Whittle, Buckelew, Satterfield, Lum, & O'Sullivan, 2015) with positive results, but not all used reliable measures to code trainee behaviors with SPs.

The effectiveness of using SPs as a means of teaching and evaluating social work students needs further exploration, and this study hopes to add to the limited research available. Specifically, the main purpose of this study was to evaluate the effectiveness of a 15-hr stand-alone SBIRT course with the use of standardized patients. The hypotheses were as follows:

1. MSW students who have completed the stand-alone SBIRT course would show increases in knowledge and confidence in SBIRT skills and maintain these gains over time;
2. MSW students would report using SBIRT skills more frequently in their practice settings and field practicum after SBIRT training.
3. MSW students would demonstrate improvement and more behavioral adherence in using SBIRT skills after taking the course as evaluated using pre- and post-SP interactions.

METHOD

Participants

The sample in this study included four classes of MSW students who enrolled in a stand-alone SBIRT course. There were 83 total participants enrolled in the class that was offered four times over the course of two academic years (2014–2015 and 2015–2016), cotaught by the same two instructors. The course was an optional elective and made available to all students in the MSW program. One credit was awarded to students who took the course. Fifty students completed training in April and June 2015 and another 33 students completed training in January and April 2016. All 83 students completed preassessment measures, 71 students (85.6%) completed postassessment measures at a 30-day follow-up, and 37 students (44.5%) completed 6-month follow-up assessments.

Procedures

After institutional review board approval was secured, MSW students were recruited through the school's "Daily Bulletin" announcements, as well as through the online course catalog. A 15-hr course was offered to eligible students at no cost, and students were accepted into the course until the

maximum enrollment of 30 was reached. Four cohorts of students participated. Students provided informed consent and could elect to not have their
data used for research; however, all students participated in 20-min SP interviews pre- and posttraining. In between the SP interviews, participants
received didactic instruction with SAMHSA's SBIRT training modules specially
adapted for MSW students. In addition to instruction, students interacted in a
number of role-play and experiential exercises designed to familiarize them
with the intervention, build behavioral skills, and foster positive attitudes
about individuals who display at-risk substance use patterns.

The SPs were trained by the principal investigator and research team
members using specific cases that were created to mimic real situations in
which clients received services from social workers. The pre- and posttest
case were similar in terms of the client's substance use severity (e.g., a client
being referred by an employer to an Employee Assistance Program social
worker due to concerns with work productivity impacted by alcohol use). SP
training entailed meetings to discuss the cases, how to portray the client (e.g.,
demeanor, responses), and how to respond to hypothetical behaviors from
the social worker in a standardized manner. For example, if the social work
student labeled or confronted the client, the client would react negatively with
denial or minimization, or become engaged and forthcoming if treated with
respect and empathy. SPs were professionals provided by the Clinical Education and Evaluation Lab (CEEL), a training facility dedicated to the evaluation,
assessment, and teaching of clinical skills that is supported jointly by the
university's School of Nursing and School of Medicine. All SP interviews
were videotaped and student participants' videos were identified by an ID
number.

In addition, to evaluate training effectiveness, participants completed
questionnaires before the training, at 30 days posttraining and 6 months afterward, using a unique identification code they created for tracking and
confidentiality. Participants were compensated with a $10 Amazon.com gift
card for completing the 6-month follow-up survey. All follow-up surveys were
conducted via Qualtrics, a Web-based survey platform.

Measures

SBIRT CONFIDENCE, KNOWLEDGE, AND BEHAVIORS

Students completed a self-report questionnaire assessing SBIRT confidence,
knowledge, and behaviors at pretraining, 30 days, and 6 months posttraining. Nine items assessed students' confidence to perform SBIRT activities,
using an 11-point Likert-type scale ranging from *not at all confident* to
extremely confident. For the confidence measure, Cronbach's α values
were between .95 at pretest and .87 at the 6-month follow-up. The knowledge portion included 10 multiple-choice questions addressing the SBIRT

steps, risky drinking limits, referral procedures, and other SBIRT-related facts. Reliability for this measure was fair to poor ($\alpha = .32–.66$), suggesting that knowledge items had relatively poor consistency. In addition to knowledge questions about SBIRT, students were provided with a case example and asked a series of 20 true–false questions to assess familiarity with SBIRT-adherent responses. Specifically, students were presented with a series of provider responses to a sample case (e.g., "You should know that smoking during pregnancy is dangerous") and asked to state whether the responses would motivate change (*true*) or not (*false*). These case-based questions displayed better reliability, in the excellent range (see Table 1). The behaviors portion of the assessment consisted of 20 questions that queried students about the frequency with which they screened for substance use (12 items), conducted brief interventions (8 items), and referred for treatment (16 items). Each component of the behaviors instrument included separate questions for alcohol, tobacco, illicit drugs, and prescription drug use, and questions used a 5-point Likert-type response scale ranging from *never* to *always*. Similar to other scales, the reliability of SBIRT behavior

TABLE 1 Intervention Target Variables

Variable	n	M	SD	Theoretical Range	Actual Range	Alpha	ICC
Confidence				1–11			0
Pretest	83	6.15	1.87		1.11–10.00	.95	
30-day	70	9.03	1.11		6.78–11.00	.90	
6-month	37	8.88	.99		7.22–10.88	.87	
Knowledge				0–1			.27
Pretest	83	.58	.16		.20–.90	.32	
30-day	71	.74	.13		.40–1.00	.66	
6 month	37	.70	.16		.30–1.00	.47	
Sample cases				0–1			.18
Pretest	83	.91	.07		.70–1.00	.95	
30-day	71	.92	.13		0–1.00	.96	
6-month	37	.92	.06		.75–1.00	.96	
Screening				1–5			.68
Pretest	76	2.80	1.19		1–5	.96	
30-day	58	3.02	1.10		1–5	.96	
6month	33	3.07	1.17		1–5	.95	
Brief intervention				1–5			.70
Pretest	76	2.28	1.11		1–5	.96	
30-day	58	2.60	1.18		1–5	.96	
6-month	34	2.45	1.06		1–5	.95	
Referral for treatment				1–5			.62
Pretest	76	1.84	1.03		1–5	.95	
30-day	58	2.13	1.16		1–5	.95	
6-month	34	2.08	.98		1–4.33	.95	
SP-SBIRT adherent				0–∞			.07
Pretest	81	11.59	4.04		0–22		
Posttest	74	15.50	3.94		5–24		

Note: SP = standardized patient; SBIRT = Screening, Brief Intervention, and Referral for Treatment.

subscales, Screening (.95–.96), Brief Intervention (.95–.96), and Referral for Treatment (.95) were all excellent (see Table 1).

MD3 SBIRT CODING SCALE

Students' 20-min SP interactions were videotaped and coded using the MD3 SBIRT Coding Scale (DiClemente et al., 2015), which evaluates 14 SBIRT-adherent ("desirable") behaviors, seven SBIRT-nonadherent ("undesirable") behaviors, and two global skills, communication and empathy. The scale was developed to evaluate SBIRT fidelity for the purpose of assessing training or evaluation outcomes and has produced high interrater reliability in previous studies (DiClemente et al., 2015; Giudice et al., 2015). Adherent behaviors coded include skills such as "open-ended questions," "reflections," "assess readiness to change," "respectful advice giving," and "goal setting and/or developing a plan," which are coded on a 3-point Likert-type scale based on frequency and quality of the behavior. Nonadherent behaviors are coded as behavior counts and include such items as "warning/threatening," "untimely or disrespectful advice giving," and "lecturing and/or using jargon." The two global ratings, collaboration and empathy, are coded on a 5-point Likert-type scale. For this study, only adherent behaviors were used in analysis, as nonadherent behaviors were rare at pretest and posttest.

Two trained graduate-level research assistants coded the videos using a detailed coding guide (DiClemente et al., 2015) that includes scale anchors, behavioral descriptions, and examples. Twenty percent of videos were double-coded to assess interrater reliability. Videos were covered during coding and only audio was used to ensure confidentiality. Coders were blinded to whether each video was pretraining or posttraining and whether the video was double-coded.

Interrater reliability was estimated using a two-way random model intraclass correlation coefficient (ICC), which measures rater consistency while adjusting for both chance agreement and systematic differences between raters, and is therefore a more conservative estimate than Cronbach's alpha or the Pearson product–moment correlation. ICCs were estimated separately for ratings of adherent behaviors (.92), nonadherent behaviors (.86), total points (.96; adherent minus nonadherent points), and global ratings (.82). ICCs were all in the "excellent" range (Cicchetti, 1994).

SOCIODEMOGRAPHIC AND SUBSTANCE USE CORRELATES

Age in years, race, undergraduate major, year in the program, field of practice, and field placement setting were based on self-report per the categories listed in Table 2. Questions focused on smoking were based on 100 cigarettes (lifetime use) and use of cigarettes in the past 30 days (current use). An individual was considered to have a positive family history or substance problems if they endorsed a family member having a problem with alcohol, illicit drugs, or prescription drugs. Individuals who reported drinking at least 1 day per week in college were considered frequent drinkers, and any past use of illicit or nonmedical use of prescription drugs was considered a positive for college drug use. If a student reported that most of his or her friends or all

TABLE 2 Participant Sociodemographic and Substance Use

Variable	M or %	n
Age, M (SD)	31.4 (8.8)	83
Female gender	91.6	76
Race		
Black or African American	32.5	27
White	54.2	45
Asian or Pacific Islander	7.2	6
Biracial or multiracial	4.8	4
Ethnicity		
Hispanic or Latina/o	4.8	4
Undergraduate major		
Social work	27.7	23
Psychology	26.5	22
Sociology	6.0	5
Psychology & sociology	2.4	2
Other	37.3	31
Year in the program		
First year foundation	19.3	16
First year advanced standing	9.6	8
Second year	71.1	59
Current field of practice		
Behavioral health	60.2	50
Families and children	21.7	18
Community action and social policy	7.2	6
Health	6.0	5
Aging	3.6	3
Current field placement setting		
Medical (e.g., inpatient)	14.5	12
Mental health	30.1	25
Employee assistance program	6.0	5
School or educational facility	8.4	7
Social service agency (government)	9.6	8
Social services (community-based)	14.5	12
Other	7.2	6
Smoking status		
Current smoker	6.1	5
Lifetime smoker	15.9	13
Substance use		
Family history of substance problems	45.8	38
Frequent college drinker (1+ week)	44.6	37
Peer college alcohol use (most friends drank)	85.5	71
Any college drug use	54.2	45

Note: n = 83.

of his or her friends drank, the student was categorized as having a college peer network with extensive alcohol use.

Data Analysis

Data analyses were conducted in two steps. First, univariate analyses were conducted to describe the sample of students in the class, and mean values were derived for repeated measures as a preliminary analysis for models of change over time. Specifically, we calculated ICCs, and measures of central tendency for all repeated measures.

Following descriptive analyses, regression models were used to assess the effectiveness of the training on various aspects of student knowledge, confidence, and behaviors. To assess changes in SBIRT knowledge, confidence, frequency of behaviors, and demonstrated SBIRT fidelity using SPs, we used multilevel linear regression modeling (MLM). Also called hierarchical linear models or mixed models, MLMs are used in analysis where sampling design violates the assumption of independence necessary in standard linear regression. In repeated measures analysis, observations are nested within person, in that the same person is measured repeatedly over time (in this analysis, two or three times, depending on the measure). When using MLM, model standard errors are corrected for this so-called dependency in the data. Moreover, MLM has the advantage of modeling missing data on dependent variables under the assumption of missing at random. In these analyses, we used SAS PROC MIXED (SAS Institute, 2008) specifying a correlated error structure using either an unstructured or compound symmetry structure (Moser, 2004) based on measures of model fit including the Akaike's information criterion (AIC) and the Bayesian information criterion (BIC). This approach allows for adjustment of standard errors for autocorrelation.

Specific models were constructed using time as a dummy-coded variable, with the pretest as the reference category. These time points were then regressed on knowledge, confidence, and behavior measures. Using this method, change from pre- to posttest and pretest to 6-month follow-up can be compared separately. Coefficients and adjusted means were computed to display level of change at 30 days and at 6 months. Once data were analyzed, Cohen's d statistics were calculated for each time point predictor (e.g., posttest and 6-month follow-up) as a measure of effect size (see Table 3).

RESULTS

Characteristics of the Sample

Consistent with the sociodemographic makeup of MSW education (Council on Social Work Education, 2014), our sample was largely female (91.6%) and young adult (M age = 31). Students primarily specialized in behavioral health

TABLE 3 Multilevel Modeling of 30-Day Posttest and 6-Month Follow-Up Variables

	Posttest (30 Day)					6 Month					Model Fit		
	b	SE	t	p	d	b	SE	t	p	d	$^{LR}\chi^2$	df	p
Confidence	2.85	.18	16.20	<.001	1.53	2.92	.21	14.01	<.001	1.57	81.86	5	<.001
Knowledge	.16	.02	8.60	<.001	1.02	.11	.02	4.50	<.001	.68	28.98	5	<.001
Sample cases	.01	.01	.49	.63	.07	.02	.02	.96	.34	.18	2.46	1	.11
Screening	.18	.10	1.85	.07	.06	.41	.18	2.32	.02	.28	66.04	5	<.001
Brief intervention	.34	.11	3.15	.002	.30	.36	.13	2.74	.007	.33	66.87	1	<.001
Referral for treatment	.34	.12	2.93	.004	.32	.35	.14	2.40	.02	.32	48.81	1	<.001
SP-SBIRT adherent	3.56	.68	5.25	<.001	.74	—	—	—	—	—	3.43	1	.06

Note. SP = standardized patient; SBIRT = Screening, Brief Intervention, and Referral for Treatment.

(60.2%) and most were in their second year of the program (71.1%) or entered the program with advanced standing status (9.6%). The locations where students did their field placements varied and were most commonly mental health settings (30.1%). In terms of substance use history among students, 45.0% reported some family history of alcohol or drug problems and more than half of the students reported peer alcohol use in college. Table 2 highlights additional sociodemographic, educational, and substance use information about the sample.

Information on repeated measures is provided in Table 1. Consistent with the short-term nature of the SBIRT training, change tended to occur at the 30-day follow-up and then leveled off. Based on ICC measures, some variables showed more stability over time than others. For instance, a null model of the Confidence scale across the three time points estimated 0% proportion of variance explained at the person level. The Knowledge (.27) and Sample Cases (.18) showed a moderate between-person level of variability, suggesting that 27% of the variance in the Knowledge scale and 18% of the Sample case questions can be explained by person-level differences. ICC values for the SBIRT behavior measures were much higher, ranging from .62 to .70, meaning that a high proportion of the variance in these scales can be explained by between-person variance. In terms of behaviors observed for pre- and post-SP exercises, 7% of the variance is attributable to between-person variance. See Table 1 for a complete listing of ICC values by repeated measures.

Multilevel Change Models

Separate multilevel linear regression models were conducted using a dummy-coded time variable with pretest as the reference category. For the Confidence scale, confidence increased substantially from pretest to posttest ($b = 2.85$, $t = 16.20$ $p < .001$; $d = 1.53$), and leveled off, remaining significantly higher than pretest ($b = 2.92$, $t = 14.01$ $p < .001$; $d = 1.57$). See Figure 1 for a graphical display showing change in adjusted means with standard errors.

Changes in the knowledge measure were also significant, but less pronounced than change in confidence (see Figure 1). At 30 days postintervention, students' scores on the knowledge test improved ($b = .16$, $t = 8.60$, $p < .001$; $d = 1.02$), but improvement leveled off at the 6-month follow-up ($b = .11$, $t = 4.50$, $p < .001$; $d = .68$). For the questions focused on a sample case, there were no changes from pretest through 6-month follow-up. This is likely a result of ceiling effects on the measure, as scores were greater than 90% at all time points.

The specific questions about self-reported SBIRT-related behaviors (see Figure 1) showed significant but relatively small increases in screening, but only at 6 months ($b = .41$, $t = 2.32$, $p < .02$; $d = .28$). Use of brief interventions increased in frequency at both 30 days ($b = .34$, $t = 3.15$,

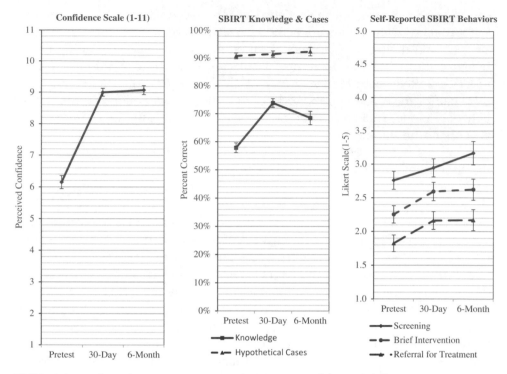

FIGURE 1   Adjusted means at pretest, 30-day posttest, and 6-month follow-up. *Note*: SBIRT = Screening, Brief intervention, and Referral to Treatment.

$p < .002$; $d = .30$) and 6 months ($b = .36$, $t = 2.74$, $p < .007$; $d = .32$). Changes in referral for treatment were similar in that they were significant, but modest (30-day: $b = .34$, $t = 2.93$, $p = .004$; $d = .32$; 6 month: $b = .35$, $t = 2.40$, $p = .02$; $d = .32$)

Measures of standardized patient SBIRT adherence showed moderate changes in SBIRT behaviors from pretest to posttest (Figure 2) at the end of the training ($b = .36$, $t = 2.74$, $p < .007$; $d = .32$). Students displayed an increase in approximately three SBIRT behaviors following the training. Although SBIRT nonadherence behaviors were also counted, we did not include them because they showed floor effects. Few students displayed even one non-adherent behavior, even at pretest.

DISCUSSION

Alcohol misuse is indeed a Grand Challenge for social workers, due to its consequences to individuals, families, and society (Begun et al., 2016). To respond effectively, the profession needs tools that are flexible enough to apply across practice settings and populations (Bliss & Pecukonis, 2009).

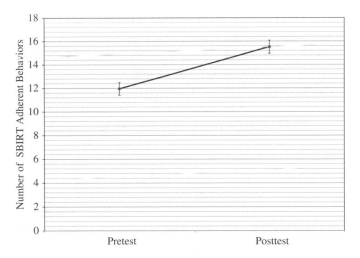

FIGURE 2 Adjusted means at pretest and posttest of Screening, Brief Intervention, and Referral to Treatment (SBIRT)-adherent behaviors.

SBIRT offers a potential avenue for responding to this Grand Challenge. This intervention strategy is useful in multiple settings and has been shown to be effective in responding to risky drinking as well as alcohol abuse or dependence (SAMHSA, 2015b).

Our findings suggest that specific stand-alone training in SBIRT can lead to the development of SBIRT competencies by social work students and support the Grand Challenge of preventing alcohol misuse and its consequences (Begun et al., 2016). Moreover, we found evidence of increased use of SBIRT techniques in practice posttraining. This is an important first step to addressing the Grand Challenge; by making SBIRT training available to any MSW student, we hope to show that this method can be disseminated broadly rather than just to those in specialty substance use settings.

Consistent with existing literature on transfer of learning, our findings demonstrate that attitudes and intentions are more immediately malleable than actual behavior (Austin, Weisner, Schrandt, Glezos-Bell, & Murtaza, 2006). In our case, we found that postsession behavioral competency and increases in students' confidence were large compared to relatively modest changes in self-reported SBIRT behaviors at 30 days and 6 months. However, motivation to apply a behavior is a moderator of behavior change itself (Blume, Ford, Baldwin, & Huang, 2010) and a precursor to intentions to implement a new behavior (Yamkovenko & Holton, 2010). Attitudes toward behavior are part of a complex interplay between learning and doing (Weisweiler, Nikitopoulos, Netzel, & Frey, 2013).

The use of SPs is believed to enhance learning transfer by providing practice opportunities (Nestel, Groom, Eikeland-Husebo, & O'Donnell, 2011). It could be that the confidence increases are driven by gains in perceived self-efficacy following student interactions with SPs. The SP, therefore, appears to be functioning as intended with respect to growth in competence. Through the SP interactions, MSW students showed that they were able to learn and apply SBIRT's elements in a structured setting.

MSW students might face challenges to immediate implementation of SBIRT in their practice due to features outside their control. For example, they might lack access to appropriate clients in field placements, or they could be limited in their authority to implement new practices. Also, given the timing of some trainings (e.g., end of the spring semester), students might not have been in field placement with access to clients within the 30-day follow-up period. Future research can employ longer follow-up periods to determine whether MSW graduates are able to implement SBIRT when they move from the student role to practitioner status. The ability to demonstrate beginning proficiency in simulation is encouraging, nonetheless.

STRENGTHS AND LIMITATIONS

Overall, this study's strengths include the use of valid measures and innovative assessment of student learning using standardized patients and behavioral coding. The SBIRT curriculum developed by SAMHSA and adapted by the research team reflects best practices in this intervention, and the outcomes suggest that students can carry out the SBIRT intervention with fidelity. Nonetheless, this project has a number of limitations. Sample size at 6 months was low, in part because the most recent class of students had not yet received their 6-month follow-up assessments. Although methods were used to model data with a missing time point, it is possible that surveys of nonresponders at 6 months were distinct from responders and not missing at random. Similarly, standardized patient assessments were conducted at pretest and posttest only, so there were no data to determine behavioral competency at 6 months posttraining. It is possible that competencies erode over time after SBIRT training, especially without further practice of skills or additional supervision or training; however, because of the evaluation design, we were not able to answer this question.

Additionally, because students volunteered for this training, it is possible that those who took part in the class might be distinct (e.g., greater interest in alcohol and other substance use, or higher levels of knowledge or confidence in this area). Therefore, they might not be typical MSW students, and generalizability cannot be assumed. Reliability of certain measures (specifically the knowledge subscale) was poor, which is a measurement issue that future research should address. Finally, this study was not designed as a randomized trial of SBIRT implementation and as such, did not include a comparison or control group.

CONCLUSIONS

To effectively meet the Grand Challenge and respond to alcohol misuse, social workers will need a complex set of tools. SBIRT offers a clear advantage in that it can be applied universally in direct practice. The evidence supporting SBIRT's effectiveness at reducing alcohol misuse is encouraging (Babor et al., 2007). SBIRT is an ideal tool for social workers who serve diverse client groups and do not necessarily specialize in substance abuse. Additionally, SBIRT has the benefit of addressing risky alcohol use, rather than simply responding to abuse or dependence. This study suggests that social work students can learn SBIRT skills and gain confidence in their ability to apply these skills. Moreover, SBIRT can be integrated into an MSW curriculum as a one-credit stand-alone course.

The question of how to integrate SBIRT more comprehensively into the curriculum remains. MSW education requires a broad set of generalist and specialist skills, and SBIRT training requires some allocation of student and instructor time. Standardized patients are a valuable but resource-intensive addition to the curriculum. Future research can explore whether similar success follows a shorter exposure across sections of a foundation course, and whether standardized patients are substantially superior to in-class role-play experiences, as well as whether practice change is initiated postgraduation.

FUNDING

This article was supported by Grant 1U79TI025379-01 from the Center for Substance Abuse Treatment.

ORCID

Paul Sacco ⓘ http://orcid.org/0000-0002-2800-9571

REFERENCES

Agerwala, S. M., & McCance-Katz, E. (2012). Integrating Screening, Brief Intervention, and Referral to Treatment (SBIRT) into clinical practice settings: A brief review. *Journal of Psychoactive Drugs, 44*, 307–317. doi:10.1080/02791072.2012.720169
Austin, M. J., Weisner, S., Schrandt, E., Glezos-Bell, S., & Murtaza, N. (2006). Exploring the transfer of learning from an executive development program for human services managers. *Administration in Social Work, 30*(2), 71–90. doi:10.1300/J147v30n0206

Babor, T. F., McRee, B. G., Kassebaum, P. A., Grimaldi, P. L., Ahmed, K., & Bray, J. (2007). Screening, Brief Intervention, and Referral to Treatment (SBIRT): Toward a public health approach to the management of substance abuse. *Substance Abuse, 28*(3), 7–30. doi:10.1300/J465v28n03_03

Baer, J. S., Rosengren, D. B., Dunn, C. W., Wells, E. A., Ogle, R. L., & Hartzler, B. (2004). An evaluation of workshop training in motivational interviewing for addiction and mental health clinicians. *Drug and Alcohol Dependence, 73*, 99–106. doi:10.1016/j.drugalcdep.2003.10.001

Barwick, M. A., Bennett, L. M., Johnson, S. N., McGowan, J., & Moore, J. E. (2012). Training health and mental health professionals in motivational interviewing: A systematic review. *Children and Youth Services Review, 34*, 1786–1795. doi:10.1016/j.childyouth.2012.05.012

Begun, A. L., Clapp, J. D., & The Alcohol Misuse Grand Challenge Collective. (2016). Reducing and preventing alcohol misuse and its consequences: A Grand Challenge for social work. *The International Journal of Alcohol and Drug Research, 5*(2), 73–83. doi:10.7895/ijadr.v5i2.223

Bernstein, E., Topp, D., Shaw, E., Girard, C., Pressman, K., Woolcock, E., & Bernstein, J. (2009). A preliminary report of knowledge translation: Lessons from taking screening and brief intervention techniques from the research setting into regional systems of care. *Academic Emergency Medicine, 16*, 1225–1233. doi:10.1111/j.1553-2712.2009.00516.x

Bliss, D. L., & Pecukonis, E. (2009). Screening and brief intervention practice model for social workers in non-substance-abuse practice settings. *Journal of Social Work Practice in the Addictions, 9*(1), 21–40. doi:10.1080/15332560802646604

Blume, B. D., Ford, J. K., Baldwin, T. T., & Huang, J. L. (2010). Transfer of training: A meta-analytic review. *Journal of Management, 36*, 1065–1105. doi:10.1177/0149206309352880

Cicchetti, D. V. (1994). Guidelines, criteria, and rules of thumb for evaluating normed and standardized assessment instruments in psychology. *Psychological Assessment, 6*(4), 284–290. doi:10.1037/1040-3590.6.4.284

Council on Social Work Education. (2014). *Annual statistics on social work education in the United States*. Washington, DC: Author. Retrieved from http://www.cswe.org/file.aspx?id=82845

DiClemente, C. C., Crouch, T. B., Norwood, A. E., Delahanty, J., & Welsh, C. (2015). Evaluating training of Screening, Brief Intervention, and Referral to Treatment (SBIRT) for substance use: Reliability of the MD3 SBIRT Coding Scale. *Psychology of Addictive Behaviors, 29*(1), 218–224. doi:10.1037/adb0000022

Duckham, B. C., Huang, H.-H., & Tunney, K. J. (2013). Theoretical support and other considerations in using simulated clients to educate social workers. *Smith College Studies in Social Work, 83*, 481–496. doi:10.1080/00377317.2013.834756

Giudice, E. L., Lewin, L. O., Welsh, C., Crouch, T. B., Wright, K. S., Delahanty, J., & DiClemente, C. C. (2015). Online versus in-person Screening, Brief Intervention, and Referral to Treatment training in pediatrics residents. *Journal of Graduate Medical Education, 7*(1), 53–58. doi:10.4300/JGME-D-14-00367.1

Logie, C., Bogo, M., Regehr, C., & Regehr, G. (2013). A critical appraisal of the use of standardized client simulations in social work education. *Journal of Social Work Education, 49*(1), 66–80. doi:10.1080/10437797.2013.755377

Madras, B. K., Compton, W. M., Avula, D., Stegbauer, T., Stein, J. B., & Clark, H. W. (2009). Screening, brief interventions, referral to treatment (SBIRT) for illicit drug and alcohol use at multiple healthcare sites: Comparison at intake and 6 months later. *Drug and Alcohol Dependence, 99*(1–3), 280–295. doi:10.1016/j.drugalcdep.2008.08.003

Madson, M. B., Loignon, A. C., & Lane, C. (2009). Training in motivational interviewing: A systematic review. *Journal of Substance Abuse Treatment, 36*(1), 101–109. doi:10.1016/j.jsat.2008.05.005

McPherson, T. L., Goplerud, E., Derr, D., Mickenberg, J., & Courtemanche, S. (2010). Telephonic screening and brief intervention for alcohol misuse among workers contacting the employee assistance program: A feasibility study. *Drug and Alcohol Review, 29*, 641–646. doi:10.1111/j.1465-3362.2010.00249.x

Mertens, J. R., Chi, F. W., Weisner, C. M., Satre, D. D., Ross, T. B., Allen, S., … Sterling, S. A. (2015). Physician versus non-physician delivery of alcohol screening, brief intervention and referral to treatment in adult primary care: The ADVISe cluster randomized controlled implementation trial. *Addiction Science & Clinical Practice, 10*(1), 1–17. doi:10.1186/s13722-015-0047-0

Miller, W. R., Yahne, C. E., Moyers, T. B., Martinez, J., & Pirritano, M. (2004). A randomized trial of methods to help clinicians learn motivational interviewing. *Journal of Consulting and Clinical Psychology, 72*, 1050–1062. doi:10.1037/0022-006X.72.6.1050

Mitchell, S. G., Gryczynski, J., Gonzales, A., Moseley, A., Peterson, T., O'Grady, K. E., & Schwartz, R. P. (2012). Screening, Brief Intervention, and Referral to Treatment (SBIRT) for substance use in a school-based program: Services and outcomes. *American Journal on Addictions, 21*(Suppl. 1), S5–S13. doi:10.1111/j.1521-0391.2012.00299.x

Moser, E. B. (2004, May). *Repeated measures modeling with PROC MIXED*. Paper presented at the the 29th SAS Users Group International Conference, Montreal, Canada. Retrieved from http://www2.sas.com/proceedings/sugi29/toc.html

National Association of Social Workers. (2000). *Practice area*. PRN: Practice Research Network. Retrieved from http://www.socialworkers.org/naswprn/surveyOne/area.pdf

National Institute on Alcohol Abuse and Alcoholism. (2007). *Helping patients who drink too much: A clinician's guide* (NIH Publication No. 07-3769). Bethesda, MD: National Institutes of Health.

Nestel, D. P., Groom, J. P. C., Eikeland-Husebo, S. M. R. N., & O'Donnell, J. M. D. M. S. N. C. (2011). Simulation for learning and teaching procedural skills: The state of the science. *Simulation in Healthcare: the Journal of the Society for Simulation in Healthcare, 6*(Suppl. 7), S10–S13. doi:10.1097/SIH.0b013e318227ce96

Pitts, S., & Shrier, L. A. (2014). Substance abuse screening and brief intervention for adolescents in primary care. *Pediatric Annals, 43*, e248–e252. doi:10.3928/00904481-20140924-09

Prendergast, M. L., & Cartier, J. J. (2013). Screening, Brief Intervention, and Referral to Treatment (SBIRT) for offenders: Protocol for a pragmatic randomized trial. *Addiction Science & Clinical Practice, 8*(1), 16. doi:10.1186/1940-0640-8-16

Rawlings, M. A. (2012). Assessing BSW student direct practice skill using standardized clients and self-efficacy theory. *Journal of Social Work Education, 48*, 553–576. doi:10.5175/JSWE.2012.201000070

Research Society on Alcoholism. (2011). *Impact of alcoholism and alcohol induced disease on America*. Retrieved from http://www.rsoa.org/2011-04-11RSAWhitePaper.pdf

SAS Institute Inc. (2008). The mixed procedure. In SAS Institute (Ed.), *SAS/STAT user's guide* (pp. 3886–4086). Cary, NC: SAS Institute Inc.

Standards for Social Work Practice with Clients with Substance Use Disorders Work Group. (2013). *NASW standards for social work practice with clients with substance use disorders*. Washington, DC: National Association of Social Workers.

Substance Abuse and Mental Health Services Administration. (2015a). *Behavioral health trends in the United States: Results from the 2014 national survey on drug use and health* (HHS Publication No. SMA 15-4927, NSDUH Series H-50). Retrieved from https://www.samhsa.gov/data/sites/default/files/NSDUH-FRR1-2014/NSDUH-FRR1-2014.pdf

Substance Abuse and Mental Health Services Administration. (2015b). *Screening, Brief Intervention, and Referral to Treatment*. Retrieved from https://www.samhsa.gov/sbirt

Swiggart, W. H., Ghulyan, M. V., & Dewey, C. M. (2012). Using standardized patients in continuing medical education courses on proper prescribing of controlled substances. *Substance Abuse, 33*, 182–185. doi:10.1080/08897077.2011.640217

U.S. Department of Health and Human Services. (2014). *NREPP: SAMHSA's National Registry of Evidence-based Programs and Practices*. Retrieved from https://www.samhsa.gov/nrepp

Wamsley, M. A., Julian, K. A., O'Sullivan, P., Satterfield, J. M., Satre, D. D., McCance-Katz, E., & Batki, S. L. (2013). Designing standardized patient assessments to measure SBIRT skills for residents: A literature review and case study. *Journal of Alcohol & Drug Education, 57*(1), 46–65.

Weisweiler, S., Nikitopoulos, A., Netzel, J., & Frey, D. (2013). Gaining insight to transfer of training through the lens of social psychology. *Educational Research Review, 8*, 14–27. doi:10.1016/j.edurev.2012.05.006

Whittle, A. E., Buckelew, S. M., Satterfield, J. M., Lum, P. J., & O'Sullivan, P. (2015). Addressing adolescent substance use: Teaching Screening, Brief Intervention, and Referral to Treatment (SBIRT) and motivational interviewing (MI) to residents. *Substance Abuse, 36*, 325–331. doi:10.1080/08897077.2014.965292

Yamkovenko, B., & Holton, E. (2010). Toward a theoretical model of dispositional influences on transfer of learning: A test of a structural model. *Human Resource Development Quarterly, 21*, 381–410. doi:10.1002/hrdq.20054

Evaluation of Alcohol Screening, Brief Intervention, and Referral to Treatment (SBIRT) Training for Social Workers

JENNIFER M. PUTNEY, PhD, LICSW

KIMBERLY H. M. O'BRIEN, PhD, LICSW

CALI-RYAN COLLIN, LICSW

ADELE LEVINE, MPH

Social work education is well positioned for workforce development initiatives that prepare practitioners to use Screening, Brief Intervention, and Referral to Treatment (SBIRT) with people at risk for alcohol use disorders. This article presents preliminary process and outcome evaluation data from the first year of a three-year grant which suggests that the training is acceptable and results in significant changes in trainees' knowledge, attitudes, and self-perceived SBIRT skills. Training was embedded within the curricula of an urban school of social work, which includes a Bachelor of Social Work (BSW) program and a single-concentration clinical Master of Social Work (MSW). Trainees included social work students (n = 134) and field instructors (n = 38). More than 90% of students were very satisfied or satisfied with the training, and 100% of field instructors rated the training as excellent or good. Students demonstrated significant changes from pre- to posttraining in substance use knowledge, confidence in SBIRT skills, and attitudes about integrating SBIRT into practice. Field instructors reported increased confidence in screening. Integrating SBIRT training into social work curriculum is a promising method of developing a workforce that can effectively prevent and alleviate alcohol misuse.

The Grand Challenges for Social Work Initiative has identified 12 priorities for social work researchers and practitioners. The Grand Challenges were selected based on their scope and significance, the potential for solving the problem, the capacity for measurable progress, the likelihood of cross-sector stakeholder collaboration, and the potential for groundbreaking innovation (Padilla & Fong, 2016). Taken together, this initiative provides a comprehensive agenda that mobilizes social work scientists, practitioners, and educators to have a significant impact on pressing social problems. Among the Grand Challenges is a focus on preventing and reducing harm associated with alcohol misuse (Begun, Clapp, & The Alcohol Misuse Grand Challenge Collective, 2016). Social workers are uniquely situated to identify and intervene with individuals who are at risk for alcohol misuse and alcohol use disorders (AUDs). This article highlights a workforce development initiative that addresses the Alcohol Misuse Grand Challenge; specifically, the article describes a training model for developing social work students' competencies in Screening, Brief Intervention, and Referral to Treatment (SBIRT). Additionally, it provides preliminary results of the training with social work students and field instructors.

PREVALENCE AND IMPACT OF ALCOHOL MISUSE

Alcohol misuse is a leading cause of preventable death in the United States. For each year between 2006 and 2010, alcohol misuse contributed to 88,000 deaths and 2.5 million years of potential life lost (Stahre, Roeber, Kanny, Brewer, & Zhang, 2014). It contributes to physical and mental health morbidity, including accidental injury, sexual risk behaviors, fetal alcohol spectrum disorders, exposure to infectious disease, alcohol-involved driving fatalities, and chronic disease (Hingson & Rehm, 2014).

Results from the 2014 National Survey on Drug Use and Health (NSDUH; $N = 67,901$) estimate that 60.9 million people age 12 and older engaged in binge drinking, defined as consuming five or more drinks on one occasion in the past 30 days. Of those, 16.3 million people engaged in past-month heavy drinking, which consists of five or more drinks on the same occasion on 5 or more days. Furthermore, 17 million people over the age of 12 had an AUD. Among all individuals surveyed who met criteria for a substance use disorder, four out of five had an AUD. Among those who needed treatment at a specialized treatment facility, only 8.9% received it (Center for Behavioral Health Statistics and Quality, 2015).

SBIRT AS A PRACTICE TO ALLEVIATE ALCOHOL MISUSE

SBIRT involves universal screening for alcohol misuse with validated screening tools, patient education as indicated by screening results, nonjudgmental engagement to increase at-risk clients' insight and motivation to change drinking behavior, and referral to brief treatment or specialized addiction treatment for those who need more intensive services (Babor et al., 2007). SBIRT is a cost-effective, empirically supported practice that aims to prevent and alleviate alcohol misuse and its consequences (O'Donnell et al., 2014). It effectively helps individuals change unhealthy patterns of alcohol use, especially among people who are not seeking treatment (Barbosa, Cowell, Bray, & Aldridge, 2015; O'Donnell et al., 2014).

The U.S. Preventative Services Task Force (USPSTF) recommends that clinicians in primary care settings routinely screen adults age 18 and over for alcohol misuse (Moyer, 2013). For patients who screen positive for alcohol misuse, the USPSTF recommends that practitioners provide brief interventions to reduce hazardous drinking. This recommendation is based on a systematic review of current evidence concerning the accuracy of screening approaches, the efficacy of alcohol screening on health outcomes, the effectiveness of brief interventions, the potential harms of screening and brief counseling interventions, and factors within the health care system that facilitate or constrain alcohol screening and brief interventions (Moyer, 2013).

Despite SBIRT's demonstrated effectiveness, health professionals do not routinely implement screenings, conduct brief interventions, or make targeted referrals (Tanner, Wilehelm, Rossie, & Metcalf, 2012). Less than one third of all primary care patients are screened for alcohol use, despite recommendations from the USPSTF (Seale et al., 2010). Analysis of *Behavioral Risk Factor Surveillance System* data ($N = 166,753$) demonstrated that in 2011, only one in six adults in the United States had ever discussed their alcohol use with a health care professional (McKnight-Eily et al., 2014). Among a nationally representative sample of adults, less than half of participants who had seen a doctor within the past year reported being screened for alcohol use (Hingson, Heeren, Edwards, & Saitz, 2012). Among patients who were screened and exceeded the low-risk drinking limits, less than one third received a brief intervention or brief advice from a health care provider.

SUBSTANCE USE WORKFORCE DEVELOPMENT IN THE CONTEXT OF HEALTH POLICY

Changes in health policy, namely the Patient Protection and Affordable Care Act (ACA) and the Mental Health Parity and Addiction Equity Act, have created a demand for trained social workers who can provide empirically based practice strategies (Wilkey, Lundgren, & Amodeo, 2013). However, the need for qualified social workers exceeds the available behavioral health workforce, as evidenced by the national shortage of qualified providers who have training in substance use assessment and treatment (Cochran, Roll, Jackson, & Kennedy, 2014; Institute of Medicine [IOM], 2006). The Bureau of Labor Statistics (2015) estimates a 19% employment growth in behavioral health between 2014 and 2024.

Additionally, health care reform has increased the integration of primary care and behavioral health services. Given the evidence base for SBIRT, qualified social workers are well positioned to provide alcohol use screening and assessment as interdisciplinary team members in integrated primary care settings (Tai & Volkow, 2013). Changes in health policies have reshaped access to, and reimbursement for, behavioral health services while increasing access to insurance and coverage of behavioral health treatment for millions of Americans (Mechanic, 2012). The USPSTF has classified SBIRT as a Category B clinical preventative service; therefore, insurance companies cannot require a copay for alcohol use screening and brief intervention.

SBIRT TRAINING IN SOCIAL WORK EDUCATION

Student Training

The roles of social workers in health care, mental health care, and social service settings often mean that they are among the first service providers to meet with clients (Hall, Amodeo, Shaffer, & Bilt, 2000). Failure to train social workers to provide patient-centered, evidence-based interventions, such as SBIRT, has serious individual, family, and community-level consequences (IOM, 2006). Yet, most social workers receive inadequate training in substance use prevention and treatment (Wilkey et al., 2013).

The current structure of alcohol and other drug use education in social work curriculum, training, and field education is inadequate to prepare future practitioners to competently identify and treat AUDs (Richardson, 2008). Insufficient education perpetuates social workers' negative attitudes toward persons misusing alcohol and further contributes to the shortage of qualified behavioral health professionals (Hall et al., 2000). Social work education must ensure new professionals develop the skills needed to address the magnitude of alcohol misuse (Quinn, 2010). Effective training, particularly within early career development, provides the skills and confidence necessary for SBIRT implementation (Tanner et al., 2012). Trainings that positively affect social workers' knowledge and attitudes toward alcohol use are necessary to provide patient-centered, respectful, and individualized care (IOM, 2006).

Field Instructor Training

Classroom-based learning alone might not adequately support and sustain SBIRT use in clinical practice. Support and mentorship in the field, especially for younger social workers, leads to a greater fund of knowledge and improved clinical practice with those who misuse alcohol (Galvani & Hughes, 2010). Medical education research supports the value of supervision for successful SBIRT application. Trained physician faculty, who operate as field supervisors in their precepting role, are necessary for medical students' use of SBIRT in practice (Childers et al., 2012). SBIRT trainings accompanied by ongoing instruction are more successfully integrated as an alcohol use intervention when compared to one-time instructional trainings (Agerwala & McCance-Katz, 2012). Based on evidence from the medical context, it stands to reason that ongoing instruction and supervision would support social workers' successful integration of SBIRT in practice. Although social work field instructors must mentor their students as they develop SBIRT competencies, instructors might not have the requisite knowledge, confidence, and skills to supervise students in its application.

Training Model

With funding from the Substance Abuse and Mental Health Services Administration (SAMHSA) for a three-year training grant, we sought to train social work students in the SBIRT model and train social work field instructors to support SBIRT adoption and sustainability in local health care and social service settings. The conceptual framework guiding the SBIRT training program and its proposed mechanisms of action is presented in Figure 1.

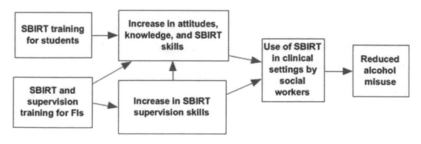

FIGURE 1 Conceptual model for screening, brief intervention, and referral to treatment (SBIRT) training.

Specifically, the training program simultaneously targeted the SBIRT attitudes, knowledge, and skills of students and field instructors, with an additional emphasis on supervision skills for field instructors. Based on the aforementioned evidence, we posit that by increasing SBIRT attitudes, knowledge, and skills, the likelihood of SBIRT use with clients will increase, which will lead to a decrease in client alcohol misuse.

STUDY AIMS AND HYPOTHESES

The aims of the study were twofold. First, we evaluated the level of student and field instructor satisfaction with the trainings. Second, we evaluated pre- to posttraining changes in SBIRT attitudes, knowledge, and skills among students and field instructors. We hypothesized that students and field instructors would be satisfied with the training, and that their SBIRT attitudes, knowledge, and skills would significantly increase from pre- to posttraining.

METHOD

Study Design

This study used a posttraining evaluation of training satisfaction among students and field instructors, and a pre–post design to assess changes in SBIRT attitudes, knowledge, and skills. Assessment of student and field instructor satisfaction occurred immediately following the training. To determine changes in SBIRT attitudes, knowledge, and skills, students completed assessments prior to training ($n = 134$), immediately following training (post$_0$, $n = 134$), and 30 days following training (post$_{30}$, $n = 128$). Field instructors completed pretraining ($n = 35$) and immediate posttraining ($n = 37$) assessments. This study was approved by the university's institutional review board.

Participants

STUDENTS

A total of 134 students from both Bachelor in Social Work (BSW, $n = 14$) and Master of Social Work (MSW, $n = 119$) degree programs completed SBIRT training. The majority of students were White ($n = 107$, 79.9%), non-Hispanic ($n = 122$, 94.6%), female ($n = 115$, 85.8%), and between ages 20 and 30 ($n = 104$, 77.6%). This gender and age distribution is consistent with social work student demographics across the United States, with the exception that this cohort contains more Whites than the national average (Council on Social Work Education, 2013). Six students were lost to follow-up (i.e., they were absent from class on the day research staff returned to classrooms to administer questionnaires). Analyses indicated that students lost to follow-up were not different from those retained in demographics; baseline hours of prior SBIRT training; or baseline ratings of SBIRT confidence, importance, or attitudes. It is also important to note that BSW students did not differ from MSW students in SBIRT attitudes, knowledge, skills, or demographics (except for age), therefore leading us to combine students in both programs in analyses.

A total of 38 field instructors from two separate training events completed the SBIRT training. Field instructor demographics mirrored social work student demographics, as a majority of participants were White ($n = 25$, 65.8%), non-Hispanic ($n = 31$, 88.6%) and female ($n = 26$, 74.2%). This is consistent with a national study of licensed social workers that showed the social work profession is disproportionately likely to identify as female and White compared to the U.S. population as a whole (Center for Health Workforce Studies, 2006). Five field instructors had incomplete data (i.e., some participants came late to the training, and some did not fill out the second page of their pretraining questionnaire). The field instructors with complete data did not differ from those with incomplete data in demographics; hours of prior SBIRT training; or posttraining ratings of SBIRT confidence, importance, or attitudes.

Student Training

Training was embedded within the curricula of an urban school of social work, which includes a BSW program and a single-concentration clinical MSW. In collaboration with classroom faculty, we integrated introductory SBIRT training into required foundation year course work. To reduce discrepancies in instruction, the director of clinical training conducted all trainings. She is a licensed independent clinical social worker with 6 years of motivational interviewing and SBIRT practice in health care and community-based settings. Students received equivalent trainings in nine sections of the master's-level assessment and diagnosis course and in one section of the bachelor's-level social work practice course.

SAMHSA provided SBIRT core curricula as a foundation for cross-disciplinary training. The core curricula are largely a compilation of trainings developed by previous grantees and focus on the following: the importance of utilizing SBIRT; universal screening using the Alcohol Use Disorders and Identification Test (AUDIT; Babor, Higgins-Biddle, Saunders, & Monteiro, 2001); brief interventions with a specific focus on motivational interviewing skills and strategies; and making referrals to specialty treatment. We adapted the curricula to reflect the needs of social workers, therefore addressing the differences in practice settings, the connection to biopsychosocial stressors, and the core values of social work. These adaptations were made in both didactic and role-play components of the training.

Students engaged in a flipped classroom model: They watched prerecorded video lectures followed by in-class, face-to-face skills practice. Online, self-paced training took approximately 1 hr to complete and included follow-up questions. The four modules included the following content: introduction to SBIRT as a public health approach, the prevalence of substance and alcohol misuse, universal screening, standardized screening tools, principles of motivational interviewing (Miller & Rollnick, 2013), and successful referrals to treatment. Special attention was given to connecting SBIRT to social work core values as well as the use of SBIRT in diverse settings. Online content featured recorded video instruction superimposed by complementary Microsoft PowerPoint slides.

Following the online didactic training, students engaged in 1.5 hr of face-to-face skills practice through standardized role-play scenarios. This included 15 min of review of online content, a 5-min SBIRT video demonstration, and 1 hr and 10 min dedicated to role-play. Trainees practiced scoring the AUDIT and providing screening feedback based on the principles and core skills of motivational interviewing (Miller & Rollnick, 2013). Students were organized into triads, and each student rotated through the roles of provider, client, and observer.

Field Instructor Training

The SBIRT training model for social work field instructors did not use a flipped classroom model; instead, it consisted of a 3-hr face-to-face seminar (for which they received free continuing education units). The seminar included the adapted SAMHSA core curriculum that students received as well as discussion about barriers to, and facilitators of, implementing SBIRT supervision into practice; a framework for mentoring students' use of SBIRT and its incorporation into field education; and guided practice on how to use the Clinical SBIRT Proficiency Checklist (Pringle, 2016). Discussion included the use of process recordings to evaluate students' fidelity to SBIRT.

Student Satisfaction

The Government Performance and Results Act (GPRA) survey was administered immediately after the in-class training to evaluate student satisfaction. Students rated their agreement with five items related to training satisfaction, skill development, and training utility on 5-point Likert-type scales with scores ranging from 1 (*very satisfied* or *strongly agree*) to 5 (*very dissatisfied* and *strongly disagree*). Survey content included quality of training components, enhancement of SBIRT skills, potential benefit to clients, and usefulness of information presented.

Field Instructor Satisfaction

One item taken from a workshop satisfaction survey developed by the university's professional development team was used to evaluate field instructor satisfaction with the training. Field instructors rated their overall training experience on a 4-point Likert-type scale ranging from 1 (*poor*) to 4 (*excellent*). The question read, "Overall, this course was …" and field instructors selected a response to complete the sentence.

SBIRT Attitudes, Knowledge, and Skills

The Attitudes, Knowledge, and Skills (AKS) survey is a 14-item tool (Sprague, Vinson, & Horwitz, 2010) that measures respondents' attitudes toward, knowledge of, and perceived skills in SBIRT on a 7-point Likert scale ranging from 1 (*strongly agree*) to 7 (*strongly disagree*). The instrument is currently undergoing validity studies for continued use as a research measure, but Sprague et al. (2010) calculated a Cronbach's alpha with adequate internal consistency ($\alpha = .730$). For this study, the Cronbach's alpha at pretest demonstrated adequate internal consistency ($\alpha = .805$). Exploratory factor analysis from the data in this study delineated three main factors within the AKS: confidence, importance, and attitudes. Pre- to posttraining outcomes on each of these three factors, as well as the composite score of the three factors, were examined. Field instructors were also asked to rate their level of confidence in supervising a practicum student or employee's use of SBIRT on a 5-point Likert scale ranging from 1 (*extremely confident*) to 5 (*not at all confident*).

ANALYTIC APPROACH

Data were collected via paper-and-pencil questionnaires and entered into SPSS 21 for data management and analysis. Training satisfaction was evaluated by a calculation of means. Differences in mean scores in SBIRT attitudes, knowledge, and skills from pre- to $post_0$ were assessed using paired t tests. To determine if the changes held 30 days after the training, we conducted a second paired t test analysis between pre- and $post_{30}$.

RESULTS

Satisfaction with Training

STUDENT SATISFACTION

Students ($n = 134$) demonstrated a high level of satisfaction on five GPRA items related to the quality and utility of the training, materials, and instruction. Specifically, 90.9% were satisfied or very satisfied with the overall quality of the training; 87.3% agreed or strongly agreed that the training enhanced their SBIRT skills; 89.6% agreed or strongly agreed that they expected to use the information from the training; 87.3% agreed or strongly agreed that they expected this training to benefit clients; and 94.8% rated the information received as useful or very useful.

FIELD INSTRUCTOR SATISFACTION

One hundred percent of field instructors ($n = 36$) reported an overall rating of excellent or good for the overall training.

SBIRT Attitudes, Knowledge, and Skills

Table 1 and Table 2 present mean differences from pre- to $post_0$- and pre- to $post_{30}$ in SBIRT attitudes, knowledge, and skills among social work students. Results are shown for individual measure items, three thematic factors, and a composite score of the three factors. In summary, students demonstrated significant mean differences from pre- to $post_0$ on 8 of 14 individual items. Significant changes from pre- to $post_0$ were evident in the confidence and importance factors, and in the three-factor composite score. Significant differences in means were noted from pre- to $post_{30}$ on 9 of 14 items, in all three factors—confidence, importance, and attitudes—and in the three-factor composite score. There was a large effect size from pre to $post_0$ in the Confidence subscale ($d = .79$), and low effect sizes for the Importance ($d = .35$) and Attitudes ($d = .15$) subscales. A medium effect size was found from pre to $post_0$ for the composite score of the AKS ($d = .67$). There was a large effect size from pre to $post_{30}$ in both the Confidence subscale ($d = .83$) and the AKS composite score ($d = .75$). Low effect sizes were found for the Importance ($d = .29$) and Attitudes ($d = .27$) subscales.

Table 3 shows mean differences from pre to posttraining in SBIRT attitudes, knowledge, and skills among field instructors. Similar to Tables 1 and 2, results are shown for individual measure items, three thematic factors, and a composite score of the three factors. Field instructors demonstrated statistically significant mean differences in 3 of 14 individual items, as well as in the confidence factors and in the three-factor composite score. There was a medium effect size from pre to post in the Confidence subscale ($d = .68$) and AKS composite score ($d = .59$). Low effect sizes for the Importance ($d = .26$) and Attitudes ($d = .16$) subscales were detected.

DISCUSSION

This article presents preliminary evaluation data from the first year of a 3-year grant, which suggests that the training is acceptable and results in significant changes in trainees' knowledge, attitudes, and self-perceived SBIRT skills,

TABLE 1 Pre- to Post-training Paired t Tests on Student Attitudes, Knowledge, and Skills.

Attitude, Knowledge, and Skills Item	Pretest M	Posttest M	M Difference	SD	t	df	Significance
1. I have a good understanding of substance use and abuse.	3.29	2.65	0.64	1.43	5.15	132	< .001
2. I want to learn effective methods for directly addressing clients' risky substance use.	1.71	1.59	0.12	1.37	1.02	132	.31
3. Learning to screen and intervene in clients' hazardous or harmful substance use is important for me in my current/future position.	1.87	1.94	−0.08	1.50	−0.58	132	.56
4. Substance use and abuse are not appropriate topics to address with clients in my current or future practice.	2.20[a]	2.05[a]	0.15	2.19	0.79	132	.43
5. There are many physicians I work with who address alcohol and drug problems skillfully and effectively.	4.21	4.05	0.17	1.45	1.33	132	.18
6. There are many nonphysician providers (social workers and others) I work with who address alcohol and drug problems skillfully.	3.19	3.14	0.05	1.34	0.39	132	.70
7. I am confident in my ability to screen patients or clients for alcohol/drug problems.	4.39	3.25	1.14	1.50	8.80	132	< .001
8. I am confident in my ability to assess patients' or clients' readiness to change their behavior.	3.62	2.85	0.77	1.31	6.81	132	< .001
9. I am confident in my ability to discuss patients' or clients' substance use and advise them to change their behavior.	3.85	3.07	0.77	1.48	5.97	132	< .001
10. I am confident in my ability to refer patients or clients with alcohol/drug problems.	3.84	2.96	0.88	1.65	6.16	132	< .001
11. It takes too much time to deal with patients' or clients' drinking/drug behavior.	2.01[a]	1.68[a]	0.32	1.34	2.78	132	< .001
12. Patients or clients will be angry if I ask questions about their substance use.	3.35[a]	3.33[a]	0.02	1.46	0.18	132	0.86
13. My interaction with a patient or client can make a difference regarding their use of substances.	2.72	2.21	0.51	1.34	4.42	132	< .001

(*Continued*)

TABLE 1 (Continued)

Attitude, Knowledge, and Skills Item	Pretest M	Posttest M	M Difference	SD	t	df	Significance
14. Incorporating SBIRT into routine medical practice is critical for meeting health care needs.	2.74	1.97	0.77	1.42	6.28	132	< .001
Factor I: Confidence (Items 7–10)	15.68	12.12	3.56	4.51	9.12	132	< .001
Factor II: Importance (Items 2, 3, 13, 14)	9.05	7.71	1.33	3.78	4.06	132	< .001
Factor III: Attitudes (Items 4, 11, 12)	7.56	7.07	0.50	3.45	1.66	132	.099
Composite score: Factor 1 + 2 + 3	32.29	26.90	5.39	8.01	7.77	132	< .001

Note: SBIRT = screening, brief intervention, and referral to treatment. Because of scaling (7 = *strongly disagree*), lower scale scores at posttest indicate higher confidence in SBIRT, belief in importance in SBIRT, and self-perceived attitudes about SBIRT.
[a]Due to negative question wording, a positive mean difference indicates more disagreement in these cases.

with a notably large effect size for confidence ratings among students. Students and field instructors reported a high level of satisfaction related to the quality and utility of the training, materials, and instruction. Results specific to changes in SBIRT attitudes, knowledge, and skills as a result of the training demonstrated significant pre- to immediate posttraining changes in students' confidence in using SBIRT skills and perceived importance of understanding and using SBIRT. These changes were sustained to 30 days posttraining, with an additional delayed mean increase in attitudes related to the use and adoption of SBIRT. Field instructors also demonstrated significant increases in confidence in using SBIRT skills and in supervising students' use of SBIRT. Although field instructors did not demonstrate significant increases in the domains of SBIRT importance and attitudes, this is likely because their starting scores were high. Taken together, these data support the feasibility, acceptability, and preliminary effectiveness of a student and field instructor training that can be implemented in MSW programs.

These findings must be interpreted with caution, however, as limitations include self-reports of skill ratings, rather than an objective observation of skills by another professional. Furthermore, although the same trainer delivered the training to all sections, enabling us to reduce training discrepancies, an additional limitation is that we were not able to account for different classroom factors (e.g., variations in students' interest in the material prior to the training), and therefore, we did not address them methodologically. During this data collection period, the field instructor training was held after the students had completed their 30-day follow-up survey. For this reason, we are unable to determine the impact of field instructor training on students' SBIRT-

TABLE 2 Pre- to $Post_{30}$ training Paired t Tests on Student Attitudes, Knowledge, and Skills

Attitude, Knowledge, and Skills Item.	Pretest M	Posttest M	M Difference	SD	t	df	Significance
1. I have a good understanding of substance use and abuse.	3.32	2.51	0.81	1.48	6.20	127	< .001
2. I want to learn effective methods for directly addressing clients' risky substance use.	1.72	1.61	0.11	1.27	0.98	127	.33
3. Learning to screen and intervene in clients' hazardous or harmful substance use is important for me in my current/future position.	1.89	1.91	−0.02	1.41	−0.13	127	.90
4. Substance use and abuse are not appropriate topics to address with clients in my current or future practice.	2.21[a]	2.06[a]	0.16	2.08	0.85	127	.40
5. There are many physicians I work with who address alcohol and drug problems skillfully and effectively.	4.18	4.10	0.08	1.45	0.61	126	.54
6. There are many nonphysician providers (social workers and others) I work with who address alcohol and drug problems skillfully.	3.18	3.23	−0.06	1.57	−0.40	127	.69
7. I am confident in my ability to screen patients or clients for alcohol/drug problems.	4.38	3.11	1.27	1.44	9.95	127	< .001
8. I am confident in my ability to assess patients' or clients' readiness to change their behavior.	3.65	2.77	0.88	1.36	7.26	127	< .001
9. I am confident in my ability to discuss patients' or clients' substance use and advise them to change their behavior.	3.82	2.96	0.86	1.45	6.73	127	< .001

(*Continued*)

TABLE 2 (Continued)

10. I am confident in my ability to refer patients or clients with alcohol/ drug problems.	3.80	2.91	0.89	1.79	5.62	127	< .001
11. It takes too much time to deal with patients' or clients' drinking/drug behavior.	2.07[a]	1.70[a]	0.37	1.32	3.16	127	.002
12. Patients or clients will be angry if I ask questions about their substance use.	3.38[a]	3.02[a]	0.36	1.41	2.89	127	.005
13. My interaction with a patient or client can make a difference regarding their use of substances.	2.73	2.26	0.47	1.42	3.74	126	< .001
14. Incorporating SBIRT into routine medical practice is critical for meeting health care needs.	2.75	2.17	0.58	1.53	4.26	125	< .001
Factor I: Confidence (Items 7–10)	15.64	11.75	3.89	4.70	9.37	127	< .001
Factor II: Importance (Items 2, 3, 13,14)	9.08	7.94	1.14	3.99	3.22	125	.002
Factor III: Attitudes (Items 4, 11, 12)	7.66	6.78	0.88	3.28	3.04	127	.003
Composite score: Factor 1 + 2 + 3	32.44	26.44	6.01	8.07	8.34	125	< .001

Note: SBIRT = screening, brief intervention, and referral to treatment. Because of scaling (7 = *strongly disagree*) lower scale scores at posttest indicate higher confidence in SBIRT, belief in importance in SBIRT, and self-perceived attitudes about SBIRT.
[a]Due to negative question wording, a positive mean difference indicates more disagreement in these cases.

related attitudes, knowledge, and skills. Also important to consider in this study is whether or not it should be considered a good outcome that our students scored in the middle of the scale for the SBIRT attitudes, knowledge, and skills items at the end of the training. Although this might reflect a realistic aspect of student trainings, as students in general tend to report lower confidence in skills than professionals, it nevertheless stimulates thinking about the implications of the findings with respect to the readiness of students to practice with individuals at risk for substance misuse after the training.

As these data were gathered at the end of the first year of a 3-year grant, the results must inform adaptations to enhance the effects of the training. Many students wanted more time for skills practice in class to allow for increased comfort and competence in SBIRT-related skills. This requires instructors' willingness to

TABLE 3 Pre- to Post-training Paired t Tests on Field Instructor Attitudes, Knowledge, and Skills.

Attitude, Knowledge, and Skills Item	Pretest M	Posttest M	M Difference	SD	t	df	Significance
1. I have a good understanding of substance use and abuse.	2.53	2.12	0.41	0.86	2.80	32	.008
2. I want to learn effective methods for directly addressing clients' risky substance use.	1.50	1.65	−0.15	0.82	−1.04	33	.30
3. Learning to screen and intervene in clients' hazardous or harmful substance use is important for me in my current/ future position.	1.91	1.62	0.29	1.17	1.47	33	.15
4. Substance use and abuse are not appropriate topics to address with clients in my current or future practice.	1.38[a]	1.41[a]	−0.03	0.46	−0.37	33	.71
5. There are many physicians I work with who address alcohol and drug problems skillfully and effectively.	4.33	3.97	0.36	1.19	1.75	32	.09
6. There are many nonphysician providers (social workers and others) I work with who address alcohol and drug problems skillfully.	2.97	2.94	0.03	1.68	0.11	30	.092
7. I am confident in my ability to screen patients or clients for alcohol/drug problems.	3.10	2.13	0.97	1.05	5.14	30	< .001
8. I am confident in my ability to assess patients' or clients' readiness to change their behavior.	2.61	2.10	0.52	0.85	3.38	30	.002
9. I am confident in my ability to discuss patients' or clients' substance use and advise them to change their behavior.	2.74	2.45	0.29	1.24	1.30	30	.20
10. I am confident in my ability to refer patients or clients with alcohol/drug problems.	2.68	2.36	0.32	1.13	1.58	30	.13
11. It takes too much time to deal with patients' or clients' drinking/drug behavior.	1.87[a]	1.68[a]	0.19	1.30	0.83	30	.41
12. Patients or clients will be angry if I ask questions about their substance use.	3.32[a]	3.19[a]	0.13	1.36	0.53	30	.60
13. My interaction with a patient or client can make a difference regarding their use of substances.	2.27	2.15	0.12	1.36	0.51	32	.61

(*Continued*)

TABLE 3 (Continued)

Attitude, Knowledge, and Skills Item	Pretest M	Posttest M	M Difference	SD	t	df	Significance
14. Incorporating SBIRT into routine medical practice is critical for meeting health care needs.	2.52	2.09	0.42	1.25	1.95	32	.06
Factor I: Confidence (Items 7–10)	11.13	9.03	2.10	3.09	3.78	30	.001
Factor II: Importance (Items 2, 3, 13, 14)	8.24	7.55	0.70	2.71	1.48	32	.15
Factor III: Attitudes (Items 4, 11, 12)	6.58	6.29	0.29	1.85	0.88	30	.39
Composite score: Factor 1 + 2 + 3	25.61	22.71	2.90	4.90	3.30	30	.002

Note: SBIRT = screening, brief intervention, and referral to treatment. Because of scaling (7 = *strongly disagree*) lower scale scores at posttest indicate higher confidence in SBIRT, belief in importance in SBIRT, and self-perceived attitudes about SBIRT.
[a]Due to negative question wording, a positive mean difference indicates more disagreement in these cases.

devote additional time to SBIRT training and practice in their classes, and they have agreed to do so. Therefore, we have made changes to the training protocol accordingly. Also in regard to training effects, it is important to consider how and when to disseminate the training, and to whom, to take it to scale. There are many potential barriers to dissemination and implementation (e.g., heavy faculty work-load, difficulty getting institutional buy-in, cost of implementation), which need to be considered once the training is in its final form and ready to be distributed.

With respect to improving the field instructor training, we will offer on-site technical assistance to field instructors. This will include additional guidance about how to accurately assess students' skills using the proficiency checklist and process recordings. Integration of SBIRT into a required, foundation-level course addresses, in part, the need to educate social workers in an evidence-informed practice designed to address and alleviate alcohol misuse. Although this might not ade-quately prepare students to implement substance use screening and treatment, it provides foundational knowledge, which should (combined with field instructor training) be reinforced and supported in the field. To do this, classroom and field faculty must have favorable attitudes toward its inclusion and become proficient in teaching the material. Faculty would benefit from access to SBIRT curriculum materials. The Council on Social Work Education SBIRT Consortium provides one vehicle for this information dissemination (Berger & Di Paolo, 2015).

Because self-rating of skills, such as motivational interviewing in SBIRT, does not necessarily translate to skill competency (Miller, Yahne, Moyers, Martinez, & Pirritano, 2004), future research must evaluate training effectiveness by assessing skill change through observation of behavior rather than self-reports. Role-plays have limitations, and teacher observation of students can be burdensome for the professor. The development and testing of technology-based SBIRT skill assessments, such as computerized simulations, is warranted. As technological advances continue to aid instructional practices in social work programs, it will become increasingly important to test the feasibility, acceptability, and added effect of computerized simulation training, as well as other innovative teaching methods, on outcomes for students and field instructors. In addition, future studies should test the effectiveness of SBIRT training on patient outcomes, specifically with respect to the reduction of harm associated with alcohol misuse. Although the importance of training social workers in these skills is not debatable, the extent to which these trainings directly affect their clients requires future inquiry.

CONCLUSION

To more effectively ameliorate the burden of alcohol misuse, social work programs must continue to develop innovative, yet feasible, ways to train social workers to intervene with clients at risk for substance misuse. The SBIRT training model presented in this article is feasible, is acceptable, and results in significant changes in trainees' knowledge, attitudes, confidence, and self-perception of skills, with a notably large effect size for confidence ratings. Self-rating might or might not align with skill competency; therefore, the effectiveness of training must be further evaluated by systematic observational assessment and ultimately by clients' outcomes.

FUNDING

This article was supported by Grant 1H79TI025970-01 from the Substance Abuse and Mental Health Services Administration.

REFERENCES

Agerwala, S. M., & McCance-Katz, E. F. (2012). Integrating screening, brief intervention, and referral to treatment into clinical practice settings: A brief review. *Journal of Psychoactive Drugs, 44*, 307–317. doi:10.1080/02791072.2012.720169

Babor, T. F., Higgins-Biddle, J. C., Saunders, J. B., & Monteiro, M. G. (2001). *The Alcohol Use Disorders Identification Test: Guidelines for use in primary care* (2nd ed.). Geneva, Switzerland: Department of Mental Health and Substance Dependence, World Health Organization.

Babor, T. F., McRee, B. G., Kassebaum, P. A., Grimaldi, P. L., Ahmed, K., & Bray, J. (2007). Screening, brief intervention, and referral to treatment (SBIRT): Toward a public health approach to the management of substance abuse. *Substance Abuse, 28*(3), 7–30. doi:10.1300/J465v28n0303

Barbosa, C., Cowell, A., Bray, J., & Aldridge, A. (2015). The cost-effectiveness of alcohol screening, brief intervention, and referral to treatment (SBIRT) in emergency and outpatient medical settings. *Journal of Substance Abuse Treatment, 53,* 1–8. doi:10.1016/j.jsat.2015.01.003

Begun, A. L., Clapp, J. D., & The Alcohol Misuse Grand Challenge Collective. (2016). Reducing and preventing alcohol misuse and its consequences: A Grand Challenge for social work. *International Journal of Alcohol and Drug Research, 5*(2), 73–83. doi:10.7895/ijadr.v5i2.223

Berger, L., & Di Paolo, M. (2015). Screening, Brief Intervention, and Referral to Treatment (SBIRT): An interview with Scott Caldwell, MA, and Darla Spence Coffey, PhD. *Journal of Social Work Practice in the Addictions, 15,* 219–226. doi:10.1080/1533256X.2015.1029418

Bureau of Labor Statistics, U.S. Department of Labor. (2015). Social workers. In *Occupational outlook handbook* (2016–17 ed.). Retrieved from http://www.bls.gov/ooh/community-and-social-service/social-workers.htm

Center for Behavioral Health Statistics and Quality. (2015). *Behavioral health trends in the United States: Results from the 2014 National Survey on Drug Use and Health* (HHS Publication No. SMA 15-4927, NSDUH Series H-50). Retrieved from http://www.samhsa.gov/data/

Center for Health Workforce Studies & NASW Center for Workforce Studies. (2006). Who are licensed social workers? In *Licensed social workers in the United States, 2004* (Chapter 2). Retrieved from http://workforce.socialworkers.org/studies/supplemental/supplement_ch2.pdf

Childers, J. W., Broyles, L. M., Hanusa, B. H., Kraemer, K. L., Conigliaro, J., Spagnoletti, C., … Gordon, A. J. (2012). Teaching the teachers: Faculty preparedness and evaluation of a retreat in screening, brief intervention, and referral to treatment. *Substance Abuse, 33,* 272–277. doi:10.1080/08897077.2011.639686

Cochran, G., Roll, J., Jackson, R., & Kennedy, J. (2014). Health care reform and the behavioral health workforce. *Social Work Practice in the Addictions, 14,* 127–140. doi:10.1080/1533256X.2014.902244

Council on Social Work Education. (2013). *2013 statistics on social work education in the United States.* Retrieved from http://www.cswe.org/file.aspx?id=74478

Galvani, S., & Hughes, N. (2010). Working with alcohol and drug use: Exploring the knowledge and attitudes of social work students. *British Journal of Social Work, 40,* 946–962. doi:10.1093/bjsw/bcn137

Hall, M. N., Amodeo, M., Shaffer, H. J., & Bilt, J. V. (2000). Social workers employed in substance abuse treatment agencies: A training needs assessment. *Social Work, 45,* 141–155. doi:10.1093/sw/45.2.141

Hingson, R., Heeren, T., Edwards, E., & Saitz, R. (2012). Young adults at risk for excess alcohol consumption are often not asked or counseled about drinking alcohol. *Journal of General Internal Medicine, 27,* 179–184. doi:10.1007/s11606-011-1851-1

Hingson, R., & Rehm, J. (2014). Measuring the burden: Alcohol's evolving impact on individuals, families, and society. *Alcohol Research: Current Reviews, 35,* 117–118.

Institute of Medicine. (2006). *Improving the quality of health care for mental and substance-use conditions.* Washington, DC: National Academies Press.

McKnight-Eily, L. R., Liu, Y., Brewer, R. D., Kanny, D., Lu, H., Denny, C. H., … Collins, J. (2014). Vital signs: Communication between health professionals and their patients about alcohol use—44 states and the District of Columbia, 2011. *MMWR Morbidity & Mortality Weekly Report, 63*(1), 16–22.

Mechanic, D. (2012). Seizing opportunities under the Affordable Care Act for transforming the mental and behavioral health system. *Health Affairs, 31,* 376–382. doi:10.1377/hlthaff.2011.0623

Miller, W. R., & Rollnick, S. (2013). *Motivational interviewing: Helping people change.* New York, NY: Guilford.

Miller, W. R., Yahne, C. E., Moyers, T. B., Martinez, J., & Pirritano, M. (2004). A randomized trial of methods to help clinicians learn motivational interviewing. *Journal of Consulting and Clinical Psychology, 72,* 1050–1062. doi:10.1037/0022-006X.72.6.1050

Moyer, V. A. (2013). Screening and behavioral counseling interventions in primary care to reduce alcohol misuse: U.S. Preventive Services Task Force recommendation statement. *Annals of Internal Medicine, 159,* 210–218.

O'Donnell, A., Andersen, P., Newbury-Birch, D., Schulte, B., Schmidt, C., Reimer, J., & Kaner, E. (2014). The impact of brief alcohol interventions in primary healthcare: A systematic review of reviews. *Alcohol & Alcoholism, 49,* 66–78. doi:10.1093/alcalc/agt170

Padilla, Y. C., & Fong, R. (2016). Identifying grand challenges facing social work in the next decade: Maximizing social policy engagement. *Journal of Policy Practice, 15,* 133–144. doi:10.1080/15588742.2015.1013238

Pringle, J. (2016). *Evaluation of SBIRT training: Assessing SBIRT skills using a proficiency checklist.* Retrieved from http://www.peru.pitt.edu/resources/

Quinn, G. (2010). Institutional denial of minimization: Substance abuse training in social work education. *Substance Abuse, 31,* 8–11. doi:10.1080/08897070903442475

Richardson, M. A. (2008). Social work education: The availability of alcohol-related course curriculum and social workers' ability to work with problem drinkers. *Journal of Social Work Practice, 22*(1), 119–128. doi:10.1080/02650530701872470

Seale, J., Shellenberger, S., Velasquez, M., Boltri, J., Okosun, I., Guyinn, M., … Johnson, J. (2010). Impact of vital signs screening & clinician prompting on alcohol and tobacco screening and intervention rates: A pre–post intervention comparison. *BMC Family Practice, 11*(18). doi:10.1186/1471-2296-11-18

Sprague, D., Vinson, D. C., & Horwitz, B. (2010). *Attitudes, self-perception of skills, and knowledge survey.* Unpublished manuscript, Center for Research and Evaluation, Missouri Institute of Mental Health, University of Missouri-St. Louis, St. Louis, MO.

Stahre, M., Roeber, J., Kanny, D., Brewer, R. D., & Zhang, X. (2014). Contribution of excessive alcohol consumption to deaths and years of potential life lost in the United States. *Prevention of Chronic Disease, 11,* 130293. doi:10.5888/pcd11.130293

Tai, B., & Volkow, N. (2013). Treatment for substance use disorder: Opportunities and challenges under the Affordable Care Act. *Social Work in Public Health, 28,* 165–174. doi:10.1080/19371918.2013.758975

Tanner, T. B., Wilehelm, S. E., Rossie, K. M., & Metcalf, M. P. (2012). Web-based SBIRT skills training for health professional students and primary care providers. *Substance Abuse, 33,* 316–320. doi:10.1080/08897077.2011.640151

Wilkey, C., Lundgren, L., & Amodeo, M. (2013). Addiction training in social work schools: A nationwide analysis. *Journal of Social Work Practice in the Addictions, 13,* 192–210. doi:10.1080/1533256X.2013.785872

Complementing SBIRT for Alcohol Misuse with SBIRT for Trauma: A Feasibility Study

JAMES TOPITZES, PhD

LISA BERGER, PhD and LAURA OTTO-SALAJ, PhD

JOSHUA P. MERSKY, PhD

FIONA WEEKS, PhD

JULIAN D. FORD, PhD

Reducing alcohol misuse is a priority for U.S. health officials considering that misuse of alcohol is a leading preventable cause of morbidity and mortality. Consequently, health centers are integrating Screening, Brief Intervention, and Referral to Treatment (SBIRT) for

The authors would like to thank administrators and supervisors at agencies participating in this study. Special appreciation is extended to service providers at each site who worked diligently, creatively, and competently to implement and help test the SBIRT for trauma or T-SBIRT intervention. Last, the authors would like to recognize and honor study participants for their patience, honesty, and resilience.

alcohol misuse within usual care. Although SBIRT is well validated among general patient samples, results have not generalized to drinkers with probable alcohol use disorder; moreover, little is known about the efficacy of SBIRT with patients who are of low-income or ethnic or racial minority status. Members of these groups are of particular concern because they are at risk to experience trauma, potentially in concert with alcohol misuse. Therefore, translational approaches to delivering SBIRT particularly with these groups of interest might be needed to meet the Grand Challenge of reducing alcohol misuse. Accordingly, this study combined SBIRT with a model designed to address psychological trauma: T-SBIRT. With a sample of 112 adults, most of whom were African American or Latino/a, authors analyzed multiple indicators of feasibility. Results indicated that T-SBIRT is suitable for and acceptable to patients accessing community-based health services, and T-SBIRT can promote high referral acceptance rates to specialty treatment, particularly among patients with probable alcohol use disorder.

Alcohol misuse contributes to numerous chronic diseases and conditions while also significantly increasing risk for natural or accidental death (Shield, Parry, & Rehm, 2013). As a leading preventable cause of morbidity and mortality, it has been the target of many policy initiatives. For example, the U.S. government recently invested heavily in alcohol misuse prevention and treatment through health care reform, promoting widespread dissemination of several identified service models; chief among these selected models was Screening, Brief Intervention, and Referral to Treatment (SBIRT; Humphreys & McLellan, 2010).

Implemented typically within primary health care settings by physicians and allied health professionals, such as social workers and nurses, SBIRT protocols introduce well-validated screening procedures followed by, when indicated, a follow-up intervention. A brief intervention represents standard treatment for alcohol misuse, whereas a multisession intervention or referral to more intensive treatment is recommended for probable alcohol use disorder (Babor, Higgins-Biddle, Saunders, & Monteiro, 2001). The goal of SBIRT is to reduce unhealthy drinking patterns among medium- to high-risk drinkers and to help treat alcohol use disorder. As such, it is a low-intensity service with the potential to impact health at the population level (Babor et al., 2007). Recently, SBIRT has been used not only in hospitals but in community-based settings, and is considered an integrated health practice that crosses disciplinary boundaries to affect service recipients' physical and behavioral health (Agerwala & McCance-Katz, 2012).

Although SBIRT has been found to be effective in addressing medium to high-risk drinking, also defined as hazardous or harmful use, it does not appear to produce significant effects among those with probable alcohol use disorder (Glass et al., 2015). Furthermore, efficacy studies report positive SBIRT outcomes among middle-class White adults, but less is known about SBIRT effects with low-income, ethnic and racial minorities (O'Donnell et al., 2014). To meet the Grand Challenge of reducing widespread alcohol misuse while also extending SBIRT effects to groups at risk for comparatively poor health, Begun, Clapp, and The Alcohol Misuse Grand Challenge Collective (2016) suggested adapting SBIRT via translational processes.

This article describes such a translational project. The authors adapted, implemented, and tested the feasibility of a model based on SBIRT for substance misuse but designed to address psychological trauma, that is, T-SBIRT. Intended to be delivered with traditional SBIRT services, T-SBIRT aims to improve SBIRT outcomes for all patient groups, yet we implemented the intervention with groups at high risk for comparatively poor health outcomes such as adults with probable alcohol use disorder or low-income adults of color. We suspected that T-SBIRT could most effectively augment traditional SBIRT services for these patient groups at risk for poor health or health disparities because trauma often (a) cooccurs with and undermines resolution of risky alcohol use (McCauley, Killeen, Gros, Brady, & Back, 2012), and (b) disproportionately affects low-income adults and racial and ethnic minorities (Briere & Scott, 2015).

LITERATURE REVIEW

A robust literature supports the efficacy of traditional SBIRT for reducing alcohol use within 6 months of completing an SBIRT session (e.g., Madras et al., 2009). Significant intervention effects have emerged across emergency and primary care settings (Agerwala & McCance-Katz, 2012), and SBIRT is making its way into community-based service settings with the help of social work practitioners and scholars (Bliss & Pecukonis, 2009). However, a recent meta-analysis from Glass and colleagues (2015) reveals that SBIRT does not result in successful referral to treatment for those with probable alcohol use disorder. Moreover, in a thorough review of the literature, O'Donnell and colleagues (2014) indicated that the benefits of SBIRT for low-income, racial and ethnic minorities have not been well-studied or well-reported.

Following the recommendation to adapt SBIRT for target groups, Salvalaggio et al. (2013) proposed an enhanced SBIRT model tailored for socioeconomically disadvantaged patients. Model adaptations were designed to facilitate patient engagement and resource access, thereby addressing common barriers to health care for low-income patients. Although the authors described the model and study protocol, they have not published patient outcome results.

Aside from problems with health service engagement and resource availability, another key factor that might diminish the effectiveness of SBIRT for vulnerable populations is the presence of trauma-related comorbidity. For instance, among individuals with substance use disorders (SUDs), the rate of posttraumatic stress disorder (PTSD) has been found to range from 33% to 60% (Ford, Hawke, Alessi, Ledgerwood, & Petry, 2007; McCauley et al., 2012), and for low-income patients, rates of comorbidity in all likelihood drift toward the high end of the published range (Briere & Scott, 2015). Moreover, Kramer, Polusny, Arbisi, and Krueger's (2014) literature review suggests that trauma exposure more often than not presages substance abuse (Kramer et al., 2014) and that PTSD complicates SUD treatment (Ford et al., 2007). Clinical wisdom previously dictated that treatment for cooccurring PTSD and SUDs solely or initially target SUD symptoms, but new evidence is emerging favoring integrated treatment models (e.g., McCauley et al., 2012).

Although integrated PTSD and SUD treatment models are ascendant, little is known about the translation of these concurrent treatment approaches to brief interventions that address clinical or subclinical presentations of substance abuse and posttraumatic stress. One study revealed that college students with posttraumatic stress symptoms could benefit from a brief intervention targeting heavy episodic alcohol use (Monahan et al., 2013). Another study, set in primary health care, indicated that alcohol and trauma screening followed by indicated brief treatment could reduce alcohol consumption among problem drinkers (Israel et al., 1996). The authors concluded that addressing trauma and alcohol misuse simultaneously in a primary health care setting represents an efficient strategy to confront a common comorbidity and to promote health.

CURRENT IMPLEMENTATION PROJECT AND FEASIBILITY STUDY

The current implementation project represents a component of a parent project titled the SBIRT Training for Substance Misuse Program at the University of Wisconsin–Milwaukee. Funded by the Substance Abuse and Mental Health Services Administration (SAMHSA), the parent project aimed to disseminate SBIRT within community health clinics. The authors proposed piloting a T-SBIRT "module" at several sites based on the listed rationale and consistent with priorities that SAMHSA articulated both in a 2011 program announcement (Screening, Brief Intervention, and Referral to Treatment with a Trauma Module) and in recent program initiatives (Grants for Adult Trauma Screening and Brief Intervention or GATSBI).

T-SBIRT Model

DEVELOPMENT

A first draft of the T-SBIRT model emerged as authors reviewed the literature. Subsequently, practitioners from the T-SBIRT project pilot sites reviewed the initial draft of the protocol and provided feedback to inform model revisions. The first author then met with representatives from participating sites to establish in-clinic procedures for identifying and recruiting patients for T-SBIRT services. Last, a graduate student intern conducted trial T-SBIRT sessions, leading to protocol refinements. In sum, the protocol arose iteratively through a blend of conceptual and practical approaches. Translating insights from basic science to applied settings often involves complex processes undertaken in multiple stages, starting with adaptation and design and moving to field testing and refinement (Topitzes, Mersky, & McNeil, 2015).

STRUCTURE

The structure of the T-SBIRT protocol mimics that of traditional SBIRT. However, its purpose is to generate patient insight into trauma exposure and effects and to enhance patient motivation for behavioral or mental health services, if indicated. T-SBIRT, like traditional SBIRT, rests on motivational interviewing principles (Agerwala & McCance-Katz, 2012) and relies on the following common practice elements: seeking permission to share information, providing information and education, asking open-ended questions, reflecting and summarizing responses, and reinforcing statements that reflect motivation to change behavior.

The actual sequence of the T-SBIRT protocol unfolds as follows. Immediately after the traditional SBIRT protocol is completed, T-SBIRT is introduced with a brief statement about the known connections between stress and health. The T-SBIRT service provider then asks an open-ended question about specific stressors in the patient's life. Next, the provider queries the patient about potential traumatic events (PTEs) to which the patient might have been exposed throughout life, invoking items from the Trauma History Screen (THS; Carlson, 2001). The provider also probes for current PTSD symptoms by verbally administering the Primary Care Post-Traumatic Stress Disorder Screen (PC-PTSD; Prins et al., 2003). After covering topics of trauma exposure and traumatic stress, the provider asks the patient about "positive" and "unhelpful" strategies used to cope with trauma.

Consistent with the self-medication theory (Kramer et al., 2014), the provider next informs the patient that at times it can be difficult to eliminate alcohol or drug misuse or other unhelpful coping strategies without simultaneously addressing trauma exposure and symptoms. These steps are designed to enhance the patient's motivation to address trauma. Hence, the provider subsequently gauges the patient's motivation for a behavioral or mental health treatment referral and refers the patient to a service provider practicing either within or outside the host clinic, if indicated. When referring within the clinic, T-SBIRT providers offer ongoing services themselves or introduce the client to the prospective ongoing mental and behavioral health service providers (i.e., a warm handoff). If referring outside the clinic, T-SBIRT providers follow up referrals with patient phone calls to either ensure that patients pursued the referral or facilitate referral pursuit via problem solving. The provider concludes services by offering the patient an educational booklet on PTSD published by the National Center for PTSD if appropriate and by implementing an evidence-based calming exercise if necessary.

The Appendix displays the T-SBIRT protocol in the form of an integrity checklist that providers referenced and completed when delivering T-SBIRT services. Providers reported that completing all steps of the T-SBIRT protocol required an average of 10 to 15 min. In total, the length of time needed to complete both SBIRT protocols was approximately 20 to 25 min.

Implementation Project Procedures

PROVIDERS AND AUDIENCE

Due to the nature of the topic and time required to complete the procedure, nursing, social work, or mental health staff as opposed to primary care physicians conducted T-SBIRT services. Nevertheless, the T-SBIRT protocol is designed to be brief and present-moment focused. To specify, T-SBIRT service providers direct patients' attention to current effects of trauma exposure and traumatic stress. Exploration of the historical details of traumatic events is not clinically indicated during brief interventions (Najavits & Kanukollu, 2005).

The target audience in this initial trial was low-income primary health care patients who presented with risk factors for behavioral health problems. Identified risk factors included a positive result on an alcohol use prescreening test administered to all patients, a referral from a hospital emergency room, and physician determination of possible alcohol misuse. One of the two sites involved in the project, Site 2, focused primarily on the first criterion, yielding a lower risk patient group.

STUDY SITES

Two community-based health clinics located within a large city in the upper Midwest region of the United States participated in this T-SBIRT implementation project. Operating the first clinic, or Site 1, is a nonprofit organization that offers a menu of services such as primary health care and case management to adults who are homeless, underinsured, or uninsured. The current implementation project involved primary and behavioral health care units colocated within the agency's health clinic. Designated as a federally qualified health center, the clinic employs multiple physicians, nurses, and behavioral health specialists, and primarily serves African American patients. The T-SBIRT project coincided with clinic efforts to integrate primary and behavioral health care services. Site 2 is a community-based health clinic that offers primary health care free of charge to patients facing significant barriers to care, such as lack of insurance. Along with five nurses, the small clinic employs one full-time psychologist in an effort to address the mental and behavioral health needs of a primarily Latino patient population.

PROVIDER TRAINING AND PRACTICE

Before initiating feasibility data collection, three service providers participating in the project completed training in traditional SBIRT. Afterward, the providers—a bachelor's-level nurse functioning as a patient navigator with 3 years of practice experience, a master's-level social work intern providing behavioral health services with 1 year of practice experience, and a master's-level counseling psychology intern delivering mental health services with 1 year of practice experience—attended weekly supervision meetings with the first author. The initial aim of the meetings was to facilitate protocol mastery. To that end, providers practiced SBIRT and T-SBIRT skills in vivo prior to collecting data.

PATIENT CONTACT

During the prestudy service period, SBIRT providers worked with physicians, nurses, and medical assistants to solidify procedures whereby eligible patients would be referred to SBIRT providers before primary care visits. Per the established procedures, SBIRT providers would meet identified patients in waiting or exam rooms, ask permission to conduct SBIRT protocols, and facilitate SBIRT sessions in behavioral health unit offices or physician exam rooms. Seldom were SBIRT sessions interrupted by physicians; however, in such cases, SBIRT providers resumed services after the conclusion of the primary care appointment.

Feasibility Study Procedures

SERVICE PROVISION AND STUDY INTRODUCTION

When SBIRT service providers began collecting data for the feasibility study, they continued to (a) follow the referral and recruitment procedures outlined earlier, (b) implement both SBIRT and T-SBIRT services as designed, and (c) complete T-SBIRT integrity checklists. The checklists were meant to increase fidelity to the model and record feasibility data. After the combined SBIRT and T-SBIRT sessions were completed, the SBIRT providers introduced the feasibility study survey to assess patient acceptability of the T-SBIRT protocol. Providers asked service recipients if they were interested in completing the survey, informing patients that the survey was nine items in length and that it referred specifically to the provider–patient conversation about trauma (i.e., T-SBIRT) as opposed to the conversation about substance use (i.e., SBIRT). In addition, providers notified patients that they would receive a $5 gift card after completing the survey.

Administering and Collecting the Survey

If a patient agreed to take the feasibility study survey (102 out of 112 patients did so for a 91.1% response rate), the SBIRT provider administered the survey by handing a copy to the study participant, allowing the participant to complete the tool in private and answering questions about specific items. The participant placed the completed survey in a large envelope and exchanged the envelope for a gift card; afterward, the provider inserted the completed integrity checklist in the envelope. One study packet was generated for each participant, and the first author collected packets at supervision meetings consistent with the human subjects protection plan.

Supervision Meetings

The first author continued to hold weekly supervision meetings during data collection periods. Supervision discussions centered on provider adherence and competence. That is, the first author ensured that providers covered all steps of the protocol and recorded each completed step with a check mark (i.e., adherence). Furthermore, the first author discussed quality of service provision by referencing motivational interviewing principles, role-playing with SBIRT providers, and exploring case scenarios (i.e., competence).

Service Capacity

During the study period, Site 1 completed roughly twice the number of SBIRT and T-SBIRT service sessions compared to Site 2 (74 vs. 38) due to (a) an earlier launch date, and (b) the presence of two SBIRT service providers at Site 1 versus one at Site 2. Over a period of 4 months, Site 1 conducted an average of just under five protocols per week, whereas over a period of 2.5 months, Site 2 completed an average of just under four SBIRT and T-SBIRT protocols per week. Although the clinics pre-screened all patients for alcohol use, they devoted limited staff time to SBIRT services given the part-time schedule of interns, the myriad other duties of the interns and nurse patient navigator, and limited available resources.

Feasibility Study Purpose and Domains

This study is meant to assess the feasibility of the T-SBIRT protocol and prepare the way for an efficacy trial (see Arain, Campbell, Cooper, & Lancaster, 2010). Accordingly, the study collected and analyzed data from five distinct yet related domains relevant to formative evaluations: (a) suitability of treatment, (b) acceptability of treatment, (c) patient compliance (also known as patient adherence), (d) treatment integrity, and (e) intended outcomes (Bowen et al., 2009). Suitability, sometimes considered a subset of acceptability, refers to the goodness of fit between services and the presenting problem. Acceptability is defined as "the extent to which interventions are considered appropriate, effective, and fair" (Finn & Sladeczek, 2001, p. 176) by either service providers or service recipients; we assessed acceptability from the standpoint of the service recipients (i.e., patients). Unsurprisingly, patient perception of acceptability can contribute to compliance (e.g., acceptance and completion of services).

Treatment integrity or fidelity has been characterized as a latent construct composed of several distinct dimensions including provider adherence and competence (Sanetti & Kratochwill, 2009). Adherence denotes the thoroughness with which providers follow the steps of a treatment or intervention protocol and competence refers to the skillfulness with which providers deliver the protocol. We promoted both but collected adherence data only. Finally, Arain et al. (2010) suggested that feasibility studies collect data on intended outcomes to inform and justify future efficacy trials. We therefore gathered pilot data on one obvious intervention outcome (i.e., referral acceptance) to generate insight into the model's potential efficacy.

METHOD

Sample and Design

SAMPLE

The sample consisted of adult patients from two community health clinics identified through convenience sampling procedures. Based on a daily schedule of appointments, SBIRT providers culled in-house SBIRT referrals from medical assistants with additional input from nurses and physicians during designated SBIRT service hours. Prior to primary care visits, SBIRT providers contacted patients identified for SBIRT services while the patients sat in waiting or exam rooms, and on contact, SBIRT providers offered combined SBIRT and T-SBIRT services. Each provider devoted 2 to 5 hr per week to SBIRT during the study period.

In total, 112 patients participated in the study: 74 from Site 1 and 38 from Site 2. Of the full sample, 53.7% were African American, 36.1% identified as Latino, and 5.6% were White; 40.6% were female. The average age was 41.4 years, with a range of 18 to 74. Participants' age did not vary across sites, but the race or ethnicity and gender composition did. At Site 1, 82.9% of participants were African American, 8.6% were White and 1.4% identified as Latino; in contrast, all participants at Site 2 identified as Latino. Also, whereas 44.4% of the participants at Site 1 were female, only 32.4% of participants at Site 2 were female.

SBIRT providers completed integrity checklists for all participants. At the conclusion of SBIRT services, 5 participants from each site refused to complete treatment acceptability surveys due to a stated concern for time. Thus, the sample size for the survey is 102.

DESIGN

To test whether it is feasible to marry T-SBIRT with SBIRT in community health clinics, the authors used a nonexperimental research design to collect data on an intervention group at one time point with patient-report surveys and provider-completed integrity checklists. The authors also relied on a monitoring and interactive design to ensure that providers delivered the protocol and collected the data as planned. With these two approaches, the authors collected indicators from all five feasibility study domains identified earlier.

Measures

We collected data from self-report assessments completed by study participants and from the T-SBIRT integrity checklists completed by SBIRT service providers. From these data, we created multiple measures to assess various indicators of feasibility. To specify, measures contributing to suitability and acceptability of treatment derived from validated self-report scales were administered during patient contact and embedded within the SBIRT protocols. Measures of patient compliance, treatment integrity, and intended outcomes emerged from the integrity checklists. In the first five measures subsections that follow, we introduce the validated alcohol-misuse screener, trauma screeners, and treatment acceptability survey along with, in some cases, measures constructed from these assessments. Subsequently, in the final four subsections, we identify the way in which we created measures to assess our five feasibility constructs.

ALCOHOL USE DISORDERS IDENTIFICATION TEST

During receipt of traditional SBIRT services, patients completed a drug abuse screening test along with the Alcohol Use Disorders Identification Test (AUDIT; Babor et al., 2001). For this study, however, authors analyzed results from the AUDIT only. The AUDIT is a 10-item tool that has been shown to distinguish between safe alcohol use, hazardous and harmful use, and probable alcohol use disorder (Babor et al., 2001). Items address frequency and quantity of drinking, consequences of drinking, and specific symptoms of alcohol use disorders. Answer categories range from 0 to 4 for each item, resulting in a possible summed total ranging from 0 through 40. Total scores equaling 0 to 7 indicate low risk for alcohol misuse; scores ranging from 8 to 15 reflect hazardous use patterns (medium risk); scores from 16 to 19 represent harmful use patterns (high risk); and scores of 20 or above suggest alcohol use disorder. The instrument demonstrates good psychometric properties in primary care settings (Reinert & Allen, 2002).

We created a continuous AUDIT score variable reflecting raw AUDIT results, and from these scores, we also constructed two ordinal measures: one with three AUDIT score categories (i.e., low risk, medium and high risk combined, and alcohol use disorder), and one with two AUDIT score categories (i.e., low risk vs. all others). For the former measure, we combined medium and high-risk categories due to our conceptual interest in hazardous and harmful users as one cluster. For the latter measure, we combined all drinkers at risk for misuse or alcohol use disorder, as this is the group targeted by SBIRT.

TRAUMA HISTORY SCREEN

While delivering T-SBIRT services, providers probed for patient experiences of PTEs with the help of the THS. The THS (Carlson, 2001) assesses lifetime exposure to 14 PTEs such as natural disasters, child sexual and physical abuse, and adult physical and sexual assault. Designed to be both brief and easy to -read, the instrument has demonstrated strong construct and convergent validity along with high test–retest reliability (α = .74–.94) with health care samples (Carlson et al., 2011). Providers did not administer the THS in the conventional manner by reading all items; instead, they discussed examples of PTEs and asked patients if they had ever experienced such traumatic stressors. Although they tried to cover all items, providers essentially asked about "anchor" traumas (i.e., recent or lasting experiences), as opposed to asking for thorough reports of patients' trauma histories. In a brief interview context, providers avoided probing for historical details in a way that might be perceived as time-consuming and intrusive and was inconsistent with the protocol purpose. Therefore, we created one variable from the THS results: 1 or more PTEs.

Primary Care-PTSD Screen

In addition to assessing for PTEs, providers screened for PTSD with the PC-PTSD, a brief 4-item screening tool that asks respondents if they have experienced, within the past month, four diagnostic symptoms of PTSD: reexperiencing, avoidance, numbing, and hyperarousal (Prins et al., 2003). The tool is widely used, requires only binary responses, and demonstrates high sensitivity (0.91) and moderate specificity (0.72) using a cutoff score of 2 within a health care setting (Prins et al., 2003). Relying on this threshold to determine a positive screening result, providers administered the PC-PTSD conventionally by reading the instrument's preamble and all items verbatim to patients. In our sample, the instrument yielded a Cronbach's alpha reliability estimate of .76. We created two measures based on PC-PTSD results: number of PTSD symptoms and positive PTSD screen. The THS and PC-PTSD have been combined in past trials; together, they help detect PTSD, which is predicated on both trauma exposure and traumatic stress symptoms.

Combined AUDIT And PC-PTSD

We also created a composite measure informed by the positive PTSD screen and two AUDIT score categories measures: PTSD/AUDIT bombined. It is a categorical variable identifying four mutually exclusive patient outcomes on both the PC-PTSD and AUDIT: negative PTSD screen and low alcohol misuse risk (Group 1), negative PTSD screen and medium or higher alcohol misuse risk (Group 2), positive PTSD screen and low alcohol misuse risk (Group 3), and positive PTSD screen and medium or higher alcohol misuse risk (Group 4).

Treatment acceptability And preferences

To determine acceptability from the patient perspective, SBIRT providers administered a modified version of the 9-item Treatment Acceptability and Preferences (TAP) measure (Sidani, Epstein, Bootzin, Moritz, & Miranda, 2009). The tool was designed to assess the acceptability of behavioral health treatments delivered within health care settings. Items assess a respondent's judgment of the effectiveness, appropriateness, severity, and convenience of an intervention, and item responses range from 0 (*not at all*) to 4 (*very much*). In previous studies, the TAP measure demonstrated good psychometric properties (e.g., Houle et al., 2013; Sidani et al., 2009). With our sample, it yielded a Cronbach's alpha reliability coefficient of .86.

SUITABILITY

To measure whether the T-SBIRT protocol was well-suited for patients receiving traditional SBIRT services within community health clinics, the authors assessed four outcomes: 1 or more PTEs; positive PTSD screen; correlation between AUDIT score and number of PTSD symptoms; and percentage of participants who produced a positive PC-PTSD screening result while also judged to be at low risk for alcohol misuse, at medium to high risk for alcohol misuse (hazardous or harmful use), or at risk for alcohol use disorder, according to the three AUDIT score categories variable. We also assessed positive PTSD screen rates across the two AUDIT score categories. Results were organized by full sample and, when useful, by participating site.

ACCEPTABILITY

We calculated the overall scale mean of the TAP, after reverse coding one item in which a higher score indicated poorer acceptability, to create a simple indicator of overall acceptability. We calculated the range, mean, and standard deviation of each item and subscale, and also assessed the overall scale mean per category of the PTSD/AUDIT combined measure. We reported the percentage of respondents endorsing a score of 2 or more on each item, reported response categories corresponding to acceptable or higher, and calculated the percent of respondents selecting 0 on each item, a response category of unacceptable. Finally, we reported results by full sample and by site, and constructed an alternative measure of patient acceptability: provider report of implementing the calming exercise listed at the end of the integrity checklist.

COMPLIANCE AND TREATMENT INTEGRITY

Using the integrity checklist to document patient compliance, SBIRT providers indicated whether a patient accepted or refused SBIRT services and whether a patient completed or withdrew from SBIRT services. We calculated the percentage of patients who accepted SBIRT services on request (i.e., acceptance), along with the percentage of those who completed services after initially agreeing (i.e., completion). To create a measure of provider adherence, we calculated the percentage of required T-SBIRT protocol steps completed by providers as indicated by integrity checklists. Results were organized between and within sites.

Based on integrity checklist data, we calculated the percentage of patients who verbally accepted a referral to a behavioral or mental health specialist. A positive response on this measure indicated that a patient agreed to accept a referral near the end of the T-SBIRT protocol when providers asked patients if they wanted an onsite appointment or referral to an offsite mental or behavioral health provider. Referrals were accepted based on stated concerns about trauma exposure, trauma symptoms, and trauma-related coping mechanisms. T-SBIRT providers then capitalized on patient motivation by (a) scheduling an appointment for the patient to see the attending T-SBIRT provider for an hour-long mental or behavioral health consult session; (b) introducing the patient to a mental or behavioral health provider in the clinic who had openings if possible or scheduling a meeting with the provider if they were not available at the moment; or (c) referring the patient to an outside clinic and following up with a supportive phone call within 2 weeks. We analyzed referral acceptance rates for the full sample, for each site, and for three alcohol misuse risk categories: low, medium to high, and alcohol use disorder. In addition, we assessed referral acceptance rates per PTSD/AUDIT combined categories.

Analysis

Most analyses took the form of simple descriptive statistics or percentage calculations. We tested the relation between the AUDIT score and number of PTSD symptoms with a bivariate correlation. We employed a chi-square test to compare rates of positive PTSD screen results between the low-risk alcohol misuse group and the group scoring in the medium or higher risk categories. With a univariate analysis of variance (ANOVA), we compared overall acceptability mean scores across the PTSD/AUDIT combined categories, and with chi-square tests we compared referral acceptance rates across the three AUDIT score categories and across the four PTSD/AUDIT categories. All analyses were conducted with SPSS 22 software (IBM, 2012).

RESULTS

Suitability

Fully 92% of study participants endorsed exposure to one or more PTEs; of the participants from Site 1, 95.9% reported exposure to one or more PTEs versus 84.4% from Site 2 (see Table 1). In addition, 55.7% of the full sample produced a positive screening result on the PC-PTSD; 68.9% of the sample from Site 1 did so compared to 28.9% from Site 2 (see Table 1). All participants with positive PC-PTSD results acknowledged experiencing at least one

TABLE 1 Trauma Exposure, Trauma Symptoms, and Referral Acceptance by Study Site

Study Site	Sample Size	% Sample	% 1 or More PTEs	% PositivePTSD Screen	% Accept a Referral
Full sample	$N = 112$	100	92.0	55.4	62.5
Site 1	$n = 74$	66.1	95.9	68.9	74.3
Site 2	$n = 38$	33.9	84.4	28.9	39.5

Note: PTEs = potential traumatic events; PTSD = posttraumatic stress disorder.

TABLE 2 Trauma Exposure, Trauma Symptoms, and Referral Acceptance by AUDIT Score Category

AUDIT Score	Alcohol Misuse Risk Category	Sample Size	% Sample	% 1 or More PTEs	% PositivePTSD Screen	% Accept a Referral
Missing on AUDIT		$n = 8$	7.1	62.5	25.0	25.0
0–7	Low risk	$n = 55$	49.1	90.9	49.1	54.5
8–19	Medium and high risk	$n = 26$	23.2	96.2	65.4	73.1
20+	Alcohol use disorder	$n = 23$	20.5	100	69.6	82.6

Note: AUDIT = Alcohol Use Disorders Identification Test; PTEs = potential traumatic events; PTSD = posttraumatic stress disorder.

PTE, and over 50% reported experiencing symptoms of avoidance over the past month (53.6%); a majority (51.6%) also endorsed PTSD symptoms of hyperarousal (not shown in Table 1).

The AUDIT score and number of PTSD symptoms were correlated at the bivariate level ($r = .205$, $p = .036$). Table 2 displays the rate of exposure to 1 or more PTEs and rate of positive PTSD screen by the three AUDIT score categories. Due to administrator or provider error, AUDIT scores were not recorded for 8 participants. Of those with low risk for alcohol misuse, 90.9% were exposed to at least one PTE and 49.1% screened positive for PTSD. In contrast, of those at medium to high risk for alcohol misuse, 96.2% were exposed to one or more PTEs and 65.4% produced a positive PC-PTSD screening result. Similarly, of those with potential alcohol use disorder, 100% were exposed to at least one PTE and nearly 70% had positive PTSD screening results. Analysis of the two AUDIT score categories (not shown) indicated that of the medium or higher risk group ($n = 49$), 67.3% screened positive for PTSD, a rate that trended higher than the 49.1% positive PTSD screen result for the low group, $\chi^2 = 3.538$, $p = .060$.

TABLE 3 Results from Treatment Acceptability and Preferences (TAP) Measure

Item/Subscale	Range	Overall		Site 1		Site 2		% 2 or More		
		M	SD	M	SD	M	SD	Overall	Site 1	Site 2
1. How effective, in the short term, do you think this treatment will be in improving any problems related to trauma, stress, or both?	0–4	2.75	1.08	3.01	1.02	2.18	0.98	86.3	91.3	75.8
2. How effective, in the long term, do you think this treatment will be in improving any problems related to trauma, stress, or both?	0–4	2.96	1.01	3.12	1.02	2.61	0.92	90.0	91.3	87.1
3. How effective do you think this treatment will be in reducing problems you experience during the day as a result of trauma, stress, or both?	0–4	2.71	1.09	2.74	1.09	2.66	1.11	89.8	91.3	86.2
4. How effective do you think this treatment will be in improving your ability to perform your daily usual activities?	0–4	2.76	1.13	2.72	1.16	2.83	1.05	85.9	84.1	90.0
Effective subscale (Items 1–4)	0–4	2.78	0.89	2.90	0.89	2.53	0.86	—	—	—
5. How acceptable and reasonable does this treatment seem to you?	1–4	3.19	0.93	3.54	0.74	2.45	0.87	97.1	100	90.9
6. How suitable or appropriate does this treatment seem to be for your trauma, stress, or both?	0–4	2.88	1.04	3.06	0.98	2.52	1.06	90.2	94.2	81.8
Appropriateness subscale (Items 5–6)	0.5–4	3.03	0.89	3.30	0.78	2.49	0.88	—	—	—
7. How severe or bad do you think are the risks or side effects of this treatment? (reverse coded)	0–4	3.69	0.75	3.75	0.70	3.58	0.85	98.0	98.5	96.8
Severe indicator (Item 7 only)	—	—	—	—	—	—	—	—	—	—
8. How easy do you think it will be for you to apply recommendations or plans resulting from this treatment to your life?	0–4	2.93	1.12	3.12	1.09	2.48	1.09	86.7	89.9	79.3
9. How willing are you to comply with this treatment?	0–4	3.15	1.10	3.46	0.92	2.33	1.11	88.5	95.7	70.4
Convenience of application (Items 8–9)	0–4	3.04	1.00	3.29	0.86	2.43	1.07	—	—	—
Total TAP score (overall acceptability)	0–4	2.99	0.72	3.17	0.66	2.60	0.69	—	—	—

Note: N = 102.

Acceptability

Table 3 shows results of the TAP survey. The overall mean was 2.99, corresponding to a response category of *very acceptable*. For the full sample, the four-item average for the effectiveness subscale was 2.78, reflecting a rating between *effective* and *very effective*. The mean of the appropriateness subscale for the full sample was 3.03, or just above *very appropriate*. The item indicating severity of treatment, which was reverse coded, yielded a full sample mean of 3.69, approaching a rating of *not severe at all*, and all respondents rated, on average, the convenience of application just above *very convenient*, a 3.04 subscale mean.

The overall scale mean varied across PTSD/AUDIT combined categories (not shown in tables): 2.70 for Group 1 or those with a negative PTSD screen and low alcohol misuse risk ($n = 28$), 2.97 for Group 2 or those with a negative PTSD screen and medium or higher alcohol misuse risk ($n = 16$), 3.07 for Group 3 or those with a positive PTSD screen and low alcohol misuse risk ($n = 26$), and 3.17 for Group 4 or the group with a positive PTSD screen and medium or higher alcohol misuse risk ($n = 32$). ANOVA results indicated that the overall contrasts between groups was not statistically significant ($p = .074$) but that Group 4 differed significantly from Group 1 ($p = .011$) on overall acceptability.

The percentage of participants who rated any one item 2 or above, response categories signifying acceptable or better, ranged from 85.9 to 98.0 (see column five of results in Table 3). Conversely, participants coded items 0 or unacceptable at rates ranging from 0.0% to 4.5% (not shown). No respondent rated Item 5 as unacceptable, an item that addresses general acceptability and reasonableness of the protocol. From 0.9% to 1.8% of participants rated the remaining items 0, with the exception of Items 3 and 4, which address effectiveness and garnered unacceptable ratings of 3.6% and 4.5%, respectively (not shown). Site-level results listed in Table 3 reveal that participants from Site 1 rated the T-SBIRT protocol more acceptable than participants from Site 2 on all but one item, and according to integrity checklists, in no case did providers introduce an evidence-based calming exercise to deactivate distressed patients (Briere & Scott, 2015).

Compliance and Treatment Integrity

All patients who were asked to participate in the SBIRT protocols agreed to do so, and all patients who agreed to participate in SBIRT services completed the services. In total, there are 11 mandatory steps that providers followed when implementing the T-SBIRT protocol (see Appendix). Considering all 112 participants, providers for both sites completed 97.2% of the required protocol steps, with little difference between sites.

Intended Outcome

Returning to Table 1, the last column of results displays referral acceptance rates for study participants. Of the full sample, 62.5% accepted a referral to a behavioral or mental health service provider for alcohol or trauma-related concerns. Nearly three fourths of the sample from Site 1 accepted such a referral versus about 40% from Site 2. Referral acceptance rates stratified by AUDIT results shown in Table 2 were as follows: 54.5% of the group at low risk for alcohol misuse, 73.1% of the group at medium to high risk for alcohol misuse, and 82.6% of the alcohol use disorder group. The differences are significant, $\chi^2(2) = 6.55$, $p = .038$.

Not shown are referral acceptance rates per PTSD/AUDIT combined categories; chi-square results suggest that the rates of referral acceptance also varied significantly across the four PTSD/AUDIT combined groups, $\chi^2 (3) = 38.645$, $p < .000$. Referral acceptance rates are as follows for Groups 1 through 4, respectively: 25.6%, 43.8%, 79.3%, and 93.9%.

DISCUSSION

Contributions

SUITABILITY

With a predominantly African American and Latino sample accessing community-based primary health care services for low-income patients, this study found that over 90% of participants were exposed to one or more PTEs and over 50% screened positive for PTSD. Although the prevalence of exposure to at least one PTE is very high in this sample, it has been shown that the majority of adults in the United States have experienced at least one PTE (e.g., Kilpatrick et al., 2013). However, epidemiological research suggests that PTSD rates when estimated within a previous 6-month period are approximately 4% as defined either by the fourth or fifth editions of the *Diagnostic and Statistical Manual of Mental Disorders* (*DSM–IV* or *DSM–5*; Kilpatrick et al., 2013). Furthermore, lifetime rates of PTSD appear to be 8.7% for African Americans and 7.0% for Latinos (Roberts, Gilman, Breslau, Breslau, & Koenen, 2011). Comparing our PTSD screening results to these figures from population-level studies suggests that the group of patients in our study experienced exceedingly high rates of PTSD; therefore, we conclude that trauma services such as T-SBIRT are suitable for the patient group studied.

Moreover, it appears that yoking such services to substance misuse services is reasonable given the potential correlation between PTSD symptoms and alcohol misuse. To specify, our results revealed that participants' AUDIT scores were significantly associated with number of trauma symptoms. In addition, the positive PTSD screening rates were quite high among those scoring in the medium or higher risk group for alcohol misuse categories (i.e., 67.3%), surpassing the upper limit of epidemiological estimates for comorbid trauma and substance misuse (Debell et al., 2014). Further, the rate of positive PTSD screening results were higher for those with positive alcohol misuse screening results compared to those with low alcohol misuse screening results, reinforcing Debell et al.'s (2014) suggestion to combine PTSD and alcohol misuse screening.

Our assertion regarding the suitability of combining a brief alcohol misuse intervention with a brief trauma intervention should be qualified by at least one consideration: PTSD rates were distinct across sites, recommending caution when drawing cross-site conclusions. To specify, participants at Site 2 reported lower rates of positive PTSD screening results relative to Site 1, potentially due to (a) differences in gender (e.g., 65.1% of females in the sample screened positive for PTSD vs. 52.4% of the male subsample); (b) differences in race or ethnicity composition (69.1% of African Americans in the sample screened positive for PTSD vs. 30.8% of Latino participants); and (c) slightly distinct recruitment procedures.

ACCEPTABILITY

Results from the TAP survey revealed that study participants found the T-SBIRT protocol, as implemented, acceptable. The overall mean of the survey reflected a rating of very acceptable, and the vast majority of respondents produced a rating of acceptable or better for each item. Moreover, it appeared that those at risk for cooccurring PTSD and substance misuse rated the T-SBIRT protocol higher on our acceptability metric relative to those at low risk for both, although the average rating for the low-risk group was near *very acceptable* (2.70). These results indicate that those for whom the protocol is tailored find it very acceptable, whereas those at low risk for the problems that the T-SBIRT targets are not averse to the protocol. Furthermore, no respondent rated the trademark item, Item 5, indicating general acceptability, as 0 or unacceptable, and the only items that more than 1.8% of the respondents rated as 0 were two items pertaining to effectiveness. Perhaps because Site 1 participants reported higher rates of potential PTSD relative to Site 2 participants, participants at Site 1 found the protocol to be more acceptable on average than Site 2 participants, given a total survey mean of 3.17 versus 2.60. Even so, 2.60 corresponds to a response category between acceptable and very acceptable, and compares favorably to TAP survey results from other studies. For instance, when testing the perceived acceptability of two discrete depression treatments, Houle et al. (2013) found overall TAP scale means to equate to 2.4 and 2.2, respectively. Also, in a TAP survey development study (Sidani et al., 2009), participants produced overall scale means ranging from 1.96 to 2.72 when assessing a behavioral health intervention targeting insomnia.

Finally, our finding that none of the 112 patients who completed the SBIRT protocols required a calming activity at the conclusion of services is consistent with research showing that trauma-related questionnaires generally do not prompt inordinate levels of participant distress (e.g., Black, Kresnow, Simon, Arias, & Shelley, 2006). We want to underscore that some level of reactivity to trauma assessments might be normative and even therapeutic among trauma survivors (Briere & Scott, 2015). As such, we embedded our trauma screeners within a patient-centered, motivationally based brief intervention to validate, contain, and channel patient reactions.

COMPLIANCE

Patient compliance with health, behavioral health, or mental health treatments represents a central concern for providers. Estimates of compliance are hard to come by because relatively few studies are published, but in a review of the literature, Montoya (2006) cited acceptance rates for some mental and behavioral health services as low as 38.1%. Completion rates for behavioral and mental health services can, in turn, reach lows of 50% or so among those enrolled (Topitzes et al., 2015). In this study, the combined SBIRT and T-SBIRT protocols yielded acceptance and completion rates of 100%. We surmise that these results are attributable to several key factors, some of which have been identified in the literature as potential predictors of patient compliance and adherence: (a) a focus on rapport building and motivational enhancement, (b) brief intervention translating into low patient burden, and (c) well-conceived in-clinic referral procedures (Martin, Williams, Haskard, & DiMatteo, 2005).

TREATMENT INTEGRITY

When conducting a thorough review of health behavior treatments, Borrelli and colleagues (2005) found that only 53 out of 342 studies or 15.5% of their sample reported high rates of treatment integrity; that is, instances in which providers met or exceeded a threshold of 80% adherence to an integrity checklist. By these standards, the adherence rate for T-SBIRT, 97.2%, was very high. Treatment adherence reached such a rate in our study for perhaps three reasons: (a) T-SBIRT is a brief intervention imposing minimal burden on providers; (b) the model design was easy to follow and logically sequenced, as it was founded on established theory, published research, and validated practices; and (c) providers participated in extensive prestudy training along with ongoing weekly supervision.

Intended outcome

Patient acceptance of a referral to a mental or behavioral health treatment provider represents one intended proximal outcome of the T-SBIRT model. In our study, 62.5% of all participants verbally accepted such a referral, a result that yields several lessons. First, it appears that the brief intervention succeeded in addressing a meaningful issue for the majority of participants. Second, traditional SBIRT typically generates referral to brief or specialty treatment at rates ranging from 25% to 47% (Chan, Huang, Sieu, & Unützer, 2013; Madras et al., 2009). Therefore, our findings provide preliminary indications that combining T-SBIRT with SBIRT might increase referral rates to some form of treatment for all participants.

Also, referral acceptance rates increased significantly as alcohol and PTSD risk rose among our study participants. To specify, almost 75% of our patient participants at risk for hazardous or harmful alcohol use accepted a treatment referral, suggesting that T-SBIRT could improve intended SBIRT outcomes among this category of drinkers. Rates of referral acceptance were even higher among study participants with probable alcohol use disorder (82.6%). This is noteworthy as the traditional SBIRT model has been found to confer little benefit to those at risk for alcohol use disorder and in need of specialty treatment (Glass et al., 2015). Combining SBIRT with a trauma module might help address this model weakness. Finally, rates of referral acceptance were highest among the group that produced positive PTSD and AUDIT screening results, 93.9%, providing evidence that patients at risk for cooccurring PTSD and alcohol misuse were especially likely to accept referrals. The model worked as intended in this trial.

Limitations

Although our study provides unique insights into the feasibility of complementing traditional SBIRT services with a trauma module, several limitations qualify the results. First, although we ensured confidentiality of respondents' data, service providers also administered the patient acceptability surveys, potentially resulting in socially desirable responses to items. Second, caution is needed when generalizing study results given that SBIRT and T-SBIRT were only offered to a portion of clinic patients based on service provider availability and patient alcohol misuse risk. Because SBIRT was not delivered universally as designed and the sample was not gathered through random procedures, our ability to generalize results to low-income patients of community-based health clinics or even to patients at risk for alcohol misuse is compromised.

Third, due to the date of study initiation, the PTSD screener used within the T-SBIRT protocol reflected *DSM–IV* versus *DSM–5* symptom criteria. Future iterations of T-SBIRT will integrate a *DSM–5*-based PTSD screener;

however, findings are not expected to diverge significantly considering recent epidemiological research, which indicated that PTSD prevalence rates do not vary notably if either *DSM–IV* or *DSM–5* criteria are used to determine the presence of disorder (Kilpatrick et al., 2013). Fifth, we did not analyze results from a drug abuse screening test, assessing the relevance of T-SBIRT for drug misuse; however, future research should include such explorations. Finally, our results derive from a nonexperimental feasibility study. Even our intended outcome, referral acceptance, is proximal, does not equate to a patient following through on a referral, and reflects a significant limitation of our data.

CONCLUSION

Our results indicate that it is feasible to implement T-SBIRT together with traditional SBIRT within community health clinics serving low-income minority patients. More specifically, our findings suggest that not only is T-SBIRT a suitable and acceptable service, but that it has the potential to yield high rates of referrals to mental and behavioral health treatment for low-income, minority patients presenting with substance misuse including probable alcohol use disorder, traumatic stress, or both. Results align with previous research indicating that mental health treatment might not be stigmatizing for minorities when integrated within primary care (Roberts et al., 2008). Therefore, we conclude that implementing T-SBIRT within community-based primary care clinic settings has the potential to enhance traditional SBIRT outcomes for groups at risk for health disparities who might not benefit from SBIRT alone; that is, low-income patients of color with alcohol misuse or alcohol use disorder.

Although we cannot know if our results generalize beyond settings similar to those included in this study, we would suggest that social workers implement and test T-SBIRT in multiple community-based settings and with an array of service populations. Because trauma is relevant for adults of all socioeconomic backgrounds, we believe that T-SBIRT can enhance SBIRT outcomes for patients of all economic strata and racial or ethnic identities. By improving traditional SBIRT outcomes, T-SBIRT could play a key role in meeting the Grand Challenge of reducing alcohol misuse at the population level, improving the efficacy of social workers and other allied professionals who promote integrated health care, and facilitating interdisciplinary collaboration among health professionals. Future trials should test T-SBIRT outcomes such as utilization of mental health services, engagement in primary health care, and reduction of alcohol misuse and trauma symptoms.

FUNDING

This study described herein was a component of the SBIRT Training for Substance Misuse Program at the University Wisconsin–Milwaukee (No. 1U79TI025412-01), a grant project funded by the Substance Abuse and Mental Health Services Administration through a program titled SBIRT Training (RFA: TI-13-02).

REFERENCES

Agerwala, S. M., & McCance-Katz, E. F. (2012). Integrating Screening, Brief Intervention, and Referral to Treatment (SBIRT) into clinical practice settings: A brief review. *Journal of Psychoactive Drugs*, *44*, 307–317. doi:10.1080/02791072.2012.720169

Arain, M., Campbell, M. J., Cooper, C. L., & Lancaster, G. A. (2010). What is a pilot or feasibility study? A review of current practice and editorial policy. *BMC Medical Research Methodology*, *10*(1), 67. doi:10.1186/1471-2288-10-67

Babor, T. F., Higgins-Biddle, J. C., Saunders, J. B., & Monteiro, M. G. (2001). *The Alcohol Use Disorders Identification Test (AUDIT): Guidelines for use in primary care*. Geneva, Switzerland: World Health Organization.

Babor, T. F., McRee, B. G., Kassebaum, P. A., Grimaldi, P. L., Ahmed, K., & Bray, J. (2007). Screening, Brief Intervention, and Referral to Treatment (SBIRT): Toward a public health approach to the management of substance abuse. *Substance Abuse*, *28*(3), 7–30. doi:10.1300/J465v28n03_03

Begun, A., Clapp, J. & The Alcohol Misuse Grand Challenge Collective. (2016). Reducing and preventing alcohol misuse and its consequences: A Grand Challenge for social work. *The International Journal of Alcohol and Drug Research*, *5*(2), 73–83. doi:10.7895/ijadr.v5i2.223

Black, M. C., Kresnow, M., Simon, T. R., Arias, I., & Shelley, G. (2006). Telephone survey respondents' reactions to questions regarding interpersonal violence. *Violence and Victims*, *21*, 445–459. doi:10.1891/0886-6708.21.4.445

Bliss, D. L., & Pecukonis, E. (2009). Screening and brief intervention practice model for social workers in non-substance-abuse practice settings. *Journal of Social Work Practice in the Addictions*, *9*(1), 21–40. doi:10.1080/15332560802646604

Borrelli, B., Sepinwall, D., Ernst, D., Bellg, A. J., Czajkowski, S., Breger, R., … Resnick, B. (2005). A new tool to assess treatment fidelity and evaluation of treatment fidelity across 10 years of health behavior research. *Journal of Consulting and Clinical Psychology*, *73*, 852–860. doi:10.1037/0022-006X.73.5.852

Bowen, D. J., Kreuter, M., Spring, B., Cofta-Woerpel, L., Linnan, L., Weiner, D., … Fernandez, M. (2009). How we design feasibility studies. *American Journal of Preventive Medicine*, *36*, 452–457. doi:10.1016/j.amepre.2009.02.002

Briere, J. N., & Scott, C. (2015). *Principles of trauma therapy: A guide to symptoms, evaluation, and treatment*. Los Angeles, CA: Sage.

Carlson, E. B. (2001). Psychometric study of a brief screen for PTSD: Assessing the impact of multiple traumatic events. *Assessment, 8,* 431–441. doi:10.1177/107319110100800408

Carlson, E. B., Smith, S. R., Palmieri, P. A., Dalenberg, C., Ruzek, J. I., Kimerling, R., … Spain, D. A. (2011). Development and validation of a brief self-report measure of trauma exposure: The Trauma History Screen. *Psychological Assessment, 23,* 463–477. doi:10.1037/a0022294

Chan, Y.-F., Huang, H., Sieu, N., & Unützer, J. (2013). Substance screening and referral for substance abuse treatment in an integrated mental health care program. *Psychiatric Services, 64*(1), 88–90. doi:10.1176/appi.ps.201200082

Debell, F., Fear, N. T., Head, M., Batt-Rawden, S., Greenberg, N., Wessely, S., & Goodwin, L. (2014). A systematic review of the comorbidity between PTSD and alcohol misuse. *Social Psychiatry and Psychiatric Epidemiology, 49,* 1401–1425. doi:10.1007/s00127-014-0855-7

Finn, C. A., & Sladeczek, I. E. (2001). Assessing the social validity of behavioral interventions: A review of treatment acceptability measures. *School Psychology Quarterly, 16,* 176–206. doi:10.1521/scpq.16.2.176.18703

Ford, J. D., Hawke, J., Alessi, S., Ledgerwood, D., & Petry, N. (2007). Psychological trauma and PTSD symptoms as predictors of substance dependence treatment outcomes. *Behaviour Research and Therapy, 45,* 2417–2431. doi:10.1016/j.brat.2007.04.001

Glass, J. E., Hamilton, A. M., Powell, B. J., Perron, B. E., Brown, R. T., & Ilgen, M. A. (2015). Specialty substance use disorder services following brief alcohol intervention: A meta-analysis of randomized controlled trials. *Addiction, 110,* 1404–1415. doi:10.1111/add.12950

Houle, J., Villaggi, B., Beaulieu, M.-D., Lespérance, F., Rondeau, G., & Lambert, J. (2013). Treatment preferences in patients with first episode depression. *Journal of Affective Disorders, 147*(1–3), 94–100. doi:10.1016/j.jad.2012.10.016

Humphreys, K., & McLellan, A. T. (2010). Brief intervention, treatment, and recovery support services for Americans who have substance use disorders: An overview of policy in the Obama administration. *Psychological Services, 7,* 275–284. doi:10.1037/a0020390

IBM. (2012). *IBM SPSS statistics for Windows, Version 21.0.* Armonk, NY: IBM.

Israel, Y., Hollander, O., Sanchez-Craig, M., Booker, S., Miller, V., Gingrich, R., & Rankin, J. G. (1996). Screening for problem drinking and counseling by the primary care physician–nurse team. *Alcoholism: Clinical and Experimental Research, 20,* 1443–1450. doi:10.1111/acer.1996.20.issue-8

Kilpatrick, D. G., Resnick, H. S., Milanak, M. E., Miller, M. W., Keyes, K. M., & Friedman, M. J. (2013). National estimates of exposure to traumatic events and PTSD prevalence using DSM–IV and DSM–5 criteria. *Journal of Traumatic Stress, 26,* 537–547. doi:10.1002/jts.2013.26.issue-5

Kramer, M. D., Polusny, M. A., Arbisi, P. A., & Krueger, R. F. (2014). Comorbidity of PTSD and SUDs: Toward an etiologic understanding. In P. Ouimette & J. P. Read (Eds.), *Trauma and substance abuse: Causes, consequences, and treatment of comorbid disorders* (2nd ed., pp. 53–75). Washington, DC: American Psychological Association.

Madras, B. K., Compton, W. M., Avula, D., Stegbauer, T., Stein, J. B., & Clark, H. W. (2009). Screening, brief interventions, referral to treatment (SBIRT) for illicit drug and alcohol use at multiple healthcare sites: Comparison at intake and 6 months later. *Drug and Alcohol Dependence, 99*(1–3), 280–295. doi:10.1016/j. drugalcdep.2008.08.003

Martin, L. R., Williams, S. L., Haskard, K. B., & DiMatteo, M. R. (2005). The challenge of patient adherence. *Therapeutics & Clinical Risk Management, 1*, 189–199.

McCauley, J. L., Killeen, T., Gros, D. F., Brady, K. T., & Back, S. E. (2012). Posttraumatic stress disorder and co-occurring substance use disorders: Advances in assessment and treatment. *Clinical Psychology: Science and Practice, 19*, 283–304.

Monahan, C. J., McDevitt-Murphy, M. E., Dennhardt, A. A., Skidmore, J. R., Martens, M. P., & Murphy, J. G. (2013). The impact of elevated posttraumatic stress on the efficacy of brief alcohol interventions for heavy drinking college students. *Addictive Behaviors, 38*, 1719–1725. doi:10.1016/j.addbeh.2012.09.004

Montoya, I. D. (2006). Treatment compliance in patients with co-occurring mental illness and substance abuse. *Psychiatric Times, 23*(1), 23.

Najavits, L. M., & Kanukollu, S. (2005). It can be learned, but can it be taught? Results from a state-wide training initiative on PTSD and substance abuse. *Journal of Dual Diagnosis, 1*(4), 41–51. doi:10.1300/J374v01n04_05

O'Donnell, A., Anderson, P., Newbury-Birch, D., Schulte, B., Schmidt, C., Reimer, J., & Kaner, E. (2014). The impact of brief alcohol interventions in primary healthcare: A systematic review of reviews. *Alcohol and Alcoholism, 49*(1), 66–78. doi:10.1093/alcalc/agt170

Prins, A., Ouimette, P., Kimerling, R., Cameron, R. P., Hugelshofer, D. S., Shaw-Hegwer, J., & Sheikh, J. I. (2003). The Primary Care PTSD Screen (PC-PTSD): Development and operating characteristics. *Primary Care Psychiatry, 9*, 9–14. doi:10.1185/135525703125002360

Reinert, D. F., & Allen, J. P. (2002). The Alcohol Use Disorders Identification Test (AUDIT): A review of recent research. *Alcoholism: Clinical and Experimental Research, 26*, 272–279. doi:10.1111/acer.2002.26.issue-2

Roberts, A. L., Gilman, S. E., Breslau, J., Breslau, N., & Koenen, K. C. (2011). Race/ethnic differences in exposure to traumatic events, development of post-traumatic stress disorder, and treatment-seeking for post-traumatic stress disorder in the United States. *Psychological Medicine, 41*(1), 71–83. doi:10.1017/S0033291710000401

Roberts, K. T., Robinson, K. M., Topp, R., Newman, J., Smith, F., & Stewart, C. (2008). Community perceptions of mental health needs in an underserved minority neighborhood. *Journal of Community Health Nursing, 25*, 203–217. doi:10.1080/07370010802421202

Salvalaggio, G., Dong, K., Vandenberghe, C., Kirkland, S., Mramor, K., Brown, T., ... Wild, T. C. (2013). Enhancing screening, brief intervention, and referral to treatment among socioeconomically disadvantaged patients: Study protocol for a knowledge exchange intervention involving patients and physicians. *BMC Health Services Research, 13*, 1–11. doi:10.1186/1472-6963-13-108

Sanetti, L. M. H., & Kratochwill, T. R. (2009). Toward developing a science of treatment integrity: Introduction to the special series. *School Psychology Review, 38*, 445–459.

Shield, K. D., Parry, C., & Rehm, J. (2013). Focus on: Chronic diseases and conditions related to alcohol use. *Alcohol, 85*, 155–173.

Sidani, S., Epstein, D. R., Bootzin, R. R., Moritz, P., & Miranda, J. (2009). Assessment of preferences for treatment: Validation of a measure. *Research in Nursing & Health, 32*, 419–431. doi:10.1002/nur.v32:4

Topitzes, J., Mersky, J. P., & McNeil, C. B. (2015). Implementation of parent–child interaction therapy within foster care: An attempt to translate an evidence-based program within a local child welfare agency. *Journal of Public Child Welfare, 9* (1), 22–41. doi:10.1080/15548732.2014.983288

APPENDIX

T-SBIRT Protocol Integrity Checklist

1. Introduction of provider:

Example: "Hi, I'm (name), an intern in Behavioral Health. I'm working with (Primary Health Provider) as part of your client care team."   Done: _____

2. Ask permission to implement substance use and T-SBIRT protocols

Example: "I'd like to talk to you briefly about any alcohol or drug use, stress or related concerns—things that can affect your physical health. Is that okay?"   Done: _____

Check if patient refused: _____

3. mplement substance use SBIRT protocol   Done: _____

AUDIT Score: _____

4. Introduce stress and trauma, and their relationship to health

Example: "They say that stress from daily life or from traumatic events can have a significant impact not only on mental health but on physical health as well."   Done: _____

5. Ask about specific stressor in patient's life.

"What are the top stressors in your life right now? List them."   Done: _____

6. Ask about exposure to potential traumatic events:

Example: "How about any trauma? Anything from your adult past or your childhood?"

(Start with open-ended question, then provide examples from list, continue depending on willingness to talk. Document exposure below with an x or check for your own purposes.)

A. A really bad car, boat, train, or airplane accident   _____

B. A really bad accident at work or home   _____

C. A hurricane, flood, earthquake, tornado, or fire   _____

D. Hit or kicked hard enough to injure—as a child   _____

E. Hit or kicked hard enough to injure—as an adult   _____

F. Forced or made to have sexual contact—as a child   _____

G. Forced or made to have sexual contact—as an adult   _____

H. Attack with a gun, knife, or weapon   _____

I. During military service—seeing something horrible or being badly scared   _____

J. Sudden death of close family or friend   _____

K. Seeing someone die suddenly or get badly hurt or killed   _____

L. Some other sudden event that made you feel very scared, helpless, or horrified   _____

M. Sudden move or loss of home and possessions   _____

N. Suddenly abandoned by spouse, partner, parent, or family   _____

O. Others_____   _____

Done: _____

7. Ask about trauma symptoms

"Sometimes people can actually develop posttraumatic stress symptoms from these kinds of experiences. We can even develop posttraumatic stress symptoms from traumas we can't remember. In the past month, have you ever ..." (check all that apply):

A. ... had nightmares about an upsetting event or thought about the event when you did not want to?   _____

B. ... tried hard not to think about the upsetting event or went out of your way to avoid situations that reminded you of it?   _____

C. ... were constantly on guard, watchful, or easily startled?   _____

D. ... felt numb or detached from others, activities, or your surroundings?   _____

Done: _____

8. Ask about positive coping around stress and/or trauma:

"What have been some of your positive ways of coping with stress or trauma?"

(Reflective listening, support positive mechanisms)   Done: _____

9. Ask about coping that may have led to problems:

"What have been some unhelpful ways you may have dealt or coped with stress or trauma?"

(Reflective listening enhancing motivation to get help)   Done: _____

10. Help prepare patient for referral by highlighting connections between traumatic stress and ongoing behavioral health problems.

"Often it can be hard to stop using these sometimes unhelpful coping mechanisms unless the stress and trauma are addressed. (What do you think)?"

(Reflective listening enhancing motivation to get help)   Done: _____

11. Gauge motivation for referral if applicable (patient may not need one if no problems)

"Over the past few years, significant progress has been made in finding ways for people to deal with stress and trauma. We do offer supportive services here. Do you think you may have interest in seeing someone in order to talk further about these topics?"

Patient stated yes _____

Done: _____

12. Optional: Make a referral if applicable (patient stated yes and you will give internal or external referral)   Done: _____

13. Optional: Offer the patient the PTSD pamphlet: Done: _____

14. Please mark the line that applies:

Patient accepted SBIRT services but did not complete the T-SBIRT protocol   _____

Patient accepted SBIRT services and completed protocol   _____

15. Calming or containment exercise used: No _____

Yes _____

NIAAA and the Global Challenge: An Interview with Dr. Margaret (Peggy) Murray, Director, Global Alcohol Research Program, National Institutes of Health, National Institute of Alcohol Abuse and Alcoholism

Interview Conducted by
AUDREY L. BEGUN, MSW, PhD ⓘ

In serving as editors for this special issue related to the Grand Challenge for Social Work concerned with reducing and preventing alcohol misuse and its consequences, we thought it would be helpful for readers to hear a bit about how the National Institutes of Health (NIH) through the National Institute on Alcohol Abuse and Alcoholism (NIAAA) fits into achieving goals and objectives related to the challenge. We invited Dr. Margaret (Peggy) Murray to join us in a discussion because of her long track record of advocating for social work scholars to have a prominent place at the table where alcohol research agendas are developed, as well as championing NIAAA's development and dissemination of alcohol-related curriculum materials for MSW education. She has been working with NIAAA for more than 20 years, beginning with the Homeless Demonstration and Evaluation Branch, and subsequently heading up initiatives in health professions education about alcohol and alcohol use disorders, K–12 science education, and college drinking. Dr. Murray currently heads up the Global Research Program and serves as NIAAA's representative to the NIH Collaborative Research on Addictions (CRAN), which includes the (large) Alcohol Brain and Cognitive Development (ABCD) study and other major transinstitute initiatives.

Begun: As a senior official at the National Institute on Alcohol Abuse and Alcoholism (NIAAA), please clarify for readers NIAAA's roles and goals in reducing and preventing alcohol misuse and its consequences.

Murray: Essentially, NIAAA focuses on supporting, conducting, and disseminating research on the identification, prevention, and treatment of both alcohol use disorders and the health problems that come from the abuse of alcohol. These include, but are not limited to fetal alcohol spectrum disorders (FASD), alcohol-related liver and pancreatic diseases, and alcohol-related injury, such as traffic crashes and alcohol-related violence. This is a tall order, as you are well aware that alcohol affects every part of the body, as well as every aspect of society. Our research areas cover everything from the neuroscience of addiction to alcohol (which is leading to the development of exciting new medications to treat alcohol disorders); metabolism and health effects of alcohol; efficacy and effectiveness of both pharmacological and behavioral treatments and their combination; effective strategies for prevention of underage drinking, including policies that deal with enforcement of underage drinking laws; and clinical and environmental interventions to reduce alcohol-related violence. We also have a substantial portfolio on alcohol and HIV that spans biomedical and behavioral research. Aside from being the largest funder of alcohol research in the world, NIAAA works very hard to disseminate research findings to a large and diverse audience, which includes the general public, health professionals from a variety of fields, policymakers, and even specialized audiences such as teens and pregnant women.

Begun: Since publication of NIAAA's 40 Years of Research Reports in 2010 (see http://pubs.niaaa.nih.gov/publications/arh40/5-17.pdf), what do you see as the major scientific developments achieved and emerging that have the greatest implications for social workers as we continue to address the challenge of preventing and reducing alcohol misuse and its consequences?

Murray: I think that science does not work by "major scientific developments" as it generally moves along pretty incrementally. That said, I think we are making good progress in a number of important areas and we use these findings to formulate our major initiatives at NIAAA. Some of these initiatives are the following:

- Collaborative Research on Addictions at NIH (CRAN), which is a joint effort of NIAAA, the National Institute on Drug Abuse (NIDA), and the National Cancer Institute (NCI). Social work researchers especially should be aware of funding opportunities under the heading of CRAN at NIH (see https://addictionresearch.

nih.gov/). These are focused on substance use, abuse, and addiction in combination (i.e., alcohol, marijuana, and nicotine), as they so commonly present in the real world of social work practice.

- Alcohol's effects on adolescent development is another important area. As we have learned more about the effects of exposure to alcohol and other drugs on the developing brain and how that affects behavior, we find we need to know even more to develop effective prevention and treatment strategies around adolescent substance use and substance use disorders. NIAAA is a major player in a new study that is a collaboration of several NIH Institutes known as the ABCD (Adolescent Brain and Cognitive Development) Study. It is the largest long-term study of brain development and child health in the United States. The ABCD Research Consortium consists of a Coordinating Center, a Data Informatics and Analysis Center, and 19 research sites across the country, which will recruit approximately 10,000 children ages 9 and 10 and follow them longitudinally into early adulthood. Integrating structural and functional brain imaging with genetics, neuropsychological, behavioral, and other health assessments, the ABCD Study will increase our understanding of the many factors that can enhance or disrupt a young person's life trajectory. Social workers should be aware of findings from this study, which will be published throughout the 10 years of the project, and social work researchers should be ready to use the data, which will be made publicly available in very short turnaround time, to address questions of interest to the field.

- Collaborative Studies on the Genetics of Alcoholism (COGA) is a project that has been ongoing since 1989 and has provided data on more than 2,000 families and 17,000 individuals. Social work researchers have played significant roles in the inception, design, and implementation throughout this initiative. Social work practitioners can learn much about the genetics of alcohol use disorders that is important in helping individuals and families. Not only does this include potential vulnerabilities, including genetically related comorbid conditions (e.g., depression), but also potential sources of resilience.

- Medications to treat alcohol use disorders are an extremely important focus of NIAAA at this time. It is an especially good time for this, as discoveries in basic neuroscience that take advantage of the latest technologies for studying the brain (i.e., functional magnetic resonance imaging) help to inform clinical approaches and vice versa.

- FASD remains a top priority for our Institute and we fund an important international consortium (CIFASD) that is advancing diagnosis, prevention, and treatment of these rare yet debilitating conditions by collaborating with scientists, clinicians (including social workers), and populations in countries where FASD prevalence is high.

- College drinking remains an important focus, as binge drinking among teens and young adults is a persistent problem. Although we have made progress in reducing the rates of binge drinking in this population, the intensity of drinking in those who still binge appears to be increasing. The NIAAA College AIM (Alcohol Intervention Matrix) that can be found at collegedrinkingprevention.gov is an important tool for schools to help with underage and harmful drinking. Social workers who work in college and high school settings will find it a useful compendium of research-based strategies.

Begun: What major policies and initiatives are driving the federal government's role in reducing and preventing alcohol misuse and its consequences at this juncture, and how is this affecting what is happening globally as well as at state and local levels?

Murray: The strongest finding we have in alcohol research is the effectiveness of screening and brief intervention (SBI) for harmful use of alcohol in primary care health delivery. It is exciting to see so many trainings on this and initiatives to be sure it is implemented in as many places as possible, as well as the move to be sure it is covered by insurance. Federal health service delivery has taken the lead by requiring SBI as part of federally funded programs such as Medicare and the Indian Health Service. Although SBI's effectiveness has been known for 20 years, it is great to finally see efforts to make sure it is part of routine care.

Begun: We all know the saying "all politics is local," so please discuss how the federal government goes about working with the states and communities to prevent and reduce alcohol misuse and its consequences.

Murray: The Substance Abuse and Mental Health Services Administration (SAMHSA) works with the states through the administration of the Substance Abuse and Mental Health Block Grant and other activities. The regulation of alcohol content, labeling, federal taxation, and marketing are the mission of the Alcohol and Tobacco Tax and Trade Bureau (TTB), which is part of the Treasury Department, and the Federal Trade Commission. NIAAA is not directly involved in these areas, but each of these agencies calls on NIAAA to provide comments and sometimes technical support on their initiatives, based on our research. This is true for other agencies' activities around alcohol as well. For example, NIAAA provides input on what constitutes healthy alcohol consumption for adults for the

Dietary Guidelines for Americans, which is published every 5 years as a joint effort of the Department of Agriculture and the Department of Health and Human Services

The NIH (and its components such as NIAAA) are an anomaly as an agency of the Executive Branch. We are housed in the Department of Health and Human Services and are part of the Public Health Service (along with SAMHSA and the Centers for Disease Control [CDC]), but NIH does not issue policy or engage in enforcement. Our role is clearly one of supporting, conducting, and disseminating research. We like to think that policymakers at the national, state, and local levels use our research findings as they design alcohol control legislation, develop and implement public health campaigns, and deliver health services, but there is no guarantee that this always happens.

We do have an important tool available to investigators who want to conduct research on state and federal policies and their effectiveness in reducing alcohol-related harm. It is the Alcohol Policy Information System (APIS), a Web site that provides detailed information on alcohol-related public policies at both the state and federal levels. Updated annually, the APIS can be used to identify policy changes in 33 policy areas. Up to two thirds of these policies can be tracked back to 1998, and data on the remaining one third are available since 2003. More information can be found at http://alcoholpolicy. niaaa.nih.gov/Home.html.

Begun: Alcohol misuse and its consequences are also global issues. How is the federal government working with other countries to address these problems?

Murray: Alcohol has had center stage on the global policy agenda for the past 6 years, which has been a very exciting development. The World Health Organization (WHO), the Organization for Economic Cooperation and Development (OECD), and the United Nations have all had an important focus on alcohol in recent years. In 2010, the 63rd World Health Assembly in Geneva passed a resolution to adopt *Strategies to Reduce the Harmful Use of Alcohol*. This document provides nations with information about evidence-based strategies that they can adopt to address alcohol problems. NIAAA provided consultation to WHO in preparing this document, and we will continue to be involved. In addition, NIAAA worked with international experts and WHO to produce *Guidelines for the Identification and Management of Substance Use and Substance Use Disorders in Pregnancy*, which helps countries design effective programs in this area. The United Nations General Assembly on the Prevention and Control of Non-Communicable Diseases Political Declaration was the first time that all member states of the United

Nations agreed to come together and develop an agenda to reduce the risk of these diseases (UN General Assembly Resolution 66/2, 2011). "Reduction in the harmful use of alcohol" was identified as one of the four behavioral measures that member countries must focus on as part of the global plan to reduce this risk. In 2015, the OECD published a report called *Tackling Harmful Alcohol Use: Economics and Public Health Policy*, a microsimulation model that will allow OECD member countries to determine which alcohol policies are most beneficial for each of them in reducing the harms from alcohol misuse.

NIAAA provides extensive information on effective strategies for preventing underage drinking, but reducing underage drinking has proven to be an uphill battle. Because we have the means to support research on environmental interventions, we are a bit ahead of the game in the United States compared to many other nations. Because of cultural attitudes about alcohol and its use, many countries are not ready to try widespread interventions such as training about alcohol and enforcing the minimum drinking age— even though there is excellent research to support such policies. There remain myths that somehow teens in other countries are more mature, or have family traditions around alcohol that are more protective, and this is problematic, as we are now seeing high rates of binge drinking in teens and even alcoholic liver disease in young adults in some countries in Western Europe.

Begun: What innovative, cutting-edge, or exciting developments are happening at the international level or in other nations that have potential significance for how the United States addresses the challenge of preventing and reducing the consequences of alcohol misuse?

Murray: Recognition of alcohol use disorders as medical and chronic relapsing conditions and providing adequate treatment is, unfortunately, more often the case in countries outside the United States. Many countries in Western and Eastern Europe have had professional (i.e., psychiatric) services to treat alcohol addiction and widely available, covered treatment for a long time. In Russia, there has long been a specialty to treat addiction called narcology, which is a branch of psychiatry. In the United States, it was only this past fall (2015) when addiction medicine became a certified board specialty.

Aside from that, it often surprises me how similar the fight for good and even adequate handling of addiction and other alcohol use disorders is in many countries. My colleagues from other countries and I often share "war" stories of our work and it is not that different around the world.

Begun: What are the federal government's major challenges in preventing and reducing alcohol misuse and its consequences?

Murray: Lack of treatment being available to those who need and want it. This is exacerbated by the stigma that still surrounds admitting to having a problem with alcohol and getting treatment, especially through an employer-based health plan. Only around 10% of adults who meet the criteria for an alcohol use disorder get specialized treatment, and even a smaller number of these get evidence-based treatments. There is reluctance of a number of treatment programs to use medications to treat alcohol addiction, even though we are making strides in identifying good pharmacotherapies that, coupled with behavioral treatments such as cognitive behavioral therapy, are really effective.

Begun: From your perspective, what specific roles are, or should, social workers be playing in preventing and reducing alcohol misuse and its consequences?

Murray: Every social worker needs to be versed in the identification of harmful use of alcohol, and how to make a referral for evaluation and treatment, if needed. This is very important, as harmful alcohol use is a factor in so many social and developmental problems that social workers deal with in all settings. Social workers, especially in hospital settings, should know how to systematically screen and perform a brief intervention, as this is the best way to prevent harmful or hazardous use from turning into a more intractable alcohol use disorder. Unfortunately, unless a social work student is interested in substance abuse and takes an elective during his or her course work or does a field placement in a treatment setting, most do not get adequate, if any training in SBI, or the effects of alcohol on human development and societal problems.

Begun: What should social workers be doing to increase interdisciplinary progress on this grand challenge across all levels?

Murray: Join interdisciplinary teams! Bring the social work perspective to the study of any of the issues, including alcohol, that are identified in the grand challenges. More and more, health and social research is being conceived and conducted by interdisciplinary teams, and too often, social work is absent. Social workers see how alcohol affects individuals and families, and they need to be part of setting the research agenda. The conceptual frameworks of our profession add an important perspective to how problems are defined and how solutions can be implemented.

Begun: Wrapping up, what additional resources might the readers be interested in exploring?

Murray: For more information, NIAAA's goals are stated on both the NIH Web site (www.niaaa.nih.gov) and in its Strategic Plan, which will be out for public comment in late 2016.

ORCID

Audrey L. Begun ⓘ http://orcid.org/0000-0002-1672-0315

RECOMMENDED BOOKS AND MOVIES

Baumeister, R., & Tierny, J. (2011). *Willpower: Rediscovering the greatest human strength*. New York, NY: Penguin. To understand harmful use of substances and bad habits, useful given that substance use disorders may begin as bad habits and what we know about habit formation can be applied to interrupt them and change behavior.

Kahneman, D. (2011). *Thinking fast and slow*. New York, NY: Macmillan. A must read for anyone in the human services profession who wants to understand how their mind and brain works, and how to best help those they serve.

Koob, G., & Le Moal, M. (2005). *Neurobiology of addiction*. London, UK: Academic Press. Social workers do not get enough training on the human brain and how a disease like addiction begins and becomes so hard to overcome.

Spielberg, S., Kennedy, K. (Producers), & Spielberg, S. (Director). (2012). *Lincoln*. [Film] U.S.A. Amblin Entertainment and Kennedy/Marshall Company. This film is recommended for anyone who wants to understand how the U.S. federal policy system works.

Fetal Alcohol Spectrum Disorders: An Interview with Dr. Shauna Acquavita, Assistant Professor, University of Cincinnati

Interview Conducted by
DIANA M. DiNITTO, PHD

In serving as editors for this special issue related to the Grand Challenge for Social Work concerned with reducing and preventing alcohol misuse and its consequences, Dr. Audrey Begun and I thought it was important to include information on fetal alcohol spectrum disorders. We invited Professor Shauna Acquavita to join us in this discussion. Dr. Acquavita has worked in the fields of health and behavioral health care and has published on the subject of substance use among pregnant women and on neonatal outcomes. She completed a Health Resources and Services Administration Pre-Doctoral Fellowship in Maternal and Child Health at the School of Social Work, University of Maryland, Baltimore, and a Ruth L. Kirschstein Post-Doctoral Fellowship in the Behavioral Pharmacology Research Unit in the Department of Psychiatry at Johns Hopkins University. Currently, Dr. Acquavita heads one of the Substance Abuse and Mental Health Services Administration funded grants to provide interprofessional Screening, Brief Intervention, and Referral to Treatment (SBIRT) training for health professionals. Her project includes a module on pregnant women; see "Web Sites for Information" for the URL.

DiNitto: As a leader in preventing fetal alcohol spectrum disorders (FASD), thank you for discussing how these disorders relate to the social work grand challenge of closing the health gap by reducing and preventing alcohol misuse and its consequences. As the special issue editors, we felt that this was a particularly salient topic for an issue that is about preventing the consequences associated with alcohol misuse.

First, would you clarify for our readers what FASD is and what are its most significant aspects?

Acquavita: FASD is an umbrella term that refers to disabilities and complications caused by alcohol consumption during pregnancy. It is comprised of four diagnoses: fetal alcohol syndrome (FAS), partial fetal alcohol syndrome (PFAS), alcohol-related neurodevelopmental disorder (ARND), and alcohol-related birth defects (ARBD). FASD impacts IQ, physical health, working memory, abstract thinking, and adaptive behavior. PFAS, ARND, and ARBD all have different combinations of these characteristics. FAS, being the most severe diagnosis on the spectrum, is characterized by facial abnormalities, stunted growth in the brain and body, damage to the central nervous system, and small head circumference. The challenge with assessing FASD is that the severity of diagnosis could be dependent on the timing and duration of alcohol exposure during pregnancy, dose of alcohol exposure, genetics, and environmental factors.

DiNitto: What is the rate of FASD, who is most affected, and what are the trends in the rate of FASD?

Acquavita: Alcohol use during pregnancy is the number one known cause of developmental disability and birth defects in the United States. Approximately 1 in 30 women in their child-bearing years is at risk for an alcohol-exposed pregnancy (AEP; Cannon, Guo, Denny, & Floyd, 2015). Of 1,000 live births in the United States, estimates are between two and nine will have FAS (May, Baete, Russon, Elliott, & Hoyme, 2014; Muralidharan, Sarmah, Zhou, & Marrs, 2013). However, it has been estimated that the rate of FASD ranges between 24 and 48 per 1,000 live births (May et al., 2014; May, Gossage, Kalberg, & Hoyme, 2009). The most recent study suggests that FASD might be more common than previously estimated; however, it is difficult to determine if this is because of more and better screening and treatment for FASD, or if rates have actually increased. Women at greater risk for having a child with FASD are more likely to binge drink as compared to other women and drink more than the recommended amount for women prior to pregnancy. Other risk factors that may co-occur with FASD include mothers experiencing domestic violence, mental health issues, past obstetric problems, and the use of tobacco and other drugs. The highest rates of AEP are among Native American and Alaskan Native women; Indian Health Service data indicate that 47% to 56% of mothers reported drinking alcohol while pregnant (see May et al., 2014, May et al., 2009; May et al., 2004). Children who experience adverse or unstable home environments are most likely to be diagnosed with FASD. One study found the rate of FAS among foster children was 10 to 15 times the incidence of the general population (see Astley, Stachowiak, Clarren, & Clausen, 2002).

DiNitto: What are the most important reasons social workers and others should be concerned about preventing these disorders or reducing the consequences of fetal alcohol exposure as part of the alcohol misuse grand challenge?

Acquavita: Many individuals with FASD have intellectual, cognitive, or behavioral challenges. These can impact their family, social, school, and work lives. Families of children with FASD might need specific help and support to cope with these challenges. In some cases, these children might have been placed in foster care or adopted; their foster or adoptive parents might not know their child was at risk for or has FASD until problems arise. Consequences for these families can include wrongful adoption cases in the court system (Theil et al., 2011). Wrongful adoptions occur when the adoption agency or other professionals involved in the adoption process intentionally or negligently fail to make a good faith effort to discover and reveal information to the adoptive parents. Information can include medical and social background of the child. Supporting these families in processing this diagnosis and linking them to appropriate resources, as early in the child's development as possible, are needed. School-based services are often necessary, as many individuals with FASD experience challenges at school. Individuals with FASD might have a difficult time making friends and can be easily influenced by others, leading them to engage in at-risk behaviors or become a victim of crime. Past estimates of individuals with FASD being subject to crimes range between 25% and 50%; the rate of their being sexually abused ranges between 55% and 60% (see Streissguth, Barr, Kogen, & Bookstein, 1996; Sullivan & Knutson, 2000). Also, individuals with FASD may be at risk for criminal justice system involvement. Estimates are that 60% of individuals with FASD have had criminal charges, arrests, convictions, or other trouble with the law (Streissguth, Bookstein, Barr, Sampson, & O'Malley, 2004). Approximately 50% of people diagnosed with FAS have exhibited inappropriate sexual behavior (Streissguth et al., 2004). Also, individuals with FASD are more likely to have limited social and community support, leading to increased use of emergency services. Many experience problems gaining and keeping employment.

DiNitto: A lot of research and clinical attention are directed at identifying the primary effects of fetal alcohol exposure—such as the physical and neurological aftermaths. What are the secondary consequences for the children, families, and communities that should also be receiving attention, such as shame, guilt, and the effects on communities in meeting the needs of those affected by FASD?

Acquavita: Drinking during pregnancy has been looked at in the United States as a moral or legal issue, ignoring the influences that society has on alcohol consumption. The U.S. population is inundated with ads for alcohol in print, online, and via television. Many women do not know they are pregnant until the sixth week of gestation, and thus could still be drinking. Although many women stop drinking once they realize they are pregnant, some damage may have already been experienced by the fetus. In some U.S. states, women can be committed involuntarily to treatment for alcohol misuse during pregnancy, and AEP can be used as evidence of child abuse or neglect. Punitive policies around women's alcohol consumption while pregnant have made it difficult for women to be honest with health care providers about their alcohol consumption, despite the need for supportive, nonjudgmental relationships between women and their health care providers for women to discuss their behavior, concerns, and feelings and to intervene in ways that can minimize the consequences of alcohol misuse during pregnancy.

DiNitto: What policies and practices are being used in the United States to prevent FASD and reduce its consequences, and which are especially relevant to social work practice at the micro, mezzo, and macro levels? Have practices such as screening and brief intervention been effective in preventing drinking when women are seeking to become pregnant or are pregnant? Have public service announcements, warning labels on alcohol, or other practices been effective? What are communities doing to prevent and reduce FASD, especially those most affected by it? What innovative and effective primary, secondary, and tertiary prevention methods are being used in the United States?

Acquavita: Implementing Screening, Brief Intervention, and Referral to Treatment (SBIRT) is an evidence-based practice that can be used in many settings to address the risk of FASD. Providers who are working with women intending to get pregnant should also work to educate women on the hazards of AEP prior to pregnancy. Cannon and colleagues' study (2015) indicated that women who are intending to become pregnant as compared to those who are not have a higher risk of AEP, as they often continue to drink, even after stopping contraception. Therefore, settings such as family practice, obstetrics/gynecology, and fertility offices or clinics should implement SBIRT and educate women on AEP. The Substance Abuse and Mental Health Services Administration (SAMHSA) has provided funds to train students and professionals in the health care field to implement SBIRT. SAMHSA has also worked to address AEP in substance abuse treatment centers and through the Special Supplemental Nutrition Program for Women, Infants, and Children (WIC). The Health Resources and Services Administration (HRSA) also worked with SAMHSA to address FASD with SBIRT through the Healthy Start program. HRSA has also funded an initiative with community health centers for FASD prevention and identification and to support children and families addressing FASD. Specific interventions have been developed and tested to help prevent FASD. Project CHOICES (Changing High-Risk Alcohol Use and Increasing Contraception Effectiveness Study) examined the effectiveness of a brief intervention to prevent FASD in special settings including jails, substance use disorders treatment centers, and health centers. Results indicated those women who received only information were twice as likely to be at risk for AEP compared to those who received both information and a brief motivational intervention (see Project CHOICES in Web Sites for Information). Media campaigns directed to specific populations have been evaluated for their effectiveness in increasing awareness of FASD. Populations have included African Americans, Native Americans, Latinos, and women enrolled in the WIC nutrition program. Media campaigns have included television commercials, posters, and radio ads. Government warnings printed on alcoholic beverage containers are another prevention tool. According to a critical review of public health interventions to reduce alcohol consumption and increase knowledge among pregnant women, it is difficult to say these interventions have been successful overall in reducing FASD (Crawford-Williams et al., 2015). This is due to the small number of studies being conducted, with each using different methods and outcome measures (e.g., knowledge vs. self-reported alcohol consumption rates). For caregivers of those with FAS, programs have been developed to teach stress management, implement behavioral regulation techniques, and learn to use advocacy. Training programs for teachers of those children with FAS have been tested and implemented in schools. These programs include educating teachers on components of FAS and on helping those with FAS improve communications and social skills, academic performance in reading and math, and maintenance of personal safety. Some school districts are implementing specific curricula, such as those provided by the National Organization on Fetal Alcohol Syndrome (NOFAS) for educating students in grades K–12 on FASD prevention and the National Institute on Alcohol Abuse and Alcoholism (NIAAA), to teach students about FASD. On a macro level, enforcing the minimum legal drinking age, limiting where alcohol is sold, and increasing the price of alcohol are some ways for impacting FASD. In 1991, Alaska was the first U.S. state to establish a treatment center for pregnant women with substance use disorders. Since then, Alaska has implemented a coordinated approach with its Office of FASD housed at the state level. This includes diagnostic teams, community-based FASD case managers, training teachers and health professionals, and implementing programs in prevention and early intervention. In Alaska, anyone applying for a marriage license receives a brochure on FASD. Bars, liquor stores, and restaurants must post large advertisements about how drinking while pregnant can lead to birth defects. Although the initial education and intervention policies seemed to make a difference in Alaska's FASD rate when implemented in the 1990s, recent rates have been increasing as funding for these initiatives has decreased. This indicates the importance of funding efforts to combat FASD, and maintaining the efforts even after rates initially decrease.

DiNitto: What is the role of the woman's partner or others close to her in preventing FASD?

Acquavita: A woman's partner, friends, and family can help to prevent FASD by supporting and encouraging her choice not to drink alcohol prior to becoming pregnant and while pregnant. Women's social support networks can help by participating with her in activities that do not involve alcohol. It may be necessary to remove alcohol from the home, and those residing in the home will need to cooperate with this. Research suggests that women whose partners binge drink may be at greater risk to have a child with FASD (May et al., 2014). Research is currently being conducted to assess if sperm are harmed by alcohol prior to women becoming pregnant, which might affect babies' developmental outcomes. Conducting SBIRT with a woman's partner and educating both on AEP could help to prevent FASD.

DiNitto: What is happening at the international level that can help address the grand challenge as it relates to FASD prevention and reducing its consequences?

Acquavita: There are challenges in addressing FASD internationally due to different cultural norms around alcohol consumption during pregnancy. For example, U.S., Canadian, Swedish, and Australian health policies stress total abstinence during pregnancy, whereas some European countries allow for an occasional small amount of alcohol to be consumed. To confound the issue, international government definitions of standard units of alcohol vary by size and alcohol content (Drabble, Magri, Tumwesigye, Li, & Plant, 2011). Rates of FAS vary internationally by populations. For example, South Africa's FAS rate is estimated to be 20 cases per 1,000 live births, while for Russia, it is estimated to be 18 cases per 1,000 live births. However, in Russian orphanages prevalence rates have ranged from 46 to 330 cases per 1,000 live births. For some countries, such as China, research is lacking on studying alcohol consumption in the overall population (Drabble et al., 2011). Further, there is no public health system mechanism in that nation to screen and identify women at risk for FASD and health professionals are not trained in FASD, so rates of FAS are unknown (Drabble et al., 2011). Yet, strides are being made. "Too young to drink" is an international campaign sponsored by the European FASD Alliance that uses posters, social media, videos, brochures, and a Web site available in nine languages to promote FASD awareness. Research is being conducted in different countries on FASD prevention and intervention. A study by Dr. Christina Chambers in the Ukraine is evaluating the effectiveness of choline supplementation in pregnant women. Choline supplementation might reduce the severity of FASD or inhibit FASD. South Africa is targeting youth aged 10 to 18 years in locations with high FASD rates in a 2-year FASD prevention program that is integrated into sports. The International Gender, Alcohol and Culture (GENACIS) Project is a collaboration with institutions from the United States, Denmark, Canada, Australia, and Switzerland. Supported by funds from NIAAA, the World Health Organization (WHO), the European Commission Quality of Life and Management Resources Programme, and other government agencies, this collaboration has conducted studies in 39 different countries. The project reports that while women abstain from alcohol at high rates in most third-world countries, there are rapid increases in women's drinking when economic development occurs. Also, in lower income countries, women with more education and those who are employed outside the home are more likely to drink. GENACIS suggests implementing policies to prevent alcohol advertising that targets women. Overall, there is a need for international prevalence data on alcohol consumption, training for health professionals on FASD, and developing, testing, and disseminating culturally appropriate, effective interventions.

DiNitto: What are social work's particular roles in preventing FASD and reducing its consequences, and how well is the profession preparing students and practicing social workers to take on these roles?

Acquavita: There are many different roles for social work in preventing and treating FASD. Overall, social workers working with women must establish trust so that women will disclose to them information about their past and current lifestyles and any risk factors and fears about their pregnancy or child. This can aid in assessing for FASD. There is also a great need for students and social workers to know the *DSM–5* criteria for FASD. Often, FASD symptoms are mistaken for and can overlap with other disorders. These include mood disorders, attention deficit hyperactivity disorder (ADHD), conduct disorder, and substance use disorders (Pei, Denys, Hughes, & Rasmussen, 2011). Also, ARND, a new diagnosis in the *DSM–5*, is a neurodevelopmental disorder associated with prenatal alcohol exposure. It includes impaired neurocognitive functioning, self-regulation, and adaptive functioning. Students and social workers should also know how to conduct a social history and assessment with the individual (and parent or guardian if appropriate) that includes components of maternal and fetal development and questions about substance use. Early diagnosis of individuals with FASD can help to link them and their families with the proper services and support as soon as possible. This can aid in reducing their involvement in the criminal justice system. Also, developing an individualized treatment plan is needed, as the symptoms and challenges individuals with FASD face vary from person to person; there is no one treatment that works for everyone. Approaching FASD with a developmental approach is recommended. Social workers need to understand that individuals with FASD may be delayed or never meet developmental stages such as those outlined by Erik Erikson in psychosocial theory or Jean Piaget's theory of cognitive development. Unfortunately, content on substance use disorders is lacking in many social work programs. Many social work programs do not require students to complete a course in substance use disorders, or infuse enough information on this topic into their curriculum. This leads to social workers being unprepared to recognize or address substance use disorders, and specifically FASD.

DiNitto: How can social workers engage with other disciplines to address FASD as part of the challenge of reducing and preventing alcohol misuse and its consequences?

Acquavita: An interprofessional approach is necessary with social workers as part of the team. Our medical colleagues are often the first line of defense in preventing and addressing FASD, as many women see a primary care physician or their obstetrician or gynecologist at least once a year for a checkup. Pediatricians can also aid by identifying infants and children whom they suspect have been exposed to alcohol during gestation. Social workers should be available to collaborate with these professionals to set up treatments and referrals. Nurses, especially those in school-based settings, can help with identification and treatment. Social workers can also work with teachers to educate them on FASD and help with creating and implementing accommodations and individualized educational plans for children with FASD. Another aspect that is often overlooked in FASD prevention is nutrition. Research indicates that severe nutritional deficiency along with alcohol misuse could be a risk factor for FASD, especially in lower socioeconomic populations (Muralidharan et al., 2013). Individuals of any age with FASD may also have feeding issues; speech pathologists can work collaboratively with these individuals to address both swallowing and speech issues. Occupational and physical therapists aid individuals with FASD to physically or functionally adapt to their surroundings and compensate for disabilities attributable to FASD. Developing a tailored plan for an individual with FASD can mean coordinating with multiple interprofessional team members. Working with colleagues in the criminal justice system is also a way to address FASD. Fast and Conry (2009) identify several ways to help individuals with FASD. Law enforcement should be trained in how to properly interview individuals with FASD (e.g., eliminating the use of leading questions and complicated terminology). Probation officers need to know that people with FASD are often impulsive and do not link their behavior with consequences due to cognitive limitations. Judges and attorneys should be cognizant that there is federal recognition for individuals with FASD to receive special consideration when involved with the judicial system. Attorneys can utilize specific screening questions and observations to determine if an FASD diagnostic workup is needed. Victim assistance agencies should implement education and training on how to work with people with FASD (Theil et al., 2011). A strong interprofessional approach would greatly benefit those with FASD.

DiNitto: What are the most important next steps in addressing FASD as part of the grand challenges of reducing and preventing alcohol misuse and its consequences?

Acquavita: Access to free or low-cost health care can promote universal screening for alcohol use. Women should also receive education on alcohol consumption, AEP, and contraception. Health professionals should be trained to effectively screen and counsel women about alcohol use. FASD information is also needed in health professional training curricula and in continuing education. Written and oral licensing examinations for these professionals should include content on FASD. Patient-centered medical homes can also help with screening and prevention, as well as support those diagnosed with FASD. As mentioned previously, there is a great need to work interprofessonally on this issue. Interprofessional medical care group practice models need to be created. FASD system navigators and advocates should also be a part of these models to improve case management across systems of care. Individuals with FASD would also benefit from clear and consistent eligibility criteria for disability services across state agencies and insurance plans. Greater funding for research on FASD is also needed. Some promising research avenues are being explored. Animal studies are making strides in addressing FASD. For example, slow wave sleep, the deeper sleep whereby the day's events are turned into permanent memories, is fragmented in individuals who have been exposed to high levels of alcohol while in utero. Addressing slow wave sleep might be a way to help with memory impairment for individuals with FASD (see Tayade, 2015). Focusing on nutrients, such as choline supplementation, vitamin E, and other antioxidants alone or in combination with other therapeutic agents, might aid in preventing and treating defects. Stem cell research, albeit controversial, has also indicated promising results in addressing memory and social recognition. And, pre- and postnatal supplementation is being explored in human studies, as well. More development of interventions targeting the specific age groups of infants, toddlers, and teens impacted by FASD is needed. Early intervention programs and educational assistance programs are needed for children. Vocational programs are needed for adults. Physical and mental health therapy services from professionals trained in FASD would also be helpful. Better assessment tools (including the use of biomarkers) and specifically tailored interventions are also needed. Interventions that are culturally appropriate for specific populations need to be developed, such as those for Native Americans. Longitudinal studies on individuals and families affected by FASD should be conducted to determine long-range impacts and improve services. These are just some of the ways in which we can address FASD.

DiNitto: Finally, what are some resources about FASD and its prevention and treatment that can be helpful to social workers?

Acquavita: There are a range of resources available to social workers about FASD. Social workers can participate in FASD Awareness Day. This began on September 9, 1999, and is held annually on the ninth day of the ninth month (see http://www.fasday.com/). The Catalyst Learning Center Series on Fetal Alcohol Spectrum Disorders is a free eight-course series that offers online training relating to FASD (http://attcppwtools.org/LearnASkill/OnlineCourses. aspx). There are also Web sites (see list below) that provide general information about FASD, a blog, a toolkit offered through the American Academy of Pediatrics, a documentary, and an app.

WEB SITES FOR INFORMATION

- CDC: https://www.cdc.gov/ncbddd/fasd/
- National Organization on Fetal Alcohol Syndrome: http://www.nofas.org/about-fasd/
- Substance Abuse and Mental Health Services Administration: http://www.samhsa.gov/fetal-alcohol-spectrum-disorders-fasd-center
- American Bar Association: https://apps.americanbar.org/litigation/committees/childrights/content/articles/fall2012-0912-fasd-identification-advocacy.html
- List of questions for attorneys: http://qcba.org/wp-content/uploads/2013/05/QCBA-Feb-08-Bar-Bul-lo-res1.pdf
- IRETA (Institute for Research, Education & Training in Addictions) blog: http://ireta.org/2015/06/08/alcohol-exposure-affects-fetal-brain-development/?utm_source=all+IRETA +communications&utm_campaign=f6e08927f4-Social_Media_Mashu-p_8_19_168_19_2016&utm_medium=email&utm_term=0_5cec8dc768-f6e08927f4-102817985&mc_cid=f6e08927f4&mc_eid=49c393eaf8
- Project CHOICES: http://www.cdc.gov/ncbddd/fasd/previous-projects.html
- Toolkit from the American Academy of Pediatrics: https://www.aap.org/en-us/advocacy-and-policy/aap-health-initiatives/fetal-alcohol-spectrum-disorders-toolkit/Pages/default.aspx
- CDC's FASD app: https://itunes.apple.com/us/app/fetal-alcohol-spectrum-disorders/id517058288?mt=8&ls=1
- Documentary "Moment to Moment: Teens Growing Up with FASDs": http://www.ntiupstream.com/

- Module information: University of Cincinnati School of Social Work (2017) SBIRT and Pregnant Women Online Module: http://cahsmedia2.uc.edu/host/PregnancyModule/story.html

REFERENCES

Astley, S., Stachowiak, J., Clarren, S. K., & Clausen, C. (2002). Application of the fetal alcohol syndrome facial photographic screening tool in a foster care population. *The Journal of Pediatrics, 141*, 712–717. doi:10.1067/mpd.2002.129030

Cannon, M. J., Guo, J., Denny, C. H., & Floyd, R. L. (2015). Prevalence and characteristics of women at risk for an alcohol-exposed pregnancy (AEP) in the United States: Estimates from the National Survey of Family Growth. *Maternal Child Health, 19*, 776–782. doi:10.1007/s10995-014-1563-3

Crawford-Williams, F., Fielder, A., Mikocka-Walus, A., & Esterman, A. (2015). A critical review of public health interventions aimed at reducing alcohol consumption and/or increasing knowledge among pregnant women. *Drug and Alcohol Review, 34*, 154–161. doi:10.1111/dar.2015.34.issue-2

Drabble, L., Magri, R., Tumwesigye, N., Li, Q., & Plant, M. (2011). Conceiving risk, divergent responses: Perspectives on the construction of risk of FASD in six countries. *Substance Use & Misuse, 46*, 943–958. doi:10.3109/10826084.2010.527419

Fast, D. K. & Conroy, J. (2009). Fetal alcohol spectrum disorders and the criminal justice system. *Developmental Disabilities Research Reviews, 15*, 250–257. doi:10.1002/ddrr.66

May, P. A., Baete, A., Russon, J., Elliott, A. J., & Hoyme, H. E. (2014). Prevalence and characteristics of fetal alcohol spectrum disorders. *Pediatrics, 134*, 855–866. doi:10.1542/peds.2013-3319

May, P. A., Gossage, J. P., Kalberg, W. O., & Hoyme, H. E. (2009). Prevalence and epidemiologic characteristics of FASD from various research methods with an emphasis on recent in-school studies. *Developmental Disabilities Research Reviews, 15*, 176–192. doi:10.1002/ddrr.68

May, P. A., Gossage, J. P., White-Country, M., Goodhart, K. A., Decoteau, S., Trujillo, P. M., & Hoyme, H. E. (2004). Alcohol consumption and other maternal risk factors for fetal alcohol syndrome among three distinct samples of women before, during and after pregnancy: The risk is relative. *American Journal of Medical Genetics: Part C, Seminars in Medical Genetics, 127C*(1), 10–20. doi:10.1002/ajmg.c.30011

Muralidharan, P., Sarmah, S., Zhou, F. C., & Marrs, J. A. (2013). Fetal alcohol spectrum disorder (FASD) associated neural defects: Complex mechanisms and potential therapeutic targets. *Brain Sciences, 3*, 964–991. doi:10.3390/brainsci3020964

Pei, J., Denys, K., Hughes, J., & Rasmussen, C. (2011). Mental health issues in fetal alcohol spectrum disorder. *Journal of Mental Health, 20*, 438–448. doi: 10.3109/09638237.2011.577113.

Streissguth, A. P., Barr, H. M., Kogen, J., & Bookstein, F. L. (1996). *Understanding the occurrence of secondary disabilities in clients with Fetal Alcohol Syndrome*

(FAS) and Fetal Alcohol Effects (FAE). Washington, DC: Centers for Disease Control and Prevention.

Streissguth, A. P., Bookstein, F. L., Barr, H. M., Sampson, P. D., & O'Malley, K. (2004). Risk factors for adverse life outcomes in Fetal Alcohol Syndrome and Fetal Alcohol Effects. *Developmental and Behavioral Pediatrics, 25*, 228–238.

Sullivan, P., & Knutson, J. (2000). Maltreatment and disabilities: A population-based epidemiological study. *Child Abuse & Neglect, 24*(10), 1257–1273.

Tayade, M. C. (2015). Fetal alcohol spectrum disorders (FASD) and slow wave sleep. *Pravara Medical Review, 7*(4), 4–5.

Theil, K. S., Baladerian, N. J., Boyce, K. R., Cantos, O. D., Davis, L. A., Kelly, K., … Sream, J. (2011). Fetal alcohol spectrum disorders and victimization: Implications for families, educators, social services, law enforcement, and the judicial system. *Journal of Psychiatry & Law, 39*(1), 121–157. doi:10.1177/009318531103900105

Index

Note: Page numbers in *italics* refer to figures
Page numbers in **bold** refer to tables